1992
YEAR BOOK OF
ORTHOPEDICS®

The 1992 Year Book® Series

Year Book of Anesthesia and Pain Management: Drs. Miller, Abram, Kirby, Ostheimer, Roizen, and Stoelting

Year Book of Cardiology®: Drs. Schlant, Collins, Engle, Frye, Kaplan, and O'Rourke

Year Book of Critical Care Medicine®: Drs. Rogers and Parrillo

Year Book of Dentistry®: Drs. Meskin, Currier, Kennedy, Leinfelder, Matukas, and Rovin

Year Book of Dermatologic Surgery: Drs. Swanson, Salasche, and Glogau

Year Book of Dermatology®: Drs. Sober and Fitzpatrick

Year Book of Diagnostic Radiology®: Drs. Federle, Clark, Gross, Madewell, Maynard, Sackett, and Young

Year Book of Digestive Diseases®: Drs. Greenberger and Moody

Year Book of Drug Therapy®: Drs. Lasagna and Weintraub

Year Book of Emergency Medicine®: Drs. Wagner, Burdick, Davidson, Roberts, and Spivey

Year Book of Endocrinology®: Drs. Bagdade, Braverman, Horton, Kannan, Landsberg, Molitch, Morley, Odell, Rogol, Ryan, and Sherwin

Year Book of Family Practice®: Drs. Berg, Bowman, Davidson, Dietrich, and Scherger

Year Book of Geriatrics and Gerontology®: Drs. Beck, Abrass, Burton, Cummings, Makinodan, and Small

Year Book of Hand Surgery®: Drs. Amadio and Hentz

Year Book of Health Care Management: Drs. Heyssel, Brock, King, and Steinberg, Ms. Avakian, and Messrs. Berman, Kues, and Rosenberg

Year Book of Hematology®: Drs. Spivak, Bell, Ness, Quesenberry, and Wiernik

Year Book of Infectious Diseases®: Drs. Wolff, Barza, Keusch, Klempner, and Snydman

Year Book of Infertility: Drs. Mishell, Paulsen, and Lobo

Year Book of Medicine®: Drs. Rogers, Bone, Cline, Braunwald, Greenberger, Utiger, Epstein, and Malawista

Year Book of Neonatal and Perinatal Medicine®: Drs. Klaus and Fanaroff

Year Book of Nephrology: Drs. Coe, Favus, Henderson, Kashgarian, Luke, Myers, and Strom

Year Book of Neurology and Neurosurgery®: Drs. Currier and Crowell

Year Book of Neuroradiology: Drs. Osborn, Harnsberger, Halbach, and Grossman

Year Book of Nuclear Medicine®: Drs. Hoffer, Gore, Gottschalk, Sostman, Zaret, and Zubal

Year Book of Obstetrics and Gynecology®: Drs. Mishell, Kirschbaum, and Morrow

Year Book of Occupational and Environmental Medicine: Drs. Emmett, Brooks, Harris, and Schenker

Year Book of Oncology®: Drs. Young, Longo, Ozols, Simone, Steele, and Weichselbaum

Year Book of Ophthalmology®: Drs. Laibson, Adams, Augsburger, Benson, Cohen, Eagle, Flanagan, Nelson, Reinecke, Sergott, and Wilson

Year Book of Orthopedics®: Drs. Sledge, Poss, Cofield, Frymoyer, Griffin, Hansen, Johnson, Simmons, and Springfield

Year Book of Otolaryngology–Head and Neck Surgery®: Drs. Bailey and Paparella

Year Book of Pathology and Clinical Pathology®: Drs. Gardner, Bennett, Cousar, Garvin, and Worsham

Year Book of Pediatrics®: Dr. Stockman

Year Book of Plastic, Reconstructive, and Aesthetic Surgery: Drs. Miller, Cohen, McKinney, Robson, Ruberg, and Whitaker

Year Book of Podiatric Medicine and Surgery®: Dr. Kominsky

Year Book of Psychiatry and Applied Mental Health®: Drs. Talbott, Frances, Freedman, Meltzer, Perry, Schowalter, and Yudofsky

Year Book of Pulmonary Disease®: Drs. Bone and Petty

Year Book of Sports Medicine®: Drs. Shephard, Eichner, Sutton, and Torg, Col. Anderson, and Mr. George

Year Book of Surgery®: Drs. Schwartz, Jonasson, Robson, Shires, Spencer, and Thompson

Year Book of Transplantation: Drs. Ascher, Hansen, and Strom

Year Book of Ultrasound: Drs. Merritt, Mittelstaedt, Carroll, and Nyberg

Year Book of Urology®: Drs. Gillenwater and Howards

Year Book of Vascular Surgery®: Dr. Bergan

Roundsmanship®: '92–'93: A Student's Survival Guide to Clinical Medicine Using Current Literature: Drs. Dan, Feigin, Quilligan, Schrock, Stein, and Talbott

Editor
Clement B. Sledge, M.D.
Chairman, Department of Orthopaedic Surgery, Brigham and Women's Hospital; Professor of Orthopaedic Surgery, Harvard Medical School, Boston, Massachusetts

Co-Editor
Robert Poss, M.D.
Vice Chairman, Department of Orthopaedic Surgery, Brigham and Women's Hospital; Professor of Orthopaedic Surgery, Harvard Medical School, Boston, Massachusetts

Associate Editors
Robert H. Cofield, M.D.
Professor of Orthopedic Surgery, Mayo Medical School; Vice-Chairman, Department of Orthopedics, Mayo Clinic, Rochester, Minnesota

John W. Frymoyer, M.D.
Interim Dean of the College of Medicine, Professor of Orthopedic Surgery, University of Vermont; Director, McClure Musculoskeletal Research Center, Burlington, Vermont

Paul P. Griffin, M.D.
Professor of Orthopedic Surgery, Medical University of South Carolina, Charleston, South Carolina

Sigvard T. Hansen, Jr., M.D.
Professor of Orthopaedics, University of Washington School of Medicine, Seattle, Washington

Kenneth A. Johnson, M.D.
Professor of Orthopedic Surgery, Mayo Clinic Scottsdale; Past President, American Orthopaedic Foot and Ankle Society

Barry P. Simmons, M.D.
Chief, Hand Surgery Service, Brigham and Women's Hospital; Associate Professor of Orthopaedic Surgery, Harvard Medical School, Boston, Massachusetts

Dempsey S. Springfield, M.D.
Associate Professor of Orthopaedic Surgery, Harvard Medical School; Visiting Orthopaedic Surgeon, Massachusetts General Hospital, Boston

Assistant Editor to Dr. Johnson
Robert D. Teasedall, M.D.
Foot and Ankle Fellow, Mayo Clinic, Scottsdale, Arizona

1992

The Year Book of ORTHOPEDICS®

Editor
Clement B. Sledge, M.D.

Co-Editor
Robert Poss, M.D.

Associate Editors
Robert H. Cofield, M.D.
John W. Frymoyer, M.D.
Paul P. Griffin, M.D.
Sigvard T. Hansen, Jr., M.D.
Kenneth A. Johnson, M.D.
Barry P. Simmons, M.D.
Dempsey S. Springfield, M.D.

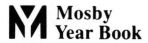
Mosby
Year Book

St. Louis   Baltimore   Boston   Chicago   London   Philadelphia   Sydney   Toronto

Editor-in-Chief, Year Book Publishing: Kenneth H. Killion
Sponsoring Editor: Linda Steiner
Manager, Literature Services: Edith M. Podrazik
Senior Information Specialist: Terri Santo
Senior Medical Writer: David A. Cramer, M.D.
Assistant Director, Manuscript Services: Frances M. Perveiler
Associate Managing Editor, Year Book Editing Services: Connie Murray
Senior Production/Desktop Publishing Manager: Max F. Perez
Proofroom Manager: Barbara M. Kelly

Editorial Office:
Mosby–Year Book, Inc.
200 North LaSalle St.
Chicago, IL 60601

International Standard Serial Number: 0276-1092
International Standard Book Number: 0-8151-7809-3

Table of Contents

JOURNALS REPRESENTED ix
PUBLISHER'S PREFACE. xi
INTRODUCTION. xiii
1. Pediatrics, *edited by* PAUL P. GRIFFIN, M.D. 1
   Introduction 1
      NEUROVASCULAR CONDITION 1
      SPINE. 10
      LOWER EXTREMITY. 13
      HIP. 20
      FRACTURE OF UPPER EXTREMITIES 31
      MISCELLANEOUS 37
2. Shoulder, Arm, and Elbow, *edited by*
   ROBERT H. COFIELD, M.D. 43
   Introduction 43
      IMAGING STUDIES. 45
         MAGNETIC RESONANCE IMAGING. 47
      FRACTURES 52
      INSTABILITY—ACROMIOCLAVICULAR 56
         GLENOHUMERAL 57
         ELBOW 63
      TENDON INJURY AND DISEASE 65
         SHOULDER IMPINGEMENT 70
         ROTATOR CUFF TEARING 72
      ARTHROPLASTY AND ARTHRODESIS—SHOULDER 78
         ELBOW 81
      VARIED TOPICS. 83
3. General Adult Reconstruction, *edited by*
   CLEMENT B. SLEDGE, M.D. 87
   Introduction 87
      DIAGNOSIS AND MANAGEMENT OF KNEE INJURIES. 89
      CRUCIATE LIGAMENTS. 99
      MISCELLANEOUS CONDITIONS 108
      CARTILAGE RESEARCH 115
      INFECTION 119
      OSTEOARTHRITIS 123
      TECHNIQUES OF TOTAL KNEE ARTHROPLASTY. 127
      UNICOMPARTMENTAL KNEE REPLACEMENT 135
      RESULTS OF TOTAL KNEE ARTHROPLASTY 141
      PATELLAR PROBLEMS. 146
      POLYETHYLENE WEAR 148
      COMPLICATIONS OF TOTAL KNEE ARTHROPLASTY 150

4. **Hip Reconstruction, Osteoporosis, and Related Research,**
   edited by Robert Poss, M.D. 155
   Introduction 155
5. **Spine,** *edited by* John W. Frymoyer, M.D. 203
   Introduction 203
      Cervical Spine: Neural Compression Syndromes 204
         Trauma 210
      Thoracic Spine 217
      Pathophysiology of Degeneration 220
      Occupation Injury and Epidemiology 224
      Lumbar Spine: Treatment, Degenerative Conditions 231
         Segmental Instability 247
         Internal Fixation 251
6. **Foot and Ankle,** *edited by* Kenneth A. Johnson, M.D.
   and Assistant Editor Robert D. Teasedall, M.D. 255
   Introduction 255
      Trauma and Its Sequelae: Osseous Injuries 256
      Trauma and Its Sequelae: Soft Tissue Injuries 268
      Problems of the Forefoot 273
      Miscellaneous Topics 279
7. **Musculoskeletal Neoplasia,** *edited by*
   Dempsey S. Springfield, M.D. 285
   Introduction 285
      Ewing's Sarcoma 286
      Osteosarcoma 294
      Soft Tissue Sarcomas 296
      Treatments 299
      Metastatic Disease 306
8. **Hand,** *edited by* Barry P. Simmons, M.D. 313
   Introduction 313
9. **Trauma and Amputation,** *edited by*
   Sigvard T. Hansen, Jr., M.D. 345
   Introduction 345
      General Traumatology 345
      Pelvic and Acetabular Fractures 356
      Amputation Topics 358
      Stimulation of Healing 365
      Soft Tissue Management 370
      Rehabilitation 374
      Complications 376
      New Technology and Implant Designs 378

Subject Index 383
Author Index 403

Journals Represented

Mosby–Year Book subscribes to and surveys nearly 900 U.S. and foreign medical and allied health journals. From these journals, the Editors select the articles to be abstracted. Journals represented in this YEAR BOOK are listed below.

Acta Orthopaedica Scandinavica
Acta Radiologica
American Journal of Public Health
American Journal of Roentgenology
American Journal of Sports Medicine
American Journal of Surgery
Anesthesia and Analgesia
Annals of Hand Surgery
Annals of Plastic Surgery
Annals of Rheumatic Diseases
Annals of Surgery
Annals of the Royal College of Surgeons of England
Archives of Internal Medicine
Archives of Orthopaedic and Trauma Surgery
Archives of Surgery
Arthritis and Rheumatism
Calcified Tissue International
Canadian Journal of Surgery
Cancer
Clinical Orthopaedics and Related Research
Clinical Radiology
Contemporary Orthopaedics
Developmental Medicine and Child Neurology
European Journal of Obstetrics, Gynecology and Reproductive Biology
Foot and Ankle
French Journal of Orthopaedic Surgery
Injury
International Journal of Radiation, Oncology, Biology, and Physics
International Orthopaedics
Italian Journal of Orthopaedics and Traumatology
Journal of Arthroplasty
Journal of Biomechanics
Journal of Bone and Joint Surgery (American Volume)
Journal of Bone and Joint Surgery (British Volume)
Journal of Bone and Mineral Research
Journal of Clinical Oncology
Journal of Computer Assisted Tomography
Journal of Hand Surgery (American)
Journal of Hand Surgery (British)
Journal of Neurology, Neurosurgery and Psychiatry
Journal of Neurosurgery
Journal of Orthopaedic Research
Journal of Orthopaedic Trauma
Journal of Pediatric Orthopedics
Journal of Reproductive Medicine
Journal of Trauma
Journal of Western Pacific Orthopaedic Association
Journal of the American Medical Association

Journal of the Royal College of Surgeons of Edinburgh
Lancet
Microsurgery
Neurosurgery
New England Journal of Medicine
Orthopaedic Review
Orthopedics
Plastic and Reconstructive Surgery
Prosthetics and Orthotics International
Radiology
Reviews of Infectious Diseases
Scandinavian Journal of Rheumatology
Skeletal Radiology
Spine
Sports Medicine
Surgery, Gynecology and Obstetrics
Thrombosis and Haemostatis
Western Journal of Medicine

STANDARD ABBREVIATIONS

The following terms are abbreviated in this edition: acquired immunodeficiency syndrome (AIDS), the central nervous system (CNS), cerebrospinal fluid (CSF), computed tomography (CT), electrocardiography (ECG), human immunodeficiency virus (HIV), and magnetic resonance (MR) imaging (MRI).

Publisher's Preface

As Publishers, we feel challenged to seek ways of presenting complex information in a clear and readable manner. To this end, the 1992 YEAR BOOK OF ORTHOPEDICS now provides structured abstracts in which the various components of a study can be identified easily through headings. These headings are not the same in all abstracts, but rather are those that most accurately designate the content of each particular journal article. We are confident that our readers will find the information contained in our abstracts to be more accessible than ever before. We welcome your comments.

Introduction

The orthopedic literature of 1992 presents information that brings us to a crossroad in our understanding and treatment of many of the problems of the musculoskeletal system. In some areas, we now see a consolidation of knowledge about many of the changes of the last decade. For example, a better assessment can now be made regarding the relative advantages and disadvantages of cemented and uncemented arthroplasties and regarding which of the many technical and material innovations of the past decade are withstanding the test of time.

Clinimetrics can be defined as the science of measuring clinical results. It is a discipline that has existed within internal medicine for some years and has been heavily used by rheumatologists in evaluating the effectiveness of medical management of arthritis. Only recently have orthopedic surgeons become interested and involved in this field. When the measurement of clinical results is coupled with the patient's own evaluation of the success of treatment, the clinical outcome can be determined. As health care expenses increase, some form of rationing becomes inevitable. If rationing is to be rational, then we must have some idea of the effectiveness of the treatments that we offer for problems of the musculoskeletal system; as long as the taxpayer or purchaser of health care insurance is financing the system, patient satisfaction will be an important criterion of the success of treatment. Several articles this year are examples of the emerging interest of orthopedic surgeons in validated methods of assessment, visual analogue scales for pain, and randomized clinical trials. An excellent example of the latter technique is the paper by Andersson, Odensten, and Gillquist comparing surgical and nonsurgical treatment for acute ruptures of the anterior cruciate ligament; the authors asked whether extraarticular repair is necessary at the time of intra-articular repair and whether synthetic materials can substitute for the anterior cruciate ligament. They also explored the major issue of what levels of function can be expected after any of several types of surgical and nonsurgical management of these injuries.

A provocative paper by Barrett examines the role of proprioception after knee injuries and suggests that an important determinant of patient satisfaction is the degree to which proprioception is restored after treatment.

There have been further refinements in certain treatment modalities, both surgical and medical, that considerably refine and enhance our care of patients in the perioperative period.

Exciting papers from basic science laboratories concerning cartilage biology, osteoinduction and osteoconduction point the way to a proliferation of knowledge on this subject and to a new era in joint preservation or replacement—the era of biologic replacement of tissues.

Finally, there is increasing recognition that the large body of orthopedic literature can only be made more meaningful by a constant nomenclature and a system of reporting of results that includes patient assessment of outcome. The results of total hip replacement are the first to be subjected to a constant nomenclature. In the next few years, we will see the results of other procedures reported in such a manner.

We are pleased to present the 1992 YEAR BOOK OF ORTHOPEDICS. These are exciting times in orthopedic surgery, and we believe that the editors of this volume have chosen exciting and important contributions from that literature to keep the reader abreast of the ever changing and expanding orthopedic landscape.

Robert Poss, M.D.
Clement B. Sledge, M.D.

1 Pediatrics

Introduction

The pediatric section has been divided into 5 subsections of related topics plus a miscellaneous section. There were many studies on neurovascular conditions published this year. We have selected 9 of the most interesting ones to put in this edition. Of particular interest are the papers on treatment options for cerebral palsy and for brachial plexus injuries in the newborn. Answers to some questions about appropriate procedures and their affect are clear, but many questions still exist.

As always, hip problems continue to be of great interest. The 10 articles selected are mostly about diagnosis and treatment of developmental dislocation, but we have included articles on slipped capital femoral epiphysis and Legg-Calvé-Perthes disease, 2 subjects where there is still controversy about treatment and cause.

In addition to neurovascular disease and the hip, we have included articles on the spine, the upper and lower extremity, and the medical and psychological aspects of the Ilizarov Method, as well as a miscellaneous section.

These articles are stimulating and informative. Some support well accepted concepts, others have new ideas that may or may not withstand the trials of time.

Paul P. Griffin, M.D.

Neurovascular Condition

Persistent Brachial Plexus Birth Palsies

Jahnke AH, Bovill DF, McCarroll HR Jr, James P, Ashley RK (Letterman Army Med Ctr; Univ of California; Shriners Hosp, San Francisco)
J Pediatr Orthop 11:533–537, 1991   1–1

Background.—Brachial plexus injuries remain a significant problem. A small proportion of affected patients will have significant morbidity and disability. Patients with persistent brachial plexus palsy were examined.

Patients.—Patients were 64 children (34 boys and 30 girls) with birth-related traumatic brachial plexus palsy diagnosed during a 15-year period. Of the 64 patients, 2 had bilateral injury. At birth 38 patients had shoulder dystocia, 10 had umbilical cord strangulation, 10 underwent forceps delivery, 5 had birth fractures, and 4 had breech presentation. Birth weight averaged 10 pounds 2½ ounces. Twenty-four children had moderate upper palsies, and 27 had severe, global palsies. Only 3 instances of isolated lower plexus injury were noted. Average time to resolution or plateau of objective findings was 4.5 months. Twenty-seven patients had flaccid extremities at birth, and 10 had Horner's syndrome. At final follow-up hypoplastic upper extremity was found in 53 of 66 extremities, internal rotational shoulder contractures were seen in 42, elbow flexion contractures were found in 36, and dislocated radial head was seen in 2. All patients had initial treatment with simple range-of-motion exercises. Operation was done in 26 patients, and most commonly involved tendon transfers for absent wrist or finger dorsiflexion or biceps tendon rerouting for forearm supination deformities.

Conclusions.—This group of patients with persistent brachial plexus palsies generally had little symptomatic improvement after age 6 months. Overall function is rarely improved by reconstructive surgery, but the patients appreciate even minor improvements. Controlled, clinical examination of the role of surgical exploration and microsurgical repair is warranted.

▶ This study emphasizes the range of residual deformity after brachial plexus injuries when nerve function does not recover. Fortunately, recovery of function occurs in most brachial plexus injuries in newborns (1).—P.P. Griffin, M.D.

Reference

1. Hoffer MM, et al: *J Bone Joint Surg* 60-A:691, 1978.

Brachial Plexus Microsurgery in Children
Hentz VR, Meyer RD (Stanford Univ; Univ of Alabama, Birmingham)
Microsurgery 12:175–185, 1991   1–2

Background.—The application of microsurgical techniques to problems involving the peripheral nervous system has provided an opportunity to use these general microsurgical techniques in the treatment of obstetric palsy. A review of the literature was undertaken to evaluate the role of brachial plexus microsurgery in children.

Analysis.—The typical obstetric palsy is a traumatic lesion caused by forced lowering of the shoulder during delivery. Complete spontaneous recovery is possible, but only if biceps and deltoid have recovered by the second month. If the biceps have not recovered within 3 months, the results will be unsatisfactory. It is at this period, between 2 and 4 months, that surgery should be considered an option. The clinical examination is the most important single determining factor in the decision to perform surgery. Obstetric palsy may involve all the roots. The upper roots are usually ruptured, whereas the lower roots, if involved, are almost always avulsed. No isolated injury to the lower roots without injury to the upper roots has been found. Surgical repair is usually by grafting. In children who reach the age of 3 months without evidence of recovery of the biceps, surgical repair offers better functional results compared with spontaneous recovery. In a series of patients who had not recovered biceps function by 3 months, two thirds had nearly normal shoulders after grafting C5 and C6 lesions, compared with none of the patients who were allowed to recover spontaneously. Surgical decisions can be difficult when treating patients with several avulsions; sacrifices have to be made and priorities must be established to obtain optimal function. Among patients who have contractures and other effects of birth palsy, palliative treatment is often difficult and results are rarely totally satisfactory.

Conclusion.—The decision to perform surgery on children with brachial plexus palsy should be made as quickly as possible before neuroplasticity is diminished and joint contractures have occurred.

▶ The authors present a strong argument for early grafting of brachial plexus lesions. Their guidelines for selection are precise, and the article should be studied closely.—P.P. Griffin, M.D.

Surgical Treatment of Brachial Plexus Birth Palsy
Gilbert A, Brockman R, Carlioz H (Institut Français de la Main; Hôpital Trousseau, Paris)
Clin Orthop 264:39–47, 1991   1–3

Background.—The consequences of brachial plexus birth palsy result from extensive paralysis with muscular imbalance and muscle contractures secondary to an anarchic reinnervation. The shoulder is the joint most often involved in paralytic results, 3 with internal rotation contracture being the most common problem.

Methods.—Between 1977 and 1988 1,000 infants with brachial plexus birth palsy were examined. Clinically, the infants had paralysis of the upper roots with the extremity held in internal rotation and pronation or with complete paralysis with a flaccid arm. Surgical exploration and repair were performed in 241 infants. The indication for surgery was the lack of clinical recovery of the biceps by age 3 months.

Results.—At 3 years after operation, shoulders of class III, IV, or V (based on the Mallet scale) were noted in 81% of 96 C5–6 repairs and 76% of 81 C5, C6, C7 repairs. Among the 64 shoulders in patients with complete paralysis, results of class IV were found in 22.5%, of class III in 42%, and of class II in 35.5%. Partial or complete recovery of the intrinsic muscles of the hand was observed in half the patients; 83% of hands recovered some function, and 30% recovered valuable function. Subscapular release for internal rotation contractures was followed up in 66 patients for 5 years, including 28 patients who had previous surgical repair of the brachial plexus. During more than 5 years of follow-up, average postoperative gain of external rotation was 70 degrees for patients who had release of the subscapularis tendon before age 2 years. Failures occurred in 18%, particularly among children older than age 2 years. Forty-seven percent of patients recovered active external rotation without treatment. Sixty-seven patients have had latissimus dorsi transfer; most were between ages 2 and 5 years at the time of surgery. All 44 patients with more than 1 year of follow-up gained active external rotation when there was none before operation. Among 32 children who had a coexisting deficit of abduction, there was an average gain of 35 degrees, a constant finding only when preoperative abduction was at least 90 degrees. Trapezius transfer was performed in 10 patients with flaccid shoulders, with modest results.

Conclusions.—Functional results are much improved after surgery for brachial plexus birth palsy compared with those obtained after observation only. Surgery is indicated when no clinical recovery of the biceps is apparent by the third month. Recovery is slow, at least 2 years for high lesions and 4 years for complete lesions. Follow-up examinations and physical therapy are necessary to avoid contractures, and palliative procedures can be performed from age 2 years with improved prognosis.

▶ This study has 2 important statements to make. The first is that, in upper brachial plexus injuries, if the biceps has not recovered by 3 months of age, surgical intervention gives better results than in late spontaneous recovery. The second is that, with residual internal rotation contracture, a release of the subscapularis should be done before age 2 years, but muscle transfer to improve active external rotation should not be done routinely at the same time, for active external rotation will develop in many patients after the release alone.— P.P. Griffin, M.D.

Cerebral Palsy and Rhizotomy: A 3-Year Follow-Up Evaluation With Gait Analysis
Vaughan CL, Berman B, Peacock WJ (Univ of Virginia, Charlottesville; Univ of California, Los Angeles)
J Neurosurg 74:178–184, 1991   1–4

Background.—Selective posterior rhizotomy has become a popular neurosurgical option for the reduction of spasticity in cerebral palsy. Postoperative outcome and long-term changes in gait patterns were evaluated after posterior rhizotomy in patients with cerebral palsy.

Methods.—In 1985 14 children with spastic cerebral palsy and none of the other features of cerebral palsy underwent selective posterior rhizotomy. By using a digital camera system sagittal plane gait patterns were examined before surgery and at 1 and 3 years after surgery. The range of motion at the knee and thigh, stride length, speed of walking, and cadence were measured. Mean age at time of surgery was 8 years.

Results.—The range of motion at the knee increased significantly at 1 year after surgery and further improved to a nearly normal range at 3 years. The thigh range exceeded normal values at 1 year but decreased toward normal range at 3 years. The midrange points in knee and thigh movement reflected a more extended thigh and knee position, indicating a more upright walking posture. Stride length and speed of walking also improved significantly.

Conclusions.—Patients with cerebral palsy can increase their strength and muscular control after selective posterior rhizotomy. The early functional outcome is encouraging and physical therapy may contribute further to this improvement.

▶ The improvement in gait in this small number of patients is impressive. The data presented show a more upright posture from the crouched gait that is so frequently a problem in spastic children. The study appears to be well controlled. The addition of a similar control group treated with extensive physical therapy would have been helpful in evaluating the results physical therapy contributed to the rhizotomy.—P.P. Griffin, M.D.

Posterior Transfer of the Adductors in Children Who Have Cerebral Palsy: A Long-Term Study
Aronson DD, Zak PJ, Lee CL, Bollinger RO, Lamont RL (Children's Hosp of Michigan, Detroit, Wayne State Univ, Detroit)
J Bone Joint Surg 73-A:59–65, 1991   1–5

Background.—Several trials have reported satisfactory results with adductor transfer in children with cerebral palsy. The long-term results were examined for a protocol involving the use of posterior transfer of the adductors as the primary treatment for children with spastic cerebral palsy and hip involvement.

Methods.—During a 13-year period 56 children underwent 108 posterior adductor transfers. Data on 78 operations in 42 children were available for analysis. The 28 boys and 14 girls had an average age of 5.5 years at surgery. All had cerebral palsy; 22 had spastic diplegia, and 20 had spastic quadriplegia. In 33 of the 78 operations a tenotomy of the iliopsoas tendon was also done. Clinical and radiographic follow-up averaged 5.7 years after operation. Results were assessed based on the patient's ability to walk, range of motion of the affected hip or hips, and radiographic measurements.

Results.—Stability, functional walking, abduction, and extension were improved or maintained in 88% of hips. Varus derotational osteotomy for progressive subluxation was needed in the 9 failed cases, all of which occurred in patients with spastic quadriplegia who were unable to walk. Flexion contractures improved from an average of 26 degrees to 9 degrees, and the mean arc of abduction improved from 20 degrees to 50 degrees. Iliopsoas tenotomy improved the mean range of abduction from 21 degrees to 57 degrees, compared to a mean improvement of 20 degrees to 44 degrees in patients who did not have this procedure.

Conclusions.—Posterior adductor transfer in children with spastic cerebral palsy appears to have a good long-term outcome. Iliopsoas tenotomy may be done routinely in conjunction with this operation. After using bilateral above-knee casts with a cross-bar for 4 weeks, vigorous physical therapy, with particular attention to increasing the active range of hip motion and gait training, is recommended.

▶ Most of the clinical and radiographic parameters usually measured for evaluation of results in the cerebral palsy hip were improved after treatment. The title of the article is misleading because the adductor brevis and part of the magnus also were released. The benefit of transfer, as compared to myotomy alone, appears to be the improvement in gait. There is little reason to do this more extensive procedure in patients who have no potential for walking. If the hip is dysplastic, part-time splinting for an extended period of time may be beneficial (1).—P.P. Griffin, M.D.

Reference

1. Houkom JA, et al: *J Pediatr Orthop* 6:285, 1986.

Extra-Articular Subtalar Arthrodesis With Cancellous Bone Graft and Internal Fixation for Children With Myelomeningocele
Aronson DD, Middleton DL (Univ Health Ctr, Burlington, Vt; Rush Orthopaedic Clinic, Midland, Mich)
Dev Med Child Neurol 33:232–240, 1991   1–6

Objective.—Hindfoot valgus deformities in children with myelomeningocele were treated by using extra-articular subtalar arthrodesis with cancellous bone grafts and internal fixation. The indication for surgery was progressive hindfoot valgus deformity that caused difficulty with fitting orthoses.

Methods.—Between 1982 and 1986 a total of 20 arthrodesis procedures were performed on 12 children aged 5.6–9.5 years (mean age, 7.4 years). Ankle valgus deformity was corrected at the same time in 6 patients. Average follow-up was 4.1 years.

Results.—All 20 feet had radiographic fusion after an average of 11 weeks. Postoperative complications included 2 superficial wound infections and 2 pathologic fractures that were treated successfully. At follow-up, 18 feet had achieved satisfactory results. The talocalcaneal screw provided rigid internal fixation, and no significant changes were noted in the talocalcaneal angle. The 2 feet with unsatisfactory results were undercorrected at the time of surgery. The calcaneus was not sufficiently rotated under the talus, and the postoperative radiographs showed insufficient correction of the lateral talocalcaneal angle.

Conclusions.—Extra-articular subtalar arthrodesis will correct hindfoot valgus deformity in children with myelomeningocele, and the use of internal fixation and iliac crest bone grafting contribute to improved success. An intraoperative lateral radiograph of the foot measuring the talocalcaneal angle is recommended to ensure that the hindfoot is in the desired position. Simultaneous surgical correction of concomitant ankle valgus deformity with the extra-articular subtalar arthrodesis is recommended.

▶ The use of cancellous bone plus firm fixation with a screw gave excellent correction and a higher fusion rate than other methods of grafting. There are 2 concerns with this paper. A 4.5-year average follow-up is too short to determine the outcome because loss of subtalar motion in the insensate foot can be a problem over time, and there is no mention of muscle imbalance. We know that, in a child, muscle imbalance will cause a deformity in spite of a solid arthrodesis.—P.P. Griffin, M.D.

Gait Analysis in the Treatment of the Ambulatory Child With Cerebral Palsy
DeLuca PA (Newington Children's Hosp, Conn)
Clin Orthop 264:65–75, 1991   1–7

Background.—In children with cerebral palsy surgical treatment has evolved from staged procedures to comprehensive, simultaneous bony and soft tissue corrections. Because many joint levels and planes of abnormality are treated in these operations, errors may occur when the procedure is based on clinical examination only. Spastic gait disturbances can be scientifically assessed and surgical outcomes evaluated by clinical gait analysis.

Clinical Assessment and Treatment Strategy.—Surgical outcome in cerebral palsy is inconsistent because of the complex patterns of reflex control and various combinations of primary deficiencies and secondary changes. The traditional clinical examination is limited by its static nature, and surgical results may be unpredictable because of unrecognized muscle weakness, central imbalance, and interference with reflex patterns. In addition, single-level surgery may leave untreated contractures at adjacent joints. The most important recent surgical advance for these patients is integrated tendon lengthenings or transfers, in conjunction with simultaneous or closely staged bony corrections. The precision of assessment required by these procedures necessitates the use of gait analysis.

Clinical Gait Analysis.—Computer-assisted, video-based motion analysis systems have been in use for several years. The testing procedure is quick and cost-effective. Computer tracking of retroflective markers creates kinematic plots of the pelvis, hip, knee, and ankle in the coronal, sagittal, and transverse planes. Ground-contact forces are measured by pressure-sensitive transducers, and these data are used to calculate moments of force, which can be combined with synchronous electromyographic information. When used for a period of several years, these data have identified specific patterns of pathology that help in selecting treatment methods. Abnormalities range from distal and less severe to proximal and more severe and can be managed by a general surgical and orthotic treatment protocol.

Conclusions.—Clinical gait analysis can be a useful tool in the evaluation of children with cerebral palsy, both in preoperative planning and postoperative assessment. It has allowed for definition of specific gait patterns, for which surgical protocols are described. The protocols ultimately can be tested for outcome.

▶ This is an excellent paper on the principles and philosophy of the management of patients with cerebral palsy. It deals with more than gait analysis. Gait analysis is a helpful tool in defining motion abnormalities and selecting surgical treatment. It is a very good research tool for motion disabilities and evaluating the result of treatment. The question is whether or not it is wrong for surgery to be done on a patient with cerebral palsy without the preoperative evaluation by gait analysis. I prefer to have a motion analysis with electromyography before performing surgery to correct a static or dynamic deformity in a patient with cerebral palsy, but this is not always possible. Repeated clinical observations by an experienced surgeon in most instances will define the problems that need correction.— P.P. Griffin, M.D.

Pediatric Atlantoaxial Instability Presenting as Cerebral and Cerebellar Infarcts
Bhatnagar M, Sponseller PD, Carroll C IV, Tolo VT (Johns Hopkins Univ, Baltimore; Northwestern Univ, Chicago; Children's Hosp of Los Angeles, Calif)
J Pediatr Orthop 11:103–107, 1991   1–8

Background.—Diagnosis of atlantoaxial subluxation can be difficult because of the often confusing signs and symptoms. One child with unexplained cerebral and cerebellar infarcts was subsequently found to have significant atlantoaxial instability.

Case Report.—Boy, 5½ years, had unexplained transient repeated cerebral and cerebellar signs. Areas of acute and subacute infarcts were detected by CT in the left cerebellar hemisphere, both occipital lobes, and left parietal lobes. Lateral films of the cervical spine showed an os odontoideum, and films taken with active extension showed 10 mm of posterior translation of the anterior margin of the atlas of the axis. These findings correlated with angiographic findings of narrowing and tortuosity of the left vertebral artery at the level of the axis and of diminished flow to the left posterior cerebellum. After stabilization and fusion of the cervical spine, the patient achieved normal neurologic function and remained symptom-free at 3-year follow-up.

Conclusion.—This case further illustrates the spectrum of abnormalities associated with atlantoaxial instability in children.

▶ This is a case report of a patient with cerebral and cerebellar signs. It should remind us that such symptoms may be caused by cervical abnormalities and even mild repeated injuries to the spine that result in the development of instability.— P.P. Griffin, M.D.

Use of the Green Transfer in Treatment of Patients With Spastic Cerebral Palsy: 17-Year Experience
Beach WR, Strecker WB, Coe J, Manske PR, Schoenecker PL, Dailey L (Shriners Hosps for Crippled Children, St. Louis; Washington Univ, St Louis; Brooke Army Med Ctr, Fort Sam Houston, Tex)
J Pediatr Orthop 11:731–736, 1991   1–9

Range of Motion Results

Motion	Preoperative		Postoperative	
	Mean	Arc	Mean	Arc
Dorsiflexion	−25°	49°	34°	47°
Volarflexion	74°		13°	
Supination	−16°	66°	43°ᵃ	96°
Pronation	82°		53°	

ᵃIncluded in these final results are 8 patients who had concomitant pronator release or reroutement.

(Courtesy of Beach WR, Strecker WB, Coe J, et al: *J Pediatr Orthop* 11:731–736, 1991.)

Background.—Different operative procedures have been used to correct all or part of the flexion-pronation deformity in children with cerebral palsy. The Green transfer is a standard technique used to treat forearm pronation, wrist flexion, and ulnar deviation deformities secondary to upper extremity spastic paralysis. The outcomes of the Green procedure were evaluated in 43 patients aged 3 years 5 months to 16 years 5 months.

Technique.—A single volar incision is used to expose the flexor carpi ulnaris (FCU). Either the extensor carpi radialis brevis or the extensor carpi radialis longus, or both, are used for insertion. Although Green originally described the FCU sutured in tension at 45 degrees of dorsiflexion and full supination, in this modification the transferred FCU tendon is tensioned to hold the wrist in neutral against gravity. The wrist is immobilized in 5 degrees of dorsiflexion and the forearm in 45 degrees of supination. Occupational therapy was done after casting or splinting.

Results.—On the basis of preoperative and postoperative functional ratings, 88% had cosmetic improvement, 79% improved functionally, and no patients had decreased functional rating (table). Patients older than 12 years of age showed less functional improvement. Operative results were not affected by quadriplegia athetosis or intellectual impairment. The total arc of motion (47 degrees) did not change postoperatively but was centered about neutral. Supination improved markedly after a pronator procedure. The most important prognostic factor was use of the extremity as a helper preoperatively.

Conclusions.—The Green transfer consistently corrects the volarflexion pronation, ulnar deviation deformity and improves range of motion, function, and cosmesis. The procedure does not increase the arc of flexion and extension. Patients younger than 12 years of age have greater functional improvement.

▶ The FCU transfer (Green procedure) can improve hand function, as reported here. The transfer should not be inserted with the wrist in full extension and the forearm in full supination, as an extension-supination contracture may be produced. The FCU muscle that fires in both flexion and extension was not addressed in this article. A muscle that is active during both flexion and extension will not give as good a result as one that is phasic, and it may cause an extension contracture.—P.P. Griffin, M.D.

Spine

MR of Cord Transection

Mendelsohn DB, Zollars L, Weatherall PT, Girson M (Univ of Texas, Dallas; Fairoaks Hosp, Fairfax, Va)
J Comput Assist Tomogr 14:909–911, 1990   1–10

Background.—Cord transection is uncommon after trauma. In 3 children, spinal cord transection was demonstrated with MRI after severe trauma.

Patients.—All 3 children had spinal cord transection after motor vehicle accidents. In 2 children, signs of neurologic deficit did not correlate with the level of skeletal injury. One child had a C5–6 compression fracture dislocation, but MR images showed spinal cord transection at T3–4, with no associated fracture or deformity (Fig 1–1). Another child had type II odontoid fracture, but MR imaging showed a transected cord at the C7–T1 level. The third child showed a cord transection at the C5–6 vertebral level without underlying skeletal injury.

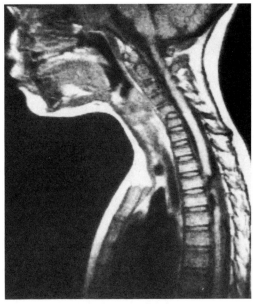

Fig 1–1.—Girl aged 4 years with C5–6 fracture dislocation. Sagittal T1-weighted image (500/40) demonstrates cord transection at T3–4 with no associated fracture or deformity within upper thoracic spine. (Courtesy of Mendelsohn DB, Zollars L, Weatherall PT, et al: *J Comput Assist Tomogr* 14:909–911, 1990.)

Conclusions.—Spinal cord transection after severe trauma in children can occur without evidence of underlying skeletal injury, or it can occur at a level remote from the site of fracture. Direct and noninvasive visualization of the traumatized spinal cord can be achieved with MRI.

▶ Spinal cord transection remote from bony injury or without bony injury is well known. Magnetic resonance imaging is the best imaging technique to show the level of cord transection.—P.P. Griffin, M.D.

Natural History of Symptomatic Isthmic Low-Grade Spondylolisthesis in Children and Adolescents: A Seven-Year Follow-Up Study

Frennered AK, Danielson BI, Nachemson AL (Sahlgrenska Hospital, Göteborg, Sweden)
J Pediatr Orthop 11:209–213, 1991   1–11

Background.—In isthmic spondylolysis or spondylolisthesis, considerable slip progression may occur during rapid growth in adolescence, although this is uncommon after age 25 years. The risk factors for this condition are well known, but the natural history is not. A series of young patients with isthmic spondylolisthesis was examined to investigate the natural history and to seek clinical and radiographic prognostic factors for slip progression.

Methods.—Records of 47 of 72 patients with spondylolysis or spondylolisthesis treated in a 10-year period were reviewed. There were 28 boys and 19 girls (mean age, 12 years at diagnosis). All patients were evaluated by questionnaire, and all but 1 were examined clinically and radiographically. Seventeen patients were treated with physical rehabilitation, physiotherapy, analgesics, or brace treatment and the other 30 had only occasional restrictions on physical activity. All 47 patients had L5 lysis. Mean follow-up time was 7 years.

Results.—Slip progressed in 2 patients (4%), and 12 patients required operative intervention after a mean observation time of 3.7 years. Results among patients not undergoing surgery were excellent in 43% of patients, good in 40%, and fair in 17%. The mean pain value was 2.8 on a scale of 1 to 10. The indication for operation was low back pain in 10 patients and presumed progression in 2. There were no significant prognostic factors for either progression of slip or need for future operative treatment.

Conclusions.—Slip progression appears to be rare in patients with low-grade spondylolisthesis. Most patients have no pain or occasional mild pain that does not interfere with their activities. Although a significant number of patients have surgery for pain or progression, or both, the natural history of the disorder appears to be benign.

▶ The data show only a 4% incidence of progression of the slip in 47 patients. The authors failed to identify prognostic signs for progression of the slip or for the development of pain requiring surgery in the future.—P.P. Griffin, M.D.

Low-Back Pain and Disk Degeneration in Children: A Case-Control MR Imaging Study

Tertti MO, Salminen JJ, Paajanen HEK, Terho PH, Kormano MJ (University of Turku, Finland; Central Hospital of Mikkeli, Finland; Public Health Care of Turku, Finland)
Radiology 180:503–507, 1991   1–12

Background.—In adults no causal relationship between disk degeneration and low-back pain can be established, mainly because of the confounding effect of physiologic, age-dependent disk degeneration. Understanding of the cause of disk degeneration can be improved by evaluation of disk degeneration in children. Magnetic resonance imaging was used to investigate lumbar disk degeneration and associated factors in matched asymptomatic children and children with low-back pain.

Methods.—Patients were selected from a population of 1,503 children aged 15 years participating in a MRI study of the lumbar spine. In this sample, the prevalence of continuous or recurrent low-back pain was 7.8%. Thirty-one of these children were selected randomly for the current investigation, along with 8 children who had sciatic low-back pain. Each of these groups of patients was matched for sex, age, and school class with an asymptomatic control. Both groups underwent MRI.

Results.—Magnetic resonance imaging detected disk degeneration in 38% of the low-back pain group and 26% of controls. The only finding that was more common in the low-back pain than in the control group was disk protrusion. The changes most commonly associated with lumbar degeneration were disk protrusion and Scheuermann-type changes. Girls with low-back pain tended to have more disk protrusion and spinal muscular atrophy than boys with low-back pain.

Conclusions.—Many children, aged 15 years, with low-back pain have disk degeneration and many asymptomatic children of this age have asymptomatic, possibly physiologic disk degeneration. There is a significant correlation between disk degeneration and disk protrusion in children with low-back pain. A long-term follow-up investigation is underway to determine whether disk degeneration associated with structural changes predisposes to low-back disorders.

▶ More studies of this type are needed to define the range of normality in young patients. The significance of the MRI findings is yet to be understood. I have seen teenagers with the complaint of severe disabling back pain who on MRI have several abnormal disks with protrusion. These children had classic conversion hysteria, and the MRI findings made it difficult to establish the correct diagnosis.—P.P. Griffin, M.D.

Low-Back Pain in Adolescent Athletes: Detection of Stress Injury to the Pars Interarticularis With SPECT

Bellah RD, Summerville DA, Treves ST, Micheli LJ (Children's Hosp, Boston)
Radiology 180:509–512, 1991   1–13

Background.—Early detection of stress injury of the pars interarticularis is vital. The ability of bone scintigraphy to localize the diagnosis is improved by single photon emission computed tomography (SPECT). The use of planar and SPECT scintigraphy in young patients referred for low-back pain was evaluated to determine whether SPECT increases detection of the pars interarticularis injury.

Methods.—A total of 162 patients were referred during a year period, including 100 females and 62 males (mean age, 16.4 years). About 130 patients were athletes, and 72% had symptoms referable to the posterior elements. All patients underwent both planar and SPECT bone scintigraphy.

Results.—Scintigraphy showed no abnormality in 56% of the patients. The abnormalities demonstrated on planar imaging also were detectable on SPECT. An abnormal focus of radiotracer uptake was found on SPECT in 71 patients, in 32 of whom the abnormality was also seen on planar scintigraphy. Single photon emission computed tomography alone demonstrated the abnormality in 39 patients. Of 56 patients with normal radiographic results, 16 had scintigraphic abnormalities that could be revealed only by SPECT.

Conclusions.—Single photon emission computed tomography is capable of detecting stress injuries that are not demonstrated by planar bone imaging or radiography. It can separate soft tissue mechanical from osseous causes of low-back pain in young athletes; this is vital for selecting the proper mode of treatment.

▶ This study further confirms that SPECT can detect stress changes in the pars interarticularis that are not seen with planar imaging or on radiographs. It can be of significant value in establishing the diagnosis of persistent low-back pain in the adolescent.— P.P. Griffin, M.D.

Lower Extremity

Leg Length Discrepancy Following Irradiation for Childhood Tumors
Robertson WW Jr, Butler MS, D'Angio GJ, Rate WR (Children's Hosp of Philadelphia; Univ of Medicine and Dentistry of New Jersey, New Brunswick; Univ of Pennsylvania)
J Pediatr Orthop 11:284–287, 1991   1–14

Background.—Ionizing radiation to the immature skeleton induces both growth abnormalities and skeletal deformities by causing arrest of chondrogenesis in the growth plate. The incidence and severity of leg length discrepancy after irradiation for childhood tumors as well as factors that may predispose patients to this complication were assessed retrospectively.

Patients.—Between 1970 and 1987 a group of 67 children was treated with radiation to the kidney, abdomen, pelvis, or lower extremities. Mean age at the time of irradiation was 7 years. Mean follow-up was 10.6 years. All children survived childhood cancer to the age of skeletal maturity.

Outcome.—Twelve children had leg length discrepancy ranging from
.6 cm to 9 cm; 7 children were symptomatic. The development of leg
length discrepancy was significantly related to the total dose of radiation
to the pelvic area, asymmetric irradiation to the pelvis, and high-dose irradiation to the leg.

Conclusion.—The quality in leg length after pelvic and long bone radiation treatment remains a significant consequence of treatment. This
complication from abdominal irradiation is directly related to iliac apo-
physeal or proximal femoral physeal growth retardation, and its severity
is dose-related.

▶ An undesirable effect of asymmetrical irradiation to the abdomen and pelvis
is the development of anisomelia in some patients. This is the result of retardation of growth of the ilium and proximal femur on the irradiated side. The number of patients was too small to correlate age with the amount of retardation of
growth. Because it is a retrospective study there is no information on either the
rate or the duration of retardation.—P.P. Griffin, M.D.

Fibular Deficiency and the Indications for Syme's Amputation
Oppenheim WL (Univ of California, Los Angeles)
Prosthet Orthop Int 15:131–136, 1991   1–15

Background.—The child with congenital fibular deficiency may
present a frustrating and anxiety-producing problem for the physician.
Few methods of management of the profoundly involved limb, except for
amputation and prosthetic fitting, have stood up over the years. Current
knowledge of fibular deficiency is evaluated, including the role of Syme's
amputation, reconstructive surgery, and prosthetic management.

Classification.—The condition may range in severity from simple hy-
poplasia to total absence of the fibula. Classification systems have been
based on ankle and foot stability and on function and overall limb
length. In the system of Coventry and Johnson, type 1 is 1 affected limb
ranging from fibular shortening to partial absence of its upper portion;
type 2 is unilateral involvement with total absence of the fibula; and type
3 is bilateral involvement sometimes in association with other malforma-
tions.

Treatment.—Type 1 feet usually need not be converted to amputations. Surgical salvage of type 2 limbs may be difficult. Syme's amputation should be thought of as a reconstructive, not ablative, procedure.
There is good evidence that it should be done as a primary, rather than a
salvage, procedure. Full activity and function may be achieved in young
children who grow up with a conversion. Indications for Syme's amputation are a deformity so severe that surgery to create a functional foot will
probably fail and a leg-length discrepancy of 7.5 cm or more by maturity.
Boyd amputation is a reasonable alternative. When ankle stability is not
a problem, the main concern becomes leg lengthening. With newer techniques, lengthening procedures are now done for severe shortening for-

merly thought to be contraindicated. Repeated procedures may be needed to keep up with the child's growth, each with a long period of recovery. Lengthening may be an attainable goal in some type 1 cases, but ankle disarticulation is still considered the procedure of choice for type 2 deformities with grossly unstable ankles.

Conclusions.—Despite many alternatives to Syme's amputation and prosthetic fitting for fibular deficiency, it is still the standard treatment against which others must be judged. Performed when the patient is young, this procedure can allow athletic and psychologic function similar to that of a nonhandicapped child. This should be the primary reconstructive procedure in a child with total congenital fibular absence.

▶ Decision making in the management of the patient with fibular deficiency involves more than our ability to lengthen the tibia. Ankle and foot function have to be assessed, and the overall effect of the prolonged treatment on the child's emotional and psychological development has to be considered. Although lengthening the limb equalizes the length, it should not be the only measure of the success of treatment.—P.P. Griffin, M.D.

Failure of Centralization of the Fibula for Congenital Longitudinal Deficiency of the Tibia

Epps CH Jr, Tooms RE, Edholm CD, Kruger LM, Bryant DD III (District of Columbia Gen Hosp, Washington, DC; Campbell Clinic, Memphis; Area Child Amputee Clinic, Grand Rapids, Mich; Shriners Hosp for Crippled Children, Springfield, Mass)
J Bone Joint Surg 73-A:858–867, 1991   1–16

Background.—Several reports of congenital longitudinal deficiency of the tibia have questioned the effectiveness of the Brown procedure, which consists of centralization of the fibula distal to the femur, a Syme-type amputation, and prosthesis fitting. Patients at 4 amputee clinics were examined to assess the value of the Brown procedure.

Methods.—Centralization of the fibula was performed on 20 knees in 14 patients with congenital longitudinal deficiency of the tibia during a 21-year period. Case histories and radiographs for each patient were examined. All had malrotation of the involved leg, leg-length discrepancy, and equinovarus deformity of the foot. Patients ranged in age from 3 months to 36 months at the time of operation, and 11 of the procedures were done on patients aged 1 year or younger. Average follow-up after the initial procedure was 12 years 4 months.

Results.—After all 20 procedures, a progressive flexion deformity of the knee developed, delaying optimal fitting of the initial prosthesis. To correct these deformities, 26 secondary procedures were performed, including disarticulation at the knee, posterior release, extension osteotomy, femorofibular arthrodesis, and biceps-to-quadriceps transfer. A second attempt at fibular centralization was made in 1 patient. In 8 limbs in 7 patients with failure of the index procedure, disarticulation at the knee had a satisfactory result. The index procedure also was considered to have failed because of flexion deformity in patients who did not have secondary disarticulation at the knee.

Conclusions.—For patients with congenital longitudinal deficiency of the tibia, knee reconstruction by centralization of the fibula is not warranted. The procedure of choice appears to be early disarticulation at the knee, fitting with a prosthesis, and close follow-up. The main problem with centralization of the fibula is a persistent, progressive flexion deformity of the knee.

▶ This article supports unequivocally the concept that reconstruction for congenital tibia deficiency by centralization of the fibula is not warranted. It is a valuable contribution to orthopedic knowledge. I have always believed that even in the best of situations, where the quadriceps appeared to be functional and could be used to extend the transferred fibula, the functional result was poor compared to early amputation of the fibula and prosthetic fitting.—P.P. Griffin, M.D.

Functional Results of Operation in Osteogenesis Imperfecta: Elongating and Nonelongating Rods

Porat S, Heller E, Seidman DS, Meyer S (Hadassah University Hospital; Alyn Children's Orthopedic Hospital, Jerusalem)
J Pediatr Orthop 11:200–203, 1991   1–17

Background.—Intramedullary nailing is the most accepted operative treatment for osteogenesis imperfecta (OI). The functional results of operation, using either the Bailey-Dubow (B-D) elongating rods or nonelongating rods, were reviewed for 20 patients with OI. Mean follow-up was 9.8 years.

Results.—Gait capacity improved in 8 patients, regressed in 3, and remained unchanged in 9. When only ambulators and nonambulators were compared, the percentage of ambulators increased markedly from 40% before operation to 75% afterward. No preoperative ambulator regressed to a nonambulatory status after operation. Gait capacity varied with each Sillence disease type. Thirty-two B-D nails and 24 nonelongating nails were inserted in the tibia of femur as the primary procedure. The complication rate was 72% for the B-D nail and 50% for the nonelongating nail. Seventy-four percent of the former and 58% of the latter were intrinsic to the type of nail used (table). The percentage of reoperation and postoperative longevity was similar for both types of nails.

Conclusions.—The treatment of a child with OI is challenging. Intramedullary nailing is an accepted treatment for these children, but the type of nail used remains the choice of the surgeons. The postoperative improvement in function and gait capacity after intramedullary nailing is encouraging, but expectations about operative intervention should be realistic and must be enhanced by a comprehensive rehabilitation program.

Details of Complications of Primary Procedure

	B-D nail			Non-elongating nail		
Complication	Reoperation	No reoperation	Total	Reoperation	No reoperation	Total
1. Migration into joint or soft tissue	5		5	5		5
2. Infection	1		1			
3. T-piece loose ***	1	3	4			
4. Failure of extension ***	1		1			
5. Disassembly of nail ***	2	6	8			
6. Disassembly with fracture of unprotected midshaft ***	4		4			
7. Outgrown nail with fracture of unprotected section †				7		7
Total	14	9	23	12		12

Abbreviation: B–D, Bailey-Dubow.
*Complication intrinsic to B–D nail.
†Complication intrinsic to nonelongating nail.
(Courtesy of Porat S, Heller E, Seidman DS, et al: *J Pediatr Orthop* 11:200–203, 1991.)

▶ Complication rates with intramedullary nailing of the long bone in OI are high, as is shown in this article. The B-D nail gives a slightly longer interval before needing to be replaced because of growth but is more difficult to insert and can break as it elongates. One complication not mentioned is severe resorption of the cortex after intramedullary fixation, which is a serious problem and one that is difficult to resolve if it occurs.—P.P. Griffin, M.D.

Treatment of Residual Clubfoot Deformity, the "Bean-Shaped" Foot, by Opening Wedge Medial Cuneiform Osteotomy and Closing Wedge Cuboid Osteotomy: Clinical Review and Cadaver Correlations

McHale KA, Lenhart MK (Walter Reed Army Med Ctr, Washington, DC)
J Pediatr Orthop 11:374–381, 1991   1–18

Background.—Residual problems after surgical treatment of clubfoot deformity are common. The "bean-shaped" foot is the result of forefoot adductus, midfoot supination, and mild hindfoot varus that produces an elongated lateral column of the foot, an internally rotated gait, and a plantigrade foot. Children who present with this deformity are usually too old for soft tissue release by itself or too young for triple arthrodesis.

Methods.—Six patients aged 4–10 years who had previous surgery for clubfoot presented with bean-shaped foot in 7 feet. Treatment consisted of opening wedge medial cuneiform and closing wedge cuboid osteotomies. A dorsal-lateral wedge was removed from the cuboid and placed in the osteotomy site in the medial cuneiform. Forefoot adductus and midfoot supination were corrected simultaneously. The procedure was repeated in fresh cadavers (8 feet) to determine how the alterations at each surgical site translated into clinical correction.

Results.—After an average follow-up of more than 2 years, all feet were markedly improved. The prominent midfoot supination resolved in all patients, and forefoot adductus was corrected in all but 1. Radiographically, there was an average improvement of 9 degrees in the talo-first metatarsal angle, whereas the second metatarsal-tarsal angle improved by 14 degrees. The change in metatarsal height was impressive, with an average decrease of 13 mm. Cadaver reproductions demonstrated consistently that the cuboid closing wedge accounted for the change in the midfoot, whereas the cuboid and cuneiform osteotomies contributed to the change in the forefoot. The changes in the forefoot were directly proportional to the size of the wedge inserted into the medial cuneiform, with 1 cm being the largest size feasible for use in a normal adult foot. These corrections were achieved without significant soft tissue dissection or release and invasion of growing areas in the foot.

Conclusions.—The combination of opening wedge medial cuneiform osteotomy with closing wedge cuboid osteotomy is a simple, direct, and reproducible procedure that addresses both residual forefoot adductus and midfoot supination in the bean-shaped foot. This procedure avoids the dangerous, extensive dissection of feet that have previously undergone operation.

▶ This is an excellent way to correct the residual clubfoot deformity described here. I prefer this procedure to a triple arthrodesis even in the teenager. A lateral closing wedge of the calcaneus can be added to the procedure to correct mild hindfoot varus.—P.P. Griffin, M.D.

Preoperative Ilizarov Frame Construction for Correction of Ankle and Foot Deformities
Rosman M, Brown K (Shriners Hosp, Montreal; McGill Univ)
J Pediat Orthop 11:238–240, 1991   1–19

Background.—Many orthopedic deformities can be corrected by means of the Ilizarov method. Because of the high complexity of ankle and foot deformities, the frames needed for such corrections are among the most difficult to construct. A technique was developed to create an exact replica of the deformity using a rubberized material.

Technique.—A standard plaster mold of the patient's leg and foot is made first. After setting, this model is filled with a firm, flexible material, Pedilen Duplicating Plastic. This model is then taken to the laboratory, and the frame is constructed at leisure. After completion of the frame, including drilling of wires through the material, the wires are removed, and the frame is taken off the model. The frame is slipped over the foot and ankle in the operating room, appropriate adjustments are made, and the wires are drilled and attached to the frame.

Conclusion.—This method allows time for accurate and creative planning for the correction of ankle and foot deformities as well as producing a replica for postoperative comparison.

▶ This appears to be an excellent contribution that will help in solving the complex problem of Ilizarov frame construction for correction of severe foot deformities. The correction of foot deformities by the Ilizarov technique is demanding and should not be attempted by one who has not had appropriate instruction in the technique.—P.P. Griffin, M.D.

Correction of Clubfoot Relapse Using Ilizarov's Apparatus in Children 8–15 Years Old

Franke J, Grill F, Hein G, Simon M (Medical Academy Erfurt, Germany; Speising Hospital, Vienna; Martin Luther University, Halle, Germany)
Arch Orthop Trauma Surg 110:33–37, 1990   1–20

Background.—Treatment of relapsed or neglected clubfeet in patients aged 8–15 years has been unsatisfactory. Correction by triple arthrodesis with wedge osteotomies is indicated only when skeletal maturity is reached. The Ilizarov external fixator allows simultaneous correction of all components of clubfoot by simultaneous guided distraction without bone resection or shortening the foot. It is not necessary to wait for completion of skeletal growth to use this apparatus.

Methods.—Thirteen feet in 12 children aged 7–15 years were treated using Ilizarov's external fixator (Fig 1–2). Duration of correction varied from 4 weeks to 10 weeks. When correction was completed, the device was retained in a fixed position for another 8–10 weeks, after which immobilization was achieved using a lower leg walking plaster for 3–4 months. Mean follow-up was 5 years.

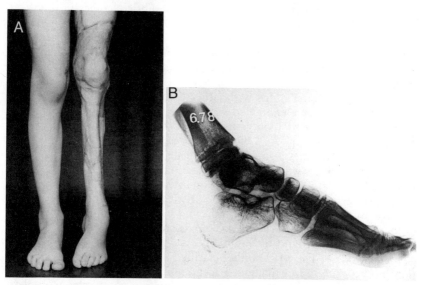

Fig 1–2.—Girl aged 9 years with posttraumatic clubfoot (A) and atrophic scarred skin (B). (Courtesy of Franke J, Grill F, Hein G, et al: *Arch Orthop Trauma Surg* 110:33–37, 1990.)

Results.—All patients achieved plantigrade feet with satisfactory radiographic appearance. All patients were able to wear ready-made shoes. As expected, stiffness of the subtalar, midtarsal, and ankle joints was not corrected. Complications included 2 severe pin-tract infections, temporary edema, and 2 relapses that were successfully treated by second corrections.

Conclusion.—Severely deformed, relapsed clubfeet in children aged 8–15 years can successfully be treated nonivasively in Ilizarov's apparatus.

▶ The construction for correcting a multiple plane deformity is complex. Exact preoperative plans are essential. Muscle imbalance, if present, must be corrected to prevent loss of correction. In my opinion, the use of the Ilizarov technique should be reserved for those deformities that cannot be corrected equally well by osteotomy, capsulotomy, and arthrodesis in the older child.—P.P. Griffin, M.D.

Hip

Magnetic Resonance Imaging in Congenital Dysplasia of the Hip
Fisher R, O'Brien TS, Davis KM (Univ of Colorado, Denver)
J Pediatr Orthop 11:617–622, 1991   1–21

Background.—Clinical examination of the newborn is the primary method of early diagnosis of congenital hip dislocation and dysplasia. Roentgenographic examination, arthrography, real-time ultrasound, and CT also offer useful information. Magnetic resonance imaging is potentially useful for providing information about subtle changes in the position of the femoral head, the soft tissue structures about the hip, cartilage, and postreduction determination of the unossified femoral head position in plaster. The usefulness of MRI in managing and predicting future developments of congenital hip dysplasia and dislocation was examined.

Methods.—Seventeen hips with either a congenital dislocation or acetabular dysplasia were examined with MRI. The results were correlated with those of standard roentgenograms. The acetabular index (AI) and the acetabular quotient (AQ) were measured. A cost analysis of the various imaging modalities also was performed.

Findings.—There was no significant difference between the bony AIs measured on plain radiographs and on MRI. Correlations between the bony and the cartilaginous AIs were statistically significant. Bony acetabular AIs of 30 degrees or greater indicated hip dysplasia, subluxation, or dislocation. It is not known whether the correlation between the bony AI and the AQ is of prognostic value.

Conclusions.—The MRI studies clarified a statistically significant relationship between the cartilaginous acetabulum and the bony acetabulum. Although MRI can provide qualitative information not available on plain films, it is not recommended for routine use in the evaluation of congenital hip dysplasia. It may be especially useful in identifying bone dysplasia with normal cartilaginous growth potential.

▶ This MRI study of hip dysplasia is important in that it demonstrates that the AI measured on a radiograph reflects the presence or absence of dysplasia. The bony acetabulum shown on a radiograph has the same contour as the nonosseous portion, and measuring it is as accurate as measuring the AI by MRI.—P.P. Griffin, M.D.

Premature Closure of the Triradiate Cartilage: A Potential Complication of Pericapsular Acetabuloplasty
Plaster RL, Schoenecker PL, Capelli AM (Shriners Hosp for Crippled Children, St. Louis)
J Pediatr Orthop 11:676–678, 1991   1–22

Background.—Normal acetabular development is dependent on both a concentric reduction of an anatomical femoral head into a true acetabulum and a viable triradiate cartilage. Premature closure has been reported secondary to fracture, injury, or postoperative complication of pericapsular acetabuloplasty. In 1 child there was growth arrest of the triradiate cartilage after open reduction and Gill acetabuloplasty.

Case Report.—Girl, 19 months, underwent a Gill acetabuloplasty for repair of a dislocated hip. After operation there was a deficiency in acetabular development and a failure of the pelvis to grow to its anticipated height. A radiograph 2 weeks after operation showed that the bone graft had been placed across the triradiate cartilage. By age 2 years a bony bridge spanned the triradiate cartilage (Fig 1–3) and by age 3 years the triradiate cartilage was narrowed at age 12 years the deformity of the hemipelvis was even more evident (Fig 1–4). A proxi-

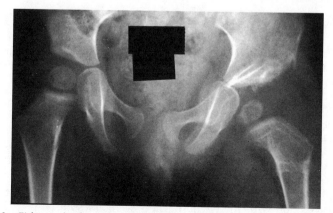

Fig 1–3.—Eight months after open reduction, Gill acetabuloplasty, and supracondylar derotational osteotomy, bony bridge is evident across left triradiate cartilage. (Courtesy of Plaster RL, Schoenecker PL, Capelli AM: *J Pediatr Orthop* 11:676–678, 1991.)

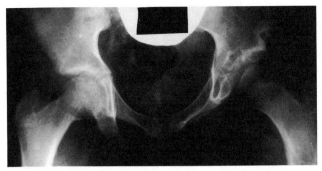

Fig 1–4.—At age 12 years, deformity of hemipelvis is even more evident. (Courtesy of Plaster RL, Schoenecker PL, Capelli AM: *J Pediatr Orthop* 11:676–678, 1991.)

mal femoral redirectional osteotomy and an innominate osteotomy improved coverage of the femoral head and hip biomechanics.

Conclusions.—The growth and development of the acetabulum may be affected by premature closure of the triradiate cartilage. The younger the patient at time of injury, the more pronounced the deformity at maturity. Injury to the triradiate cartilage during pericapsular acetabuloplasty is most likely to occur if the bone graft used to maintain fragment displacement crosses the triradiate cartilage. The Gill and Pemberton methods of pericapsular osteotomy should be performed carefully and monitored closely to avoid or detect bone graft penetration of the triradiate cartilage.

▶ The result of early closure of the triradiate cartilage results in a shallow acetabulum. Care must be taken not to place the graft across the triradiate cartilage. This is always a possibility in both the acetabuloplasty described by Pemberton and that described by Gill (1).—P.P. Griffin, M.D.

Reference

1. McKay DW: Pemberton's innominate osteotomy: Indications, technique, results, pitfalls, and complications. In Tachdjian MO (ed): *Congenital Dislocation of the Hip.* New York, Churchill Livingstone, 1982, 543–554.

Late Acetabular Dysplasia Following Early Successful Pavlik Harness Treatment of Congenital Dislocation of the Hip

Tucci JJ, Kumar SJ, Guille JT, Rubbo ER (Alfred I duPont Inst, Wilmington, Del)
J Pediatr Orthop 11:502–505, 1991   1–23

Objective.—The long-term results after treatment of congenital dislocation of the hip with the Pavlik harness were assessed.

Patients.—Sixty-one patients with 74 dislocated hips were treated with a Pavlik harness at a mean age of 6.7 weeks. All patients had either dis-

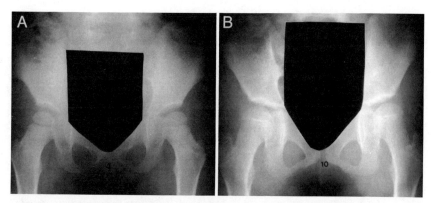

Fig 1–5.—Bilateral hip dysplasia in newborn treated with Pavlik harness. **A,** at 4-year follow-up, anteroposterior radiograph shows symmetric ossific nuclei and satisfactory acetabuli. **B,** at 10-year follow-up, there is sclerosis of acetabular roof and valgus anteverted femoral necks. (Courtesy of Tucci JJ, Kumar SJ, Guille JT, et al: *J Pediatr Orthop* 11:502–505, 1991.)

located and reducible or dislocated and irreducible hips at the beginning of treatment. The average age of the patients at follow-up was 12 years.

Results.—Interim review of radiographs at 3- and 5-year follow-up showed that all hips appeared radiographically normal. However, at the latest follow-up 17% of hips had an upward tilt of the outer portion of the acetabulum or sclerosis in this area (Fig 1–5).

Conclusions.—The long-term results of treatment of congenital dislocation of the hip successfully reduced with the Pavlik harness are superior to those after closed reduction and casting, with 83% of those using the harness expected to have normal hips. However, continued follow-up is necessary until skeletal maturity is achieved to identify those hips in which acetabular roof abnormalities may develop. The significance of this latter finding is not fully understood.

▶ There are 2 important observations in this study. The first is the importance of early treatment. The earlier the treatment was started, the less time it took for the hip to have normal radiographs. The second observation is that the end result of treatment cannot be determined until maturity. Two patients with normal radiographs at 5 years were classified as severe II and III at the 10-year follow-up. The delay in treatment allows secondary changes to occur in the capsule, labrum, and acetabulum, and these changes interfere with acetabular development.—P.P. Griffin, M.D.

Neonatal Screening and Staggered Early Treatment for Congenital Dislocation or Dysplasia of the Hip

Burger BJ, Burger JD, Bos CFA, Obermann WR, Rozing PM, Vandenbroucke JP (Univ Hosp, Leiden, The Netherlands; Elizabeth Gasthuis, Haarlem, The Netherlands)
Lancet 336:1549–1553, 1990

1–24

Background.—There is still doubt about the reliability of screening for congenital dislocation of the hip (CDH) in neonates and about the value of early treatment. A prospective follow-up investigation was done to determine whether neonatal screening and early treatment prevent dislocation only of whether they also prevent dysplasia without dislocation.

Methods.—During a 9-year period 14,264 consecutive newborn infants were screened for CDH. At the first visit the infants' hips were examined by Barlow's method and the family history of CDH was recorded. Among the screened infants 140 were Barlow positive and abduction splinting was started immediately; 133 had doubtful results on the Barlow test and were radiographed at 5 months and treated if CDH was detected; 685 were Barlow negative but with a positive family history and were also radiographed at 5 months and treated if CDH was present; 13,306 were Barlow negative with no family history of CDH. Of the Barlow negative children with no family history of CDH 596 were seen again at 5 months and 4,365 were followed-up at 2 years.

Results.—Dislocation was probably missed at primary screening in only 3 children (.02%), confirming the reliability of the screening test. Nineteen children (14%) who had equivocal Barlow test results proved to have dysplasia at 5 months. Dysplasia was also seen at 5 months in 15% of Barlow negative children with a positive family history and in 2% to 3% of reference group children. The high percentage of children with positive family histories who had dysplasia at 5 months underlines the role of hereditary factors in dysplasia. Seventeen percent of the 140 infants in whom treatment was started immediately had relapse dysplasia after withdrawal of treatment, 3% had avascular necrosis, and 78% were normal at age 2 years. When treatment was started at 5 months relapse of dysplasia did not occur, only 1% of infants had avascular necrosis, and 53% to 63% were normal at age 2 years.

Conclusions.—Although the initial 78% response to early treatment in the neonatal period seemed good compared with the 53% to 63% success rate after late treatment, avascular necrosis after earlier treatment was considerably more frequent among children treated during the neonatal period. For children with dislocatable hips, a wait-and-see treatment strategy with early ultrasonography or radiography at 5 months is recommended.

▶ This study proves that hip screening in the newborn can be effective in reducing the incidence of late diagnosis of dislocation. It also shows that early adduction splinting is not always successful, that after discontinuing treatment dysplasia can increase, and that, when family history is positive, hips should be elevated for a longer period of time. Two factors were ignored in this study: 1) the difference between the positive Ortolani hip and the hip that is dislocatable by the provocative test of Barlow and 2) the development of a pelvic obliquity from an abduction contracture that may explain the statistics of acetabular dysplasia in the different groups (1). If avascular necrosis is 3% in those splinted as newborns, I believe that abduction splinting should not be used in hips that are Ortolani negative at birth or that become negative within a week. I do not believe that the Barlow test should be part of the newborn exam, as it stretches the joint capsule.—P.P. Griffin, M.D.

Reference

1. Green NE, Griffin PP: *J Bone Joint Surg* 64-B:1273, 1982.

Neonatal Hip Stability and the Barlow Test: A Study in Stillborn Babies
Jones DA (Morriston Hosp, Swansea, Wales)
J Bone Joint Surg 73-B:216–218, 1991   1–25

Background.—It is not known why some older infants have congenital dislocation of the hip despite normal findings in the neonatal period. It has been hypothesized that performing the Barlow provocative test may contribute to neonatal hip instability.

Methods.—The Barlow test was performed in 10 hips of 5 stillborn infants within 24 hours of birth. The hips were then dissected.

Results.—None of the hips of 3 infants who underwent forcible repetition of the Barlow test 5–10 times developed subluxation or dislocation. However, in 1 infant examined after 30 forcible Barlow maneuvers both hips became lax as gas appeared in the joint spaces. In the last infant injection of 1 mL of air into the joint caused the capsule to bulge, and only slight traction was required to subluxate the hip. On dissection each femoral head was freely mobile and the posterior capsule appeared as a thin, translucent structure. Pressing the femoral head back into the acetabulum to re-establish the "suction effect" resulted in a negative Barlow test, whereas application of traction away from the acetabulum allowed air to enter the joint and restored the subluxation.

Conclusions.—It appears that the vacuum fit of the acetabulum and the proximal capsule of the femoral head is an important factor in neonatal hip stability. It is postulated that the capsule and the labrum act together as "O" rings to maintain the vacuum fit, and that repeated, forcible Barlow maneuvers, by producing an effusion, could break the seal and allow instability.

▶ This is an interesting study. It does not seem wise to dislocate the hip forcefully in a newborn to determine its stability. A properly done Ortolani test is information enough and, when complemented by ultrasound, should give guidelines for decision-making relative to treatment.—P.P. Griffin, M.D.

Why Is Congenital Dislocation of the Hip Still Missed? Analysis of 96,891 Infants Screened in Malmö 1956–1987
Sanfridson J, Redlund-Johnell I, Udén A (Lund University; Malmö General Hospital, Sweden)
Acta Orthop Scand 62:87–91, 1991   1–26

Background.—Screening of newborns for hip instability gave excellent results in the first 16 years after its introduction, but more instability eluded early diagnosis during the 1980s. An investigation was conducted to identify risk groups and improve screening routines for children who have late diagnosis of congenital dislocation of the hip (CDH).

Methods.—From 1956 to 1987, 96,891 children in Malmö, Sweden were screened. The Ortolani sign was used until 1963, after which the Barlow test was also used. Records and radiographs of children with late-diagnosed CDH were analyzed. Ninety-eight untreated newborns were controls.

Results.—In the first 16 years of screening only 4 cases of CDH were missed in a total of 58,759 children screened, a rate of .07 per 1,000. In the last 7 years 12 cases in 19,398 children were missed, a rate of .6 per 1,000. The increase could not be ascribed to any formal change in the screening program. Late diagnosis was prevented in all breech presentations and in all boys but 1. General factors such as female sex and joint laxity, appeared to imply a risk for being missed. Mechanical factors such as breech presentation and primogeniture effect appeared to facilitate early diagnosis.

Conclusions.—Risk factors for late diagnosis of CDH include joint laxity and female sex combined with normal birth weight in vertex presentation. Heredity was not a problem. Some girls with CDH have a more pronounced instability on the fifth rather than the first day of life, a condition that is not seen in boys.

▶ Screening was successful in this very large number of newborns. The percentage of cases missed was greater in the last 7 years than in the first 16 years of the program. This may be the result of the screening physicians performing the Barlow test. This test breaks the suction hold that exists between the head and acetabulum and stretches the capsule.—P.P. Griffin, M.D.

Necrosis of the Capital Femoral Epiphysis and Medial Approaches to the Hip in Piglets

Fisher EH III, Beck PA, Hoffer MM (Univ of California, Irvine)
J Orthop Res 9:203–208, 1991   1–27

Background.—The most serious complication of treatment for congenital dislocation of the hip is necrosis of the capital femoral epiphysis. Necrosis occurring after the medial approach has been blamed on vascular damage to the medial femoral circumflex vessels. Piglets were examined to determine whether damage to the medial vessels alone could cause necrosis.

Methods.—Using a medial approach, the medial femoral circumflex vessels were surgically interrupted in 11 of 13 piglet hips. Five hips underwent medial arthrotomy to dislocate the hip and transect the ligamentum teres. The other 2 animals had exposure of the hip capsule only. The femoral heads were examined an average of 4.2 months later, and evidence of necrosis was sought. Additional experiments were done using tetracycline labeling to examine postoperative blood flow, to determine if subluxated hips that underwent vessel damage were more susceptible to avascular necrosis, and to confirm that interruption of all intra-articular vessels would cause necrosis.

Results.—There were no gross, radiographic, or microscopic signs of necrosis in any of the hips with surgical damage to the medial femoral circumflex vessels. Necrosis was present in the hips that had interruption of all intra-articular vessels.

Conclusions.—Necrosis of the capital femoral epiphysis occurring after a medial approach to the hip in children does not appear to result from direct damage to the medial femoral circumflex vessels. The collateral circulation around the femoral neck probably is sufficient to provide circulation despite this damage. Postoperative positioning may be the cause of necrosis occurring with the medial approach.

▶ Position of immobilization of the hip that increases pressure on the epiphysis and physis is certainly important as a cause of necrosis of the epiphysis and physis. A combination of decreased vascular supply from obstruction to the medial circumflex artery and its branches plus pressure on the head may be cumulative, so that, with less blood flow, less pressure is needed to prevent perfusion. I believe that pressure on the head is probably the most significant factor and that the inverted labrum and other obstructions to the head seating in the acetabulum contribute to the increased pressure.—P.P. Griffin, M.D.

Biomechanical Comparison of Single- and Double-Pin Fixation for Acute Slipped Capital Femoral Epiphysis
Kruger DM, Herzenberg JE, Viviano DM, Hak DJ, Goldstein SA (Univ of Michigan, Ann Arbor)
Clin Orthop 259:277–281, 1990   1–28

Background.—The optimal number of pins required to achieve safe, secure fixation of slipped capital femoral epiphysis (SCFE) has not been established. The biomechanics of pin fixation for acute SCFE were examined in an in vitro immature canine model.

Method.—An acute SCFE was created in 24 paired mongrel dog femurs. The epiphyses were reduced and fixed with either 1 or 2 (2-mm) threaded Steinmann pins and then loaded to failure. The strength and stiffness of the paired limbs, were compared relative to the strength of the intact canine physis.

Results.—Strength and stiffness did not differ significantly between the intact physis and the fractured physis stabilized with 2 pins. In contrast, the single-pinned limbs were only 83% as strong and 78% as stiff as the intact limbs. The double-pinned limbs were 118% stronger and 112% stiffer than the single-pinned limbs.

Conclusions.—Double-pin fixation is recommended over single-pin fixation for stabilizing an acute SCFE. However, these findings may not be extrapolated to the clinical situation of chronic SCFE, wherein some inherent internal stabilization may be provided by the granulation tissue and callus.

▶ The authors proved that, in the dog, a surgically produced SCFE was more stable if pinned with 2 pins than if pinned with 1. This study was done to determine whether 1 or 2 pins should be used in the treatment of an acute SCFE. Certainly, 2 pins inserted an equal distance into the head should be stronger than 1. This study does not answer the question as to whether or not 1 large screw inserted the maximum safe distance into the center of the femoral head is sufficient fixation for an acute or chronic slip. I have had no problems with the use of 1 screw in treating an acute on chronic slip. The acute or chronic slip is probably more stable than the acute Salter Harris fracture of the normal epiphysis, which probably should be fixed with 2 screws.—P.P. Griffin, M.D.

Intertrochanteric Corrective Osteotomy in Slipped Capital Femoral Epiphysis: A Long-Term Follow-Up Study of 26 Patients
Maussen JPGM, Rozing PM, Obermann WR (Univ Hosp, Leyden, The Netherlands)
Clin Orthop 259:100–109, 1990   1–29

Background.—The treatment of moderate to severe forms of slipped capital femoral epiphysis (SCFE) remains controversial. Twenty-six patients with moderate to severe chronic SCFE were treated with intertrochanteric corrective osteotomy.

Outcome.—Arthrosis occurred in 16 hips (62%) despite satisfactory alignment. There was a direct correlation between the severity of the slip and the early occurrence of osteoarthrosis. Arthrosis occurred in 1 of 10 hips with a slippage of less than 40 degrees, compared with 15 of 16 hips with slippage exceeding 40 degrees. The difference in extremity length varied from 0 to 3.5 cm.

Conclusions.—The results of this trial and a review of previous trials suggest that intertrochanteric corrective osteotomy does not prevent degeneration in patients with SCFE with severe slippage. Good long-term results have been reported with internal fixation by pinning without realignment or with metaphyseal osteotomy and bone graft epiphysiodesis, even in patients with moderate to severe slippage. Considering all these observations, it is advocated that SCFE should be treated by fixation without realignment, accepting the deformity in moderate to severe chronic slips. Rotational osteotomy may be considered when hip joint contractures occur.

▶ There are factors that lead to progressive loss of joint space and of motion in patients with an SCFE that are yet to be explained. Severity of the slip and of the residual deformity is related to coxarthrosis, but other unknown factors exist. (See reference 1 and compare with reference 2.) It still appears that the safest treatment is in situ screw fixation and, later, rotation valgus osteotomy to improve gait if needed.—P.P. Griffin, M.D.

References

1. Boyer DW, et al: *J Bone Joint Surg* 63-A:85, 1981.
2. Carney BT, et al: *J Bone Joint Surg* 73-A:667, 1991.

The Role of Venous Hypertension in the Pathogenesis of Legg-Perthes Disease: A Clinical and Experimental Study

Liu S-L, Ho T-C (Memorial Hospital, Guangzhou, China)
J Bone Joint Surg 73-A:194–200, 1991   1 – 30

Background.—Legg-Perthes' disease is well recognized, but little is known about its cause and pathogenesis. Rather than being solely caused by arterial ischemia, the problem may have a venous origin.

Methods.—The role of venous pressure in Legg-Perthes' disease was investigated in 32 patients. Only those patients with unilateral involvement were examined, allowing comparison with the normal side. The affected joints were studied by dynamic triphasic bone imaging with ^{99m}Tc methylene diphosphonate, measurement of the intraosseous pressure of the femoral neck, intraosseous venography, and determination of intraarticular pressure and arthrography. An experiment was also done in dogs. After obstruction of venous drainage, the animals had elevation of the intraosseous pressure of the femoral head and neck by injection of 4 mL of semiliquid silicone into the femoral neck.

Results.—In the patients with Legg-Perthes' disease, there was slightly decreased arterial flow in the affected femoral head, but the difference compared with the unaffected side was not significant. However, venous drainage of the affected hip was markedly disturbed. The intraosseous pressure in the affected femoral neck and the intraarticular pressure in the affected hip also were increased compared to the other side. In the animal experiment, 11 of 20 animals had avascular necrotic areas similar to those of Legg-Perthes' disease of the femoral head.

Conclusions.—Disturbances of venous drainage and increased intraosseous pressure appear to be important factors in necrosis of the femoral head. The causal relationship is not well understood. Both disturbances may result from some condition of the bone marrow.

▶ This is another study that shows the presence of venous stasis in the hip with Legg-Perthes' disease. Its relationship to the cause of Leggs-Perthes' was not established. The arterial blood flow studies are difficult to evaluate as the radioisotope measurement of blood flow in the first phase would depend on the stage of the disease.— P.P. Griffin, M.D.

Chiari's Osteotomy in the Treatment of Perthes' Disease

Bennett JT, Mazurek RT, Cash JD (Tulane Univ)
J Bone Joint Surg 73-B:225–228, 1991   1 – 31

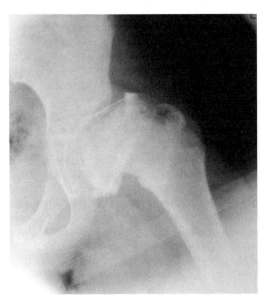

Fig 1–6.—Arthrogram demonstrates that containment of femoral head in acetabulum is no longer possible by conventional means. (Courtesy of Bennett JT, Mazurek RT, Cash JD: *J Bone Joint Surg* 73-B:225–228, 1991.)

Background.—Adolescents with Perthes' disease may require treatment for painful subluxation of the hip that may be too severe to be treated by conventional methods of containment and motion. Chiari's osteotomy has been shown to be useful in the treatment of painful subluxed hips with incongruency.

Methods.—Seventeen patients (average age, 9 years 11 months) underwent 18 Chiari's osteotomies for painful subluxation of the hips resulting

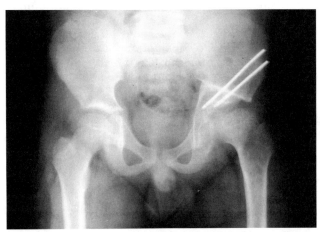

Fig 1–7.—Same case as in Figure 1–6. Containment has been achieved with Chiari's osteotomy. (Courtesy of Bennett JT, Mazurek RT, Cash JD: *J Bone Joint Surg* 73-B:225–228, 1991.)

from Perthes' disease. Radiographically, all patients fell into Catterall groups III or IV and Waldenstrom stage II or more, with progressive subluxation. Arthrography confirmed incongruency in 16 patients (Fig 1–6). Indications for surgery were severe deformity and pain. Average follow-up was 4 years 3 months.

Results.—Clinical evaluation indicated that 12 of 13 patients had fair results, and none complained of pain or instability. Radiographic evaluation revealed significant improvements in the center-edge angle and the percentage cover of the femoral head (Fig 1–7), and both measures were restored to near normal in 14 of 18 hips. There were no significant medial displacement of the femoral head. Eccentricity was reduced significantly by an average of 16%.

Conclusion.—Chiari's osteotomy is recommended for adolescents with painful subluxation of the hip resulting from Perthes' disease.

▶ The younger patients in this study might have done as well or better with a different treatment. In the adolescent with a painful deformed head, 1 option for treatment is a Chiari osteotomy, and the relief of pain in these patients supports the use of the Chiari in the selected patient for whom other osteotomies are contraindicated.—P.P. Griffin, M.D.

Fracture of Upper Extremities

Transarticular Fixation for Severely Displaced Supracondylar Fractures in Children

Archibald DAA, Roberts JA, Smith MGH (Royal Hosp for Sick Children, Glasgow, Scotland)

J Bone Joint Surg 73-B:147–149, 1991   1–32

Background.—The management of severely displaced, unstable supracondylar fractures of the humerus in children remains controversial.

Methods.—During a 20-year period 42 children with severe supracondylar humeral fractures were treated by open reduction through a medial incision and internal fixation by a single transarticular pin.

Results.—Thirty-four children were evaluated after an average follow-up period of 6.8 years (range, 9 months to 20 years). In 79% of patients excellent or good results were achieved with loss of less than 11 degrees of arc and with less than 11 degrees of change in carrying angle. All but 2 of 14 patients with nerve injuries recovered fully.

Conclusion.—Open reduction and internal fixation by transarticular pinning is a safe and reliable method for the primary management of severely displaced supracondylar fractures in children.

▶ Pin fixation after either closed or open reduction is a proven and well-accepted treatment for a supracondylar fracture of the humerus. A pin across the joint as a method of fixation seems to be an unnecessary violation of the joint and is always in danger of breaking within the joint. I am greatly concerned about the technique of fixation reported in this article and would reserve it for that case where I could not insert cross-K wires or 2 wires from the lateral condyle. The author classified an 11-degree change in the carrying angle as a good result. A child whose carrying angle is straight will be unhappy with the appearance of the arm that has an 11-degree varus.— P.P. Griffin, M.D.

Forearm Fractures in Children: Cast Treatment With the Elbow Extended
Walker JL, Rang M (Hosp for Sick Children, Toronto)
J Bone Joint Surg 73-B:299–301, 1991   1–33

Background.—Fractures of the proximal forearm in young children may be unstable with the elbow flexed but stable when the elbow is in extension. However, immobilization of these fractures in the stable, extended position has rarely been recommended because of the risk of a stiff elbow in extension and because the cast tends to slip off.

Methods.—Between 1981 and 1987, 15 children with forearm shaft fractures were treated with long-arm casts with the elbow in extension. Six patients had fractures that displaced after initial splinting with the elbow flexed. Benzoin was used to make the skin sticky under the padding, and the casts were molded in the supracondylar region. The mean immobilization period was 39 days.

Results.—Only 1 patient had more than 15 degrees of angulation at the time of bony union. All patients achieved normal elbow movement within 2 weeks, and all had full forearm rotation. No casts fell off.

Conclusions.—The extended elbow cast is a safe alternative to internal fixation for unstable forearm fractures in children. Its main disadvantage is the awkward position in which the arm is immobilized.

▶ This technique is well worth our attention.— P.P. Griffin, M.D.

Late Surgical Treatment of Lateral Condylar Fractures in Children
Roye DP Jr, Bini SA, Infosino A (Babies Hosp; Columbia Presbyterian Med Ctr; Columbia Univ, New York)
J Pediatr Orthop 11:195–199, 1991   1–34

Background.—The treatment of lateral humeral condylar fractures in children diagnosed late after the initial injury is controversial. Although late open reduction and internal fixation of nonunited fractures has been advocated, poor results have been reported after late surgical treatment. Data were reviewed on 3 children with symptomatic nonunion of lateral condylar elbow fractures who underwent successful late surgical repair.

Case 1.—Boy, 7 years, was examined 1½ years after he sustained a displaced lateral condylar fracture with disruption of the ulnohumeral articulation that was treated with cast immobilization. Nonunion of the lateral condyle was evident on the anteroposterior radiograph (Fig 1–8). He underwent open reduction with preservation of soft tissue attachment to the fragment. Because anatomical reduc-

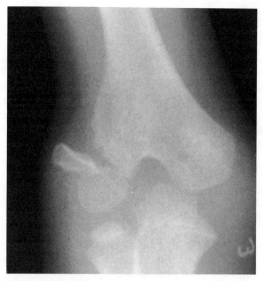

Fig 1–8.—Patient 1. Preoperative anteroposterior radiograph of the elbow. (Courtesy of Roye DP Jr, Bini SA, Infosino A: *J Pediatr Orthop* 11:195–199, 1991.)

tion was not possible, an image intensifier was used to help reduce the fragment in a position that would allow the greatest range of motion. At follow-up anteroposterior radiographs showed complete bony union. The patient had a full range of motion about the elbow with no pain or angular deformity (Fig 1–9).

Case 2.—Boy, 7 years, was seen 3 years after a lateral condylar fracture of the

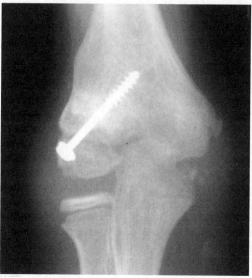

Fig 1–9.—Patient 1. Anteroposterior radiograph of the elbow 1-year follow-up. (Courtesy of Roye DP Jr, Bini SA, Infosino A: *J Pediatr Orthop* 11:195–199, 1991.)

humerus failed to unite. When the elbow showed increasing angular deformity, ulnar neuritis developed, and the ulnar nerve was transposed. As the valgus deformity continued to worsen, a closing wedge osteotomy was performed almost 5 years after initial fracture. A follow-up radiograph showed bony union, and the angular deformity was much improved. The patient was able to participate in sports.

Case 3.—Boy, 15½ years, was examined 14 years after a nondefined, right distal humeral fracture was treated in a cast. The patient had chronic pain about the elbow and numbness of the fourth and fifth digits of the dominant right hand. Anteroposterior radiographs showed nonunion of the lateral condylar fracture with epicondylar extension of the distal humerus. Open reduction and internal fixation were performed with conservation of soft tissue attachment to the fragment. A follow-up radiograph 2 years later showed complete bony union. Because of continued postlateral pain resulting from impingement of the proximal ulna in the olecranon fossa, the proximal olecranon was excised, which increased the patient's range of motion and resolved the pain.

Conclusion.—Children with a diagnosis of symptomatic nonunion and malunion of lateral condylar fractures of the humerus can benefit from late surgical treatment at the time of diagnosis.

▶ A point not made in this article is that in late nonunion the intra-articular surfaces should usually be left in their current relationship and that the surgery should be limited to obtaining an osteosynthesis between the lateral condyle and the metaphysis. Angular deformity can be corrected by an osteotomy.— P.P. Griffin, M.D.

Volkmann's Ischemic Contracture in Children: The Results of Free Vascularized Muscle Transplantation
Zuker RM, Egerszegi EP, Manktelow RT, McLeod A, Candlish S (Hospital for Sick Children, Toronto; Hôpital Sainte Justine, Montreal; University of Toronto)
Microsurgery 12:341–345, 1991   1–35

Background.—Volkmann's ischemic contracture can result in the loss of active finger motion and is a condition that should not occur in modern surgical practice. If upper extremity injuries, especially supracondylar fractures, are not monitored carefully and if the diagnosis of a compartment syndrome is made late, muscle necrosis will result. The surgical procedure for the reconstruction of the forearm in cases of severe Volkmann's contracture has been described previously. The results of free vascularized muscle transfer in children were evaluated.

Methods.—All 7 children initially had a supracondylar fracture that led to forearm muscle ischemia, necrosis, and severe Volkmann's contracture. All underwent free gracilis muscle transplantation for the reconstruction of long digital flexors, and 1 also underwent gracilis muscle transfer for reconstruction of digital extensors. Three patients required post-muscle transfer tenolysis for volar tendon adhesions. Follow-up occurred an average of 3.4 years after muscle transfer.

Results.—All transplanted muscles survived, with dramatic improve-

A

B

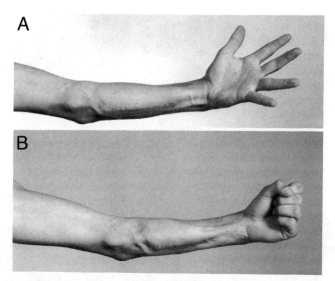

Fig 1–10.—Results of muscle transplantation after Volkmann's ischemic contracture. **A,** fingers in full extension; **B,** fingers in full flexion. (Courtesy of Zuker RM, Egerszegi EP, Manktelow RAT, et al: *Microsurgery* 12:341–345, 1991.)

ment in overall finger flexion in all children (Fig 1–10). Major gains occurred in grip and pinch strengths. All children became independent in most activities of daily living except buttoning a cuff with the affected hand, and 2 were able to participate in specific activities involving the upper extremity, such as playing the violin and baseball. Complications were minimal. In all patients, limb length discrepancies remained, and the children remained moderately disabled in fine motor activities requiring repetitive opposition.

Conclusions.—Volkmann's ischemic contracture is a generally preventable condition for which treatment—reconstruction of the forearm—is complex but can be successful. Success was based in part on the patient's perseverance with exercises. Use of the free vascularized muscle transfer seems worthy of contuation.

▶ This report is impressive, and the procedure reported should be of benefit for most patients who have a severe Volkmann's contracture but who retain median and ulnar nerve function or for whom neurolysis will give sensation and functional intrinsic muscles to the hand.—P.P. Griffin, M.D.

Operative Treatment of Congenital Pseudarthrosis of the Clavicle
Grogan DP, Love SM, Guidera KJ, Ogden JA (Shriners Hosp for Crippled Children; Florida Orthopaedic Inst, Tampa, Fla)
J Pediatr Orthop 11:176–180, 1991   1–36

Methods.—Eight children with congenital pseudarthrosis of the clavicle were treated surgically. At time of surgery, the 4 boys and 4 girls were

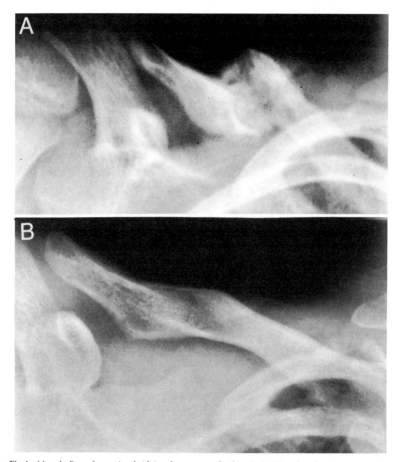

Fig 1–11.—**A,** Bone formation bridging former pseudarthrosis site 7 weeks after surgery in girl aged 5 years. **B,** appearance 4 years later. Continuous medullary cavity was evident; complete remodeling of cortices had not yet occurred, however, and small lump was still palpable. (Courtesy of Grogan DP, Love SM, Guidera KJ, et al: *J Pediatr Orthop* 11:176–180, 1991).

aged 7 months to 6 years; 6 were younger than age 3 years. In addition to a palpable prominence on the clavicle 5 patients had discomfort on compression of the area or pain on use of the arm. The operative technique involved resection of fibrous pseudarthrosis and sclerotic bone ends, careful dissection and preservation of the periosteal sleeve to maintain continuity, and approximation of bone ends. Follow-up ranged from 2 years to 14 years.

Results.—None of the patients required additional bone grafts or internal fixation. All had bridging ossification within 3 months after operation (Fig 1–11), and all appeared healed clinically within 4 months. Remodeling of the prominence occurred slowly in 2–5 years, with a palpable and radiographic "lump" evident in all patients. There was variable underdevelopment of the distal end as compared with the contralateral distal end. None of the patients had recurrence of the pseudarthrosis.

Conclusion.—For the operative treatment of congenital pseudarthrosis of the clavicle, early resection of fibrous pseudarthrosis probably does not require the extensive grafting and internal fixation that has been recommended for older children.

▶ The percentage of patients with a complaint of pain is greater than I have experienced. Also, these patients were younger than those I have treated. It is interesting that healing occurred without either graft or internal fixation. The periosteal response shown is probably related to the very young age of the patients. In older children I would prefer either fixation or graft, or both, to increase the chances of healing and would expect the prominence at the pseudarthrosis site to be less than with the technique described.—P.P. Griffin, M.D.

Miscellaneous

Magnetic Resonance Imaging in the Evaluation of Partial Growth Arrest After Physeal Injuries in Children

Havránek P, Lízler J (Thomayer University Hospital; Institute for Clinical and Experimental Medicine, Praha, Czechoslovakia)
J Bone Joint Surg 73-A:1234–1241, 1991   1–37

Background.—Children with partial growth arrest of the epiphyseal plate can have angular and longitudinal growth abnormalities. An important step in management of these children is precise delineation of the size, shape, and location of an osseous bridge. The area of growth arrest in 5 patients was examined with MRI.

Methods.—The patients (age 10–14 years) all had evidence of partial growth arrest after injury to the physis. The region of injury was the dis-

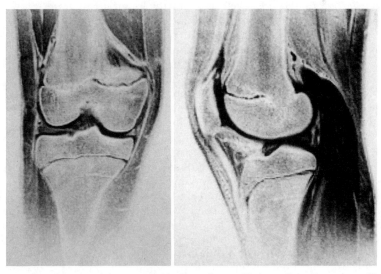

Fig 1–12.—The extent of the osseous bridge is seen better with the gradient-echo sequency (hip angle, 25 degrees; repetition time, .3 second; and echo time, 7 ms). (Courtesy of Havránek P, Lízler J: *J Bone Joint Surg* 73-A:1234–1241, 1991.)

tal femoral physis in 2 patients, the distal radial physis in 2, and the distal tibial physis in 1. The diagnosis of partial growth arrest was made with the help of conventional radiographs. All children underwent MRI in the frontal and sagittal planes (Fig 1–12).

Results.—The osseous bridge was resected with partial success in 3 patients for whom success would not have been possible without MRI. In another patient an osseous bridge resection was avoided on the basis of MRI findings. Information provided by MRI was much more precise and detailed than that provided by CT.

Conclusions.—Magnetic resonance imaging provides critical information regarding the shape, size, extent, and location of the osseous bridge in children with partial growth arrest. The surgeon can use this information to select the best treatment and to plan any necessary surgery.

▶ My experience with the use of MRI to delineate the size of an osseous bar has not been as positive. Magnetic resonance imaging is technique-dependent and theoretically should be helpful. However, at surgery I have found the area of physical closure to be larger or smaller than was demonstrated by MRI. The images presented in this article are excellent.—P.P. Griffin, M.D.

Linear Relationship Between the Volume of Hypertrophic Chondrocytes and the Rate of Longitudinal Bone Growth in Growth Plates

Breur GJ, VanEnkevort BA, Farnum CE, Wilsman NJ (Univ of Wisconsin, Madison; Cornell Univ, Ithaca, NY)
J Orthop Res 9:348–359, 1991   1–38

Background.—During skeletal maturity longitudinal bone growth is accompanied by changes in the volume of hypertrophic chondrocytes of the growth plate. The importance of the volume of hypertrophic chondrocytes as a factor in determining the rate of longitudinal bone growth was investigated. It has been hypothesized that hypertrophic cell volume varies directly with the rate of longitudinal bone growth.

Methods.—The volume of hypertrophic chondrocytes and longitudinal bone growth was measured in the proximal and distal radial growth plates and the proximal and distal tibial growth plates of hooded rats aged 21 and 35 days and of Yucatan pigs aged 21 and 35 days. The volume of hypertrophic chondrocytes was determined by using stereological techniques, and the rate of longitudinal bone growth during a 24 hour period was measured by oxytetracycline bone labeling.

Results.—There was a wide range of growth rates and volumes of hypertrophic chondrocytes in the 16 growth plates. There was a high correlation coefficient between the final volume of hypertrophic chondrocytes and the rate of longitudinal bone growth ($r = .98$ in rats; $r = .83$ in pigs). A positive linear relationship between the rate of longitudinal bone growth and the final volume of hypertrophic chondrocytes was noted (Fig 1–13). The slope of the regression line was different for rats and

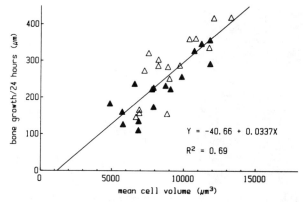

Fig 1–13.—Relationship between mean volume of hypertrophic chondrocytes and longitudinal bone growth per 24 hours in proximal and distal radial and proximal and distal tibial growth plates of 4 Yucatan pigs aged 21 days *(open triangles)* and 4 Yucatan pigs aged 35 days *(filled triangles)*. Each point represents 1 growth plate. (Courtesy of Breur GJ, VanEnkevort BA, Farnum CE, et al: *J Orthop Res* 9:348–359, 1991.)

pigs, but it was independent of the location of the growth plate and the age of the animal.

Conclusions.—The volume of hypertrophic chondrocytes appears to be an important determinant of the rate of longitudinal bone growth. It appears that mechanisms that regulate the change in volume in hypertrophic chondrocytes may exist and that the relative contribution of hypertrophy to longitudinal bone growth may be different in rats than in pigs.

▶ This is a very interesting study. It is not surprising that the growth plate of the rat and of the pig as related to volume of hypertrophic cells and longitudinal tibial growth rate were not the same, although it would seem reasonable that the volume of the hypertrophic cell column would be reflected in the rate of longitudinal growth.—P.P. Griffin, M.D.

Ultrasound in the Diagnosis and Follow-Up of Transient Synovitis of the Hip

Terjesen T, Østhus P (Trondheim University Hospital, Norway)
J Pediatr Orthop 11:608–613, 1991   1–39

Background.—Ultrasound has been used in the diagnosis of transient synovitis of the hip, but diagnostic criteria and use during follow-up have not been widely reported. A group of children with transient synovitis underwent ultrasound studies initially, during treatment, and at follow-up.

Methods.—Diagnostic criteria, the normal pattern of spontaneous regression of the hip joint effusion, and the usefulness of ultrasound in follow-up were examined based on studies of 58 children. Parameters measured on the anterior scan are shown in Figure 1–14.

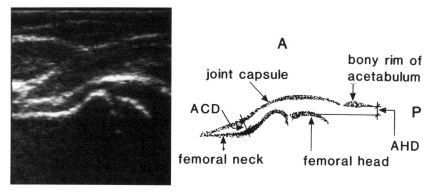

Fig 1–14.—Ultrasonogram and schematic drawing showing parameters measured on anterior scan: distance between anterior outline of femoral neck and joint capsule (anterior capsule distance, *ACD*) and distance between anterior tangent of femoral head and anterior bony acetabular rim (anterior head distance, *AHD*). *Abbreviations: A*, anterior; *P*, proximal. (Courtesy of Terjesen T, Østhus P: *J Pediatr Orthop* 11:608–613, 1991.)

Results.—The diagnostic criterion for intracapsular effusion was a side difference of at least 2 mm in the distance between the anterior joint capsule and the femoral neck. At admission the mean anterior capsule distance of the affected hip was 8.2 mm; in the unaffected hip it was 4.2 mm. Effusion persisted for more than 1 week in 58% of patients.

Conclusions.—The most important ultrasound parameter of effusion of the hip joint is the side difference in the distance between the femoral neck and the anterior joint capsule. Ultrasound is recommended as the primary imaging method in clinically suspected synovitis, septic arthritis, and hematoma of the hip because the diagnosis of fluid accumulation is rapidly and reliably obtained. It is also recommended for all children with acute or subacute pain in the hip or thigh. Radiography is indicated if Perthes' disease is suspected. Ultrasound is more useful than radiography in late follow-up because it can detect an increased lateral head distance. It is recommended as a routine examination 1 year after transient synovitis.

▶ This may be a classic study of the triumph of technology over reason. There is no doubt that ultrasound can show space densities and configurations, but the routine use of this technique to study the painful hip is extravagant and unnecessary unless the result will alter decision-making in diagnosis and treatment, which is not likely in the conditions listed.—P.P. Griffin, M.D.

The Histomorphometry of Regenerate Bone in Limb Lengthening by the Ilizarov Method
Lascombes P, Membre H, Prévot J, Barrat E (Hôpital d'Enfants de Nancy; Faculté de Médecine de Nancy, France)
French J Orthop Surg 5:115–123, 1991   1–40

Background.—The Ilizarov technique has undoubtedly advanced the surgical lengthening of long bones. The histomorphometry of regenerate bone in limb lengthening by this technique was examined.

Methods.—Eleven biopsy specimens of bone regenerated after limb lengthening by the Ilizarov technique were obtained from 10 patients (mean age, 13.5 years). At the time of biopsy the lengthening was between 14 mm and 90 mm. The interval between initial surgery and biopsy ranged from 23 days to 502 days. The undecalcified bone specimens were analyzed after embedding in methyl methacrylate resin, and the speed of mineralization was measured by double labeling with tetracycline.

Results.—Bony trabeculae were formed early, from week 3. They were disposed as a mesh—an anastomotic network that can rapidly become solid if the speed of lengthening does not exceed 1 mm per day. Ossification was of a membranous type without a cartilaginous stage. In addition, osteoblastic and osteoclastic activity were intense even 1 year after the lengthening began. The most significant point was the development of criteria of maturity of regenerate bone as early as month 4. It appears to be dangerous to change the fixation, alignment, or bone length after this point.

Conclusions.—This study outlines bone regeneration in distraction submitted to mechanical longitudinal stresses. The rate of lengthening should not exceed 1 mm per day as ischemia results if the speed of lengthening is 1.5 mm per day.

▶ This is an excellent demonstration of the process of intramembranous ossification or callotasis. The histomorphometry is well illustrated. It clearly explains the biologic process that occurs in lengthened bone.—P.P. Griffin, M.D.

2 Shoulder, Arm, and Elbow

Introduction

Imaging studies of the soft tissues of the shoulder are improving dramatically. The excitement over ultrasonography has waned, but it still has some usefulness. Perhaps it is most useful as a screening procedure or as an adjunct to follow-up assessment. It is said that arthrography is the gold standard for diagnosis of rotator cuff tearing. That may be true, but MRI is rapidly becoming the common diagnostic image of choice. Some of the studies published this year may be overly enthusiastic, as they indicate an absolutely unbelievable sensitivity and specificity for MRI. There are a few studies underway that suggest that MRI is not as perfect as one might wish. Certainly, MRI can image medium and larger rotator cuff tears quite well. One wonders whether it is as exact as one would wish for partial-thickness tears or for very small full-thickness tears. It certainly will show changes within the tendon substance, but these can be confused with the former 2 entities in many images. Whether or not MRI will be useful in imaging the labrum and capsule is still in question. Some studies suggest that it will be useful; other studies suggest that normal anatomical variation will confuse the issue enough to mitigate the value of MRI for this purpose.

Several articles this year speak of improved methods of fixation of fractures and show, not unexpectedly, that restoring anatomy often leads to excellent results. In a similar vein, a study reviews operative treatment of acute acromioclavicular dislocations. Using contemporary surgical techniques, the results are very reasonable.

Shoulder instability has received a great deal of attention. Again this year there is an article analyzing the prognosis of primary anterior shoulder dislocation. It reiterates that the recurrence rate is much lower than the classic studies would suggest. There is ongoing assessment of surgical repairs for shoulder instability. The anterior capsulolabral reconstruction may be a significant improvement for athletes with subluxation. Reviews of the Putti-Platt procedure, the Eden-Hybbinette operation, and the Bristow procedure all suggest that these operations are not as desirable in current times as they have been in the past. The recurrence rates may be higher and complications may be more frequent. Elbow instability is also receiving some attention. A diagnostic maneuver is now available to assess posterolateral rotatory instability, and more information is available on the treatment of chronic radial head dislocation.

A community survey of shoulder disorders in the elderly indicates the commonness of soft tissue problems and how they continue to increase with advancing age. Probably because of decreased physical demands, many of these patients do not seek physician care for their problems, but, indeed, the problems do exist. Studies reviewing cadaveric specimens have implied that these findings may not have been symptomatic; these studies should, in concept, be reassessed. We all are continuing to struggle with better means to assess muscle function about the shoulder. A carefully done Cybex study is another step in this direction, but it is probably too complex for office needs.

Is arthroscopy helpful for management of the frozen shoulder? Perhaps, but perhaps not. An article reviews this situation, suggesting that manipulation without arthroscopy is certainly equivalent. Unfortunately, the follow-up is not long enough to assess the long-term outcome in these patients with different modes of treatment. Arthroscopic subacromial decompression for the impingement syndrome certainly will yield quite reasonable results. It is still very difficult to address with precision the question of patient selection. Total acromionectomy has resurfaced. With meticulous technique and ample postoperative care, deltoid detachment usually can be avoided. Again though, patient selection for this procedure is uncertain. For patients with lesser amounts of rotator cuff disease, this would seem to be too extensive a procedure; for patients with severe rotator cuff disease, the support of the acromion usually would seem helpful. Finally, a report has appeared about superior humeral instability, developing after decompression for rotator cuff tears. I think we all recognize that this does occur, and an article has finally highlighted a significant potential problem.

Repairs of the rotator cuff do better if there is rotator cuff integrity after the repair. Ultrasonographic delineation has confirmed this in 2 separate studies. How are results after surgery of the rotator cuff assessed? A nice review indicates that multiple methods of assessment all have a similar value. It is, of course, not hard to believe that pain relief, strength, motion, and functional assessment after surgery are all closely interrelated.

The results are better in shoulder arthroplasty for fracture if care is given acutely. Results are not as good in the chronic setting, and they are even worse if one must reconstruct the shoulder in a chronic setting, after earlier surgery. The use of hemiarthroplasty instead of total shoulder arthroplasty for shoulder arthritis is proposed again. In certain situations, this is useful. During the upcoming years, this will be further delineated—without question. Rigid fixation for shoulder arthrodesis is a significant improvement, and this is again demonstrated in an article this year. Total elbow replacement continues to improve. Two series report quite reasonable results. However, they emphasize patient selection and rather meticulous surgical techniques. Probably, total elbow replacement still remains a somewhat more marginal procedure than many operations done in orthopedic surgery. The long-term results of elbow synovectomy in patients with rheumatoid arthritis indicate its value and its detriments. A number of patients do quite well; a number of patients progress. It is certainly a much simpler procedure than total elbow replacement and remains an important component of our armamentarium.

Interscalene brachial plexus anesthesia is now becoming more standard as an adjunct to anesthesia for shoulder surgery. Its benefits and its complications are being defined. Hemidiaphragmatic paresis is associated with this blockade. Fortunately, in many patients this has no significant effect on pulmonary function, and the paresis seems to be rather short-lived. There are, of course, some peculiar forms of disease or arthritis that affect the shoulder. Shoulder involvement in multiple epiphyseal dysplasia occurs and probably occurs almost exclusively in 2 forms: one manifests itself as a rather typical form of osteoarthritis and the other is associated with deformity (the hatchet-shaped humeral head). Pustular osteoarthropathy involves the clavicle and sternoclavicular joint. Recognizing this as an entity can prevent unnecessary biopsy in many circumstances.

All in all, this has been a productive year for the literature in this anatomical region. Diagnostic methods are continually being refined, and significant attention is being directed to the major components of injury and disease in this area: fractures, dislocations, recurrent instability, rotator cuff disease, and arthritis.

Robert H. Cofield, M.D.

Imaging Studies

Sonography for Diagnosis of Rotator Cuff Tear: Comparison With Observations at Surgery in 58 Shoulders

Kurol M, Rahme H, Hilding S (Central Hosp, Västerås, Sweden)
Acta Orthop Scand 62:465–467, 1991   2–1

Background.—Ultrasonography examination of the shoulder has been proposed to replace arthrography, but the criteria used are ambiguous. The correlation between ultrasonographic and anatomical findings was evaluated.

Methods.—A total of 58 patients with chronic subacromial pain who underwent anterior acromioplasty from 1986 to 1990 were examined. A 7.5-MHz linear-array transducer was used.

Results.—Fifteen patients had a full-thickness tear and 9 a partial tear of the rotator cuff. Fourteen ultrasound studies were negative, failing to demonstrate a thin cuff. Four of 34 patients with normal operative findings had positive ultrasound studies. When based on changes in echogenicity, 11 patients with tears had negative ultrasound studies and 6 of the normal cases were positive. Using both criteria, 8 patients with surgically proved tears had negative studies whereas 9 normal cases were positive. The study had a predictive value of .6 when positive and .8 when negative.

Conclusion.—The ultrasonographic findings do not correlate well with the presence or absence of a rotator cuff tear.

Evaluation of Degenerative Lesions of the Rotator Cuff: A Comparison of Arthrography and Ultrasonography

Misamore GW, Woodward C (Methodist Sports Med Ctr; Indiana Univ, Indianapolis)
J Bone Joint Surg 73-A:704–706, 1991   2–2

Background.—Previous reports on ultrasonography of the rotator cuff have several flaws. There are problems with study design, patient selection, and confirmation of the diagnoses. These flaws make it difficult to interpret the reports' findings. A prospective, comparative analysis of ultrasonography and arthrography was conducted.

Methods.—Thirty-two patients with a degenerative lesion of the rotator cuff were enrolled. Both arthrography and ultrasonography were done before surgery in each patient. The condition of the rotator cuff was subsequently determined during surgery.

Results.—Arthrography accurately diagnosed the lesions in 28 patients (87%). Twenty of these patients had a full-thickness tear, 7 had a partial-thickness tear, and 5 had an untorn rotator cuff and tendinitis. Ultrasonography, accurately diagnosed the lesions in only 12 patients (37%).

Conclusions.—Although ultrasonography is a relatively inexpensive and noninvasive way to assess rotator cuff lesions, it is not very accurate in diagnosing degenerative disorders. Arthrography was vastly superior to ultrasonography.

▶ Ultrasonography can certainly image the rotator cuff reasonably well. In some circumstances it will be highly accurate, and in other situations it will not be as precise as one would wish for surgical decision-making. This latter problem commonly exists, as displayed in these 2 preceding articles (Abstracts 2–1 and 2–2), when there is an intermingling of patients with small full-thickness rotator cuff tears, partial-thickness rotator cuff tears, and tendinitis. Apparently, it is difficult for ultrasonography to distinguish among these pathologic entities with a high degree of certainty.—R.H. Cofield, M.D.

MRI and Sonography of the Shoulder

Hodler J, Terrier B, von Schulthess GK, Fuchs WA (University Hospital, Zurich, Switzerland)
Clin Radiol 43:323–327, 1991   2–3

Introduction.—Arthrography remains the gold standard for the diagnosis of rotator cuff tears. The diagnostic value of sonography and MRI in suspected rotator cuff tears was compared with that of arthrography in 24 shoulders in 23 patients with suspected rotator cuff tears.

Results.—Arthrography demonstrated complete tear of the rotator cuff in 15 shoulders, whereas no pathology was evident in the remaining 9 shoulders. Sonography detected 14 of 15 tears and 7 of 9 intact rotator cuffs, whereas MRI detected 10 of 15 tears and 8 of 9 intact rotator cuffs. Signs of rotator cuff tears included complete loss of the cuff substance or focal thinning on sonography, and hyperintensity on T2-weighted images or loss of cuff substance on MRI. Retrospective analysis showed that MRI was superior to sonography in the detection of intra-articular effusion and granulation tissue. In addition, capsular hypertrophy or osteophytosis in inflammation or degeneration of the acromioclavicular joint was best depicted on MRI, whereas rotator cuff calcifications were not.

Conclusion.—Considering cost and patient compliance, sonography performed by an experienced examiner should be the initial examination in patients with suspected rotator cuff tears. However, MRI is superior in depicting additional pathology and is not operator-dependent. Magnetic resonance imaging may yet become the method of choice in noninvasive shoulder imaging.

▶ This study points out a very important fact. Sonographic assessment of the rotator cuff is very inexpensive and quite easily accomplished. It may well be a useful screening test before considering more expensive imaging modalities. So, considering this article and the 2 preceding articles, one is left with the impression that ultrasonography might still be considered as an adjunct to diagnosis. It is convenient, inexpensive, and will define many, but not all, rotator cuff tears. Please note that this study demonstrated arthrography to be the most accurate test of the 3 modalities evaluated.—R.H. Cofield, M.D.

MAGNETIC RESONANCE IMAGING

Magnetic Resonance Imaging of the Shoulder: Sensitivity, Specificity, and Predictive Value
Iannotti JP, Zlatkin MB, Esterhai JL, Kressel HY, Dalinka MK, Spindler KP (Univ of Pennsylvania, Philadelphia)
J Bone Joint Surg 73-A:17–29, 1991   2–4

Background.—Trials in small groups of patients have suggested that MRI is useful in diagnosing lesions of the rotator cuff and the glenohumeral capsule and labrum. The efficiency of MRI was evaluated in a large series of patients.

Methods.—Magnetic resonance imaging was performed on 91 patients undergoing evaluation for lesions of the rotator cuff or glenohumeral capsule and glenoid labrum and in 15 asymptomatic volunteers. A total of 127 studies were done in the 91 patients. At surgery, the rotator cuff was inspected in 73 cases and the glenohumeral capsule and glenoid labrum in 39 cases. The imaging was done with a 1.5-tesla whole-body MRI scanner, and scans were reviewed retrospectively in blinded fashion by 3 radiologists.

Results.—All of the 33 complete rotator cuff tears that were seen at operation were diagnosed with MRI; thus for complete tears the sensitivity of MRI was 100%. Specificity was 95%, and the size of the tear could be predicted consistently from the MRI scan. A correlation was seen between supraspinatus muscle atrophy seen on MRI and the size of the complete tear. In differentiating tendinitis from cuff degeneration, sensitivity was 82% and specificity 85%. In differentiating a normal tendon from one with tendinitis with signs of impingement, sensitivity was 93% and specificity 87%. There was a high correlation between formation of spurs around the acromion and acromioclavicular joint and the clinical factors of increased age and chronic rotator cuff disease. In the diagnosis of labral tears associated with glenohumeral instability, sensitivity was 88% and specificity was 93%.

Conclusion.—Magnetic resonance imaging is an excellent tool for evaluation of rotator cuff lesions and glenohumeral instability. The accuracy of MRI may depend on technical factors and on the experience of the reader. Magnetic resonance imaging may be useful in defining the spectrum of rotator cuff lesions, and it verifies the clinically suspected relationship between rotator cuff tendinitis and glenohumeral instability.

▶ This large and well-performed study clearly shows the value of MRI in the imaging of the shoulder. We must recall that these investigators had excellent equipment, and the reading was performed by experienced radiologists. One might be concerned about the ability to distinguish with great accuracy the difference between tendinitis and cuff degeneration when the histologic differences between these 2 entities are in fact quite small. The value of MRI for rotator cuff disease is becoming quite clear. The value of MRI as an adjunct to the diagnosis of instability still seems to be somewhat uncertain.—R.H. Cofield, M.D.

Alterations in the Supraspinatus Tendon at MR Imaging: Correlation With Histopathologic Findings in Cadavers

Kjellin I, Ho CP, Cervilla V, Haghighi P, Kerr R, Vangness CT, Friedman RJ, Trudell D, Resnick D (VA Med Ctr, San Diego; Univ of California, San Diego; Univ of Southern California, Los Angeles)
Radiology 181:837–841, 1991   2–5

Background.—Magnetic resonance imaging seems to be a specific and sensitive method for evaluating shoulder disorders. Some investigations of rotator cuff tears and tendinitis have shown distinct alterations in MR images, but there is recent evidence indicating that some of these alterations are present in asymptomatic persons. The clinical significance of alterations in the rotator cuff at MRI was investigated using thorough histologic correlation.

Methods.—Thirteen fresh cadaveric shoulders were studied by MRI in the coronal oblique plane at 1.5 T with proton-density– and T2 weighted spin-echo sequences. Areas in the supraspinatus tendons that corresponded to MRI alterations, judged by 2 experienced observers, were examined histologically by a pathologist who was not aware of the MR findings. No clinical data were available on the cadavers, but plain radiographs were examined to exclude shoulders with possible major abnormalities.

Results.—In 10 of the 13 cases abnormal morphological findings were seen within the supraspinatus tendon. Histologic examination showed that all tendons had some degree of degeneration, with vacuolar and mucoid degeneration within the distal portion of the rotator cuff. Fibrillary degeneration also was seen on the tendon surface, consisting of eosinophilic papillary fronds at the articular side of the rotator cuff. Scarring that suggested a relationship to a previous tear was seen in 2 cases.

Conclusions.—Areas of increased signal intensity and altered morphological characteristics of the supraspinatus tendon at MRI appear common in cadavers. These findings may not indicate active inflammation but rather degeneration. It does not seem appropriate to use the designation "tendinitis" to refer to these MRI alterations.

▶ Magnetic resonance imaging is quite sensitive to tissue changes. This review points out clearly to us all that changes may be seen within tendons that have no clinical importance.—R.H. Cofield, M.D.

Biceps Tendon Dislocation: Evaluation With MR Imaging

Chan TW, Dalinka MK, Kneeland JB, Chervrot A (Hosp of the Univ of Pennsylvania)

Radiology 179:649–652, 1991   2–6

Background.—Dislocation of the biceps tendon is a rare cause of shoulder pain, commonly associated with other shoulder abnormalities and with a clinical presentation similar to that of rotator cuff tear. Arthrographic examination can be used to diagnose medial dislocation. The effectiveness of MRI in diagnosing this entity, previously reported in only 1 case, was examined retrospectively in 6 patients.

Methods.—Two patients had surgically proven biceps tendon dislocation, and in 4 dislocation was suspected. All had MR examinations of the shoulder. The MR images were compared with those of controls for evaluation of biceps tendon diameter, width and depth of the bicipital groove, and medial wall angle of the groove.

Results.—Coronal (Fig 2–1) and axial (Fig 2–2). Four patients had fluid around the displaced biceps tendon, 3 had abnormally thick tendons, and 3 had abnormally high signal intensity within the tendon. The MR images showed abnormally shaped bicipital grooves in 2 patients, disruptures of the coracohumeral ligament in all 6 patients, disruption of thinning of the subscapularis tendon in 5 patients, and supraspinatus tendon tear in 4 patients.

Conclusions.—The nonspecific symptoms of biceps tendon dislocations make accurate diagnosis difficult, especially because these injuries often are accompanied by rotator cuff tears. Because MRI seems to result

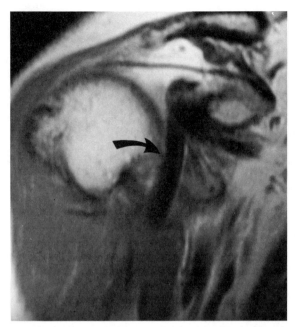

Fig 2–1.—MR image of patient who had a presumed dislocation of the biceps tendon and large tears of the supraspinatus and subscapularis tendons. Proton-density–weighted oblique coronal image (2,500/20) shows the biceps tendon medial to the groove *(arrow)*. (Courtesy of Chan TW, Dalinka MK, Kneeland JB, et al: *Radiology* 179:649–652, 1991.)

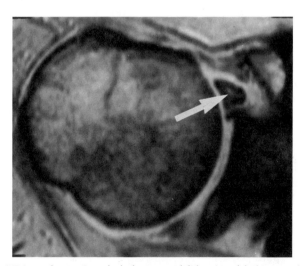

Fig 2–2.—MR image from patient who had a presumed dislocation of the biceps tendon. Axial multiplanar gradient-recalled image (800/15; flip angle, 70 degrees) shows the thickened biceps tendon *(arrow)* with a triangular shape and high signal intensity within it, mimicking an anterior glenoid labral tear. (Courtesy of Chan TW, Dalinka MK, Kneeland JB, et al: *Radiology* 179:649–652, 1991.)

in characteristic findings with this entity, the clinician's familiarity with those findings should result in accurate diagnoses.

▶ The reader of MR images of the shoulder should be aware that many pathologic changes can be seen on MRI views. As illustrated in this study, multiplane images often are necessary to be absolutely certain about these changes. With single plane views, one can be confused about what the alterations represent.— R.H. Cofield, M.D.

MR Imaging of the Labral-Capsular Complex: Normal Variations
Neumann CH, Petersen SA, Jahnke AH (San Francisco Magnetic Resonance Ctr; Letterman Army Med Ctr, San Francisco)
AJR 157:1015–1021, 1991   2–7

Background.—The appearance of normal shoulder structures on MRI has never been described. The anatomical variations of the normal labral-capsular complex as seen on MRI were reviewed.

Methods.—Magnetic resonance images were obtained of 52 shoulders in 30 asymptomatic, active, healthy volunteers (age, 21–43 years) and of 27 shoulders in 27 patients (age, 17–44 years) with clinical symptoms and surgical or arthroscopic confirmation of glenohumeral instability. All scans from the volunteers were evaluated in conference by 2 orthopedic surgeons and an experienced radiologist.

Results.—The anterior and posterior sections of the glenoid labrum in asymptomatic volunteers showed considerable morphologic variability, but several common variants were noted. A triangular labrum was the most common labral shape; it was found anteriorly in 45% and posteriorly in 73%. A round labrum was the second most common labral shape; it was found anteriorly in 19% and posteriorly in 12%. A cleaved labrum was seen in 15% and a notched labrum in 8%; these 2 patterns were seen only in the anterior labrum. A flat labrum was seen anteriorly in 7% and posteriorly in 6%. An absent labrum was seen anteriorly in 6% and posteriorly in 8%. Most anterior capsular insertions were on the labrum (47%) or on the glenoid rim (49%), whereas all posterior insertions were on the labrum. The superior, middle, and inferior thirds of the labra showed similar variability. After the analysis of normal shoulder MR scans, the interpretations of the scans obtained from patients with clinical shoulder instability improved considerably.

Conclusions.—The MR appearance of the labral-capsular complex in asymptomatic shoulders shows a wide variability. Anteriorly, labral variability was the rule. The morphology and shape of the posterior labrum was more consistent.

▶ This is an excellent example of the type of study we all value. It shows, not unexpectedly, that there is considerable variation in the structure of the anterior glenoid labrum. The implication, of course, is that differentiating normal from abnormal may be quite difficult using this imaging modality.— R.H. Cofield, M.D.

Glenoid Labrum: Evaluation With MR Imaging

Garneau RA, Renfrew DL, Moore TE, El-Khoury GY, Nepola JV, Lemke JH
(Univ of Iowa, Iowa City)
Radiology 179:519–522, 1991
2–8

Background.—Although computed arthrotomography of the shoulder remains the standard method in the evaluation of the glenoid labrum, MRI has been proposed for this purpose.

Methods.—The value of MRI in determining abnormalities of the glenoid labrum was investigated in volunteers and in 15 patients with shoulder instability. All patients underwent MRI. Two musculoskeletal radiologists interpreted the MRI images at the initial assessment and 2 years later.

Results.—In the first interpretation of results, there was a 44% sensitivity and a 7% specificity for observer A, and 78% sensitivity and a 67% specificity for observer B. The specificity for the asymptomatic volunteers was 100% for observer A and 89% for observer B. There was substantial interobserver and intraobserver variability; the observers agreed on true positive findings in only 3 of 9 patients and on true negative outcomes in 2 of 6 persons. At the end of the second assessment, observer A agreed with himself in 5 of the 9 patients and observer B agreed with himself in 7 of the 9 patients. The ability to observe correctly the occurrence of a tear was low, and the grading of the tears was even lower: observer A rightly graded the lesions in 2 of 9 patients and observer B did so in 4 of 9 patients.

Conclusions.—Although few patients underwent evaluation, MRI appears to have low sensitivity and low specificity in the assessment of labral abnormalities. In addition, MRI is invasive and costs more than computed arthrography. Computed arthrography should continue to be used to observe these abnormalities.

▶ The findings in this article confirm the suspected difficulties implied in the previous article. Even under the eyes of experienced observers, precise assessment of the glenoid labrum is not consistently possible. As we can see, there has been a great deal of activity this year in assessing the value of imaging in the shoulder, particularly the value of MRI. We all know but, perhaps, need continually to remind ourselves that the techniques of clinical evaluation, including the history, the physical examination, and plain radiographic studies, are the key items in diagnosis, and these studies are only supplementary to those most important parts of the diagnostic evaluation.—R.H. Cofield, M.D.

Fractures

Non-Union of Fractures of the Mid-Shaft of the Clavicle: Treatment With a Modified Hagie Intramedullary Pin and Autogenous Bone-Grafting

Boehme D, Curtis RJ Jr, DeHaan JT, Kay SP, Young DC, Rockwood CA Jr (Univ of Texas, San Antonio)
J Bone Joint Surg 73-A:1219–1226, 1991
2–9

Background.—Disadvantages accompany the previously recommended treatments for symptomatic nonunion of clavicular fractures. Experience with 21 patients treated by intramedullary fixation with a modified Hagie pin and autogenous bone grafting was reviewed.

Patients.—Twenty-one of 50 patients older than age 13 years were treated with the modified Hagie pin and autogenous bone grafting in 22 operations. All had a symptomatic nonunion of the mid/shaft of the clavicle. The 11 men and 10 women had a median age of 40 years; indications for operation were pain, crepitus, loss of motion, and inability to work. The graft site was the rib in 64% of patients. Follow-up averaged 35 months.

Technique.—Fragments are prepared and the intramedullary canal of the medial and lateral fragments is drilled by hand. An appropriate-sized modified Hagie pin is drilled through the distal fragment, and the pin is retracted until its end is at the site of the nonunion. The segments are aligned, and the pin is drilled into the medial fragment. If the pin does not hold, the nut is placed and tightened to achieve the desired compression (Fig 2–3). Grafts are placed superiorly, inferiorly, and posteriorly around the fracture. The patient uses a sling with only gentle motion for 2 weeks, and the pin is removed when healing is seen radiographically.

Results.—The fracture healed in all patients but 1, who had been inadvertently placed on a rehabilitation program involving overhead motion. Time to healing averaged 22 weeks. Fourteen patients were totally asymptomatic. Time to normal activities averaged 5 months. Four patients had mild symptoms; 2 continued to have pain and functional symptoms.

Conclusions.—This intramedullary fixation technique for nonunion of the midshaft of the clavicle appears superior to other methods, such as fixation with a plate and screws. The incision, which is made in the Langer line, is cosmetically acceptable, soft tissue dissection is lessened, and the pin can be removed using local anesthesia.

▶ Compression intramedullary pinning with bone grafting is an excellent form of treatment for midclavicle nonunions. Many orthopedic surgeons were intro-

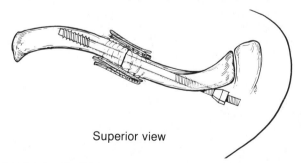

Superior view

Fig 2–3.—Superior view. If sufficient compression at site of nonunion is not obtained, Hagie nut can be applied to fine-threaded end of pin and tightened, which will produce additional compression. Bone graft is applied superiorly, inferiorly, and posteriorly about site of fracture. (Courtesy of Boehme D, Curtis RJ Jr, DeHaan JT, et al: *J Bone Joint Surg* 73-A:1219–1226, 1991.)

duced to this method by the Neviasers, who have advocated the use of a Knowles' pin. I, too, prefer this type of fixation to plating whenever possible. It is simple, the fixation is secure, and, as was demonstrated earlier and by these authors, it is quite effective.— R.H. Cofield, M.D.

Open Reduction and Internal Fixation of Two-Part Displaced Fractures of the Greater Tuberosity of the Proximal Part of the Humerus

Flatow EL, Cuomo F, Maday MG, Miller SR, McIlveen SJ, Bigliani LU (Columbia-Presbyterian Med Ctr, New York)
J Bone Joint Surg 73-A:1213–1218, 1991   2–10

Background.— There have been few reports of 2-part displaced fractures of the greater tuberosity, but they may be more common than the literature suggests. Limited motion and disability may result if the fractures are not diagnosed and treated promptly. Long-term results in 12 patients were examined.

Methods.— Of 16 patients who underwent open reduction and internal fixation for a 2-part displaced fracture of the greater tuberosity, 12 were available for follow-up interview, physical examination, and radiographs. Average follow-up was 4.5 years. The 7 men and 5 women had an average age of 53 years; 9 of the injuries resulted from a fall onto the arm. The injuries were reduced surgically because of the presence of 1 cm or more of displacement as seen on radiographs. An anterosuperior deltoid-splitting approach was used in combination with rotation of the humerus to gain exposure of the retracted tuberosity. The tuberosity was fixed with heavy, nonabsorbable sutures, and the rotator cuff was carefully repaired, allowing early passive motion.

Results.— All the fractures healed with no postoperative displacement. Six patients complained of mild pain on using the shoulder, and the other 6 had no pain. No patient was limited in activities. Active shoulder elevation averaged 170 degrees and external rotation averaged 63 degrees. The results were judged excellent in 6 patients and good in the rest, including 1 patient who had a partial, transient axillary nerve palsy.

Discussion.— Anteroposterior and outlet radiographs allow assessment of superior displacement, whereas axillary radiography is sufficient for assessment of posterior retraction. The tendon insertion should be incorporated into the suture fixation of the tuberosity.

▶ These authors nicely demonstrate that, when one reduces and sutures the tuberosity in position in association with rotator cuff repair, early passive motion can be achieved, and the results, with rare exception, will be excellent.— R.H. Cofield, M.D.

Open Reduction and Internal Fixation of Radial Head Fractures

King GJW, Evans DC, Kellam JF (University of Toronto, Ontario)
J Orthop Trauma 5:21–28, 1991   2–11

Background.—There is controversy regarding the treatment of radial head fractures. There have been relatively few reports of the results of internal fixation, and most have included only short-term follow-up.

Method.—Thirteen patients who had undergone open reduction and internal fixation for 14 radial head fractures were available for review at least 1 year after injury. Pain, motion, strength, stability, and function were assessed by the Elbow Evaluation Score. Grip strength was assessed and follow-up radiographs were taken. Average follow-up was 32 months, and mean patient age was 38 years. The usual mechanism of injury was a fall on an outstretched hand.

Results.—For Mason type II fractures, the average elbow score was 96.8 points, which corresponded to 100% good or excellent results. Flexion averaged 142.5 degrees, mean fixed flexion deformity was 3.9 degrees, and there was no loss in grip strength. In Mason type III fractures, good or excellent results were achieved in only 33% of cases. Average elbow score was 72.9 points. Results were not significantly affected by associated elbow dislocation, but fixed flexion deformity was slightly increased.

Conclusions.—Open reduction and internal fixation provide excellent results in radial head fractures if anatomical reduction, stable fixation, and early range of motion can be achieved. Because fractures may be more comminuted than they appear on radiographs, the surgeon must decide during the operation whether to reconstruct or excise the radial head. An alternative method should be considered if stable anatomical reduction cannot be achieved.

▶ Readers should note the excellent results that were obtained in these patients, particularly those with less comminuted fractures. Special comment needs to be made about the excellent results that were achieved in instances of fracture–dislocation. As one might anticipate, when the radial head fracture is comminuted, this method of treatment may not be as desirable.—R.H. Cofield, M.D.

Post-Traumatic Radioulnar Synostosis After Forearm Fracture Osteosynthesis
Bauer G, Arand M, Mutschler W (Universität Ulm, Germany)
Arch Orthop Trauma Surg 110:142–145, 1991   2–12

Background.—A synostosis between the radius and ulna after conservative forearm fracture treatment occurs in 5.5% to 9.5% of patients. Factors associated with synostosis include a fracture of the ulna and radius at the same level, interosseous membrane injury, a fracture of the hematoma, serious local trauma, and other types of injuries.

Methods.—To determine the incidence of postsurgical synostosis in patients with forearm fracture and to assess the causative factors, the records of all patients treated with plate osteosynthesis for forearm breakages in 1978–1987 were reviewed retrospectively. A prospective analysis of such patients also was conducted in 1987–1989. Patient evaluation included chart review, radiography, and physical examination. Plate osteosynthesis had stabilized 89 fractures, with a bone graft added in 22 patients.

Results.—Of the 89 patients treated, 11 (6.6%) had a radioulnar synostosis, 6 of which occurred in closed fractures and 5 in open injuries. Of the 7 2-bone fractures, 6 received a 2-plate treatment. Of the 2 synostoses associated with isolated radial breakages, 1 had an open grade 2 fracture in the proximal section of the bone, and 1 had a closed proximal-third bone fracture treated with a modified Boyd approach.

Conclusion.—Synostosis occurs more often after the Boyd approach than after other kinds of surgical procedures. Separate approaches to the radius and the ulna are recommended, and the Boyd approach should be avoided, especially when treating fractures of both bones occurring at the same level.

Instability

ACROMIOCLAVICULAR

Four-Year Outcome of Operative Treatment of Acute Acromioclavicular Dislocation
Eskola A, Vainionpää S, Korkala O, Santavirta S, Grönblad M, Rokkanen P (Helsinki Univ Central Hosp)
J Orthop Trauma 5:9–13, 1991   2–13

Introduction.—Acute traumatic complete dislocation of the acromioclavicular joint may require various treatments.

Methods.—In a prospective, randomized trial, patients were treated for acromioclavicular dislocation with 1 of 3 different operative techniques: a fixation with smooth Kirschner wires, fixation with threaded Kirschner wires, or fixation with cortical ASIF screws. Of 100 patients who were randomly assigned to 1 of the 3 surgical procedure groups, follow-up data were available for 70. Smooth Kirschner wire fixation was used to treat 29 patients, threaded Kirschner wire fixation was used to treat 20, and cortical ASIF screws were used to treat 21. The patients were asked about their views on the surgical results and pain experience.

Results.—At follow-up 67 patients rated their outcome as good, 3 patients rated their outcome as satisfactory. None of the patients had restricted joint movement. However, there was local pain in 6 patients, 2 of whom were in the screw fixation group. Stress radiographs indicated that the lateral end of the clavile was not dislocated in 56 patients. The remaining patients had significantly less subluxation at 4-year follow-up than at 1-year follow-up.

Conclusions.—These results suggest that the threaded Kirschner wire fixation method is preferable for repairing this type of injury. The holding capacity of the threaded Kirschner wires appears to be greater to than that of the smooth type, promoting less implant loosening during the fixation period.

► Recently, the emphasis on the treatment of acute acromioclavicular disloca-tions has been nonoperative with some type of external support. This article reminds us that operative treatment with acromioclavicular fixation is a reason-able option, and, when using contemporary operative techniques, a good result is the rule.—R.H. Cofield, M.D.

GLENOHUMERAL

Prognosis of Primary Anterior Shoulder Dislocation in Young Adults
Hoelen MA, Burgers AMJ, Rozing PM (Univ Hosp, Leiden, The Netherlands)
Arch Orthop Trauma Surg 110:51–54, 1990   2–14

Background.—Glenohumeral dislocation recurs in 90% of younger patients. Data on a cohort of patients were retrospectively reviewed to determine the association between the recurrence and sports activity.

Methods.—The records of all patients treated for primary traumatic shoulder dislocations in 1982–1987 were reviewed. Of the 194 pa-tients identified with 196 shoulder dislocations, 186 could be traced, 20 of whom died. Thus 166 patients with 168 dislocations partici-pated.

Results.—Of the 166 patients, 26% had at least 1 recurrence, and 13% had repeated (3 or more) recurrences. The average age of these patients was 50 years (37.5 years for men, 65 years for women). Age was associated with the time of injury and the recurrence rate. Of the 96 men and 72 women participating, 40% of the men and 8% of the women had a recurrence. An unspecified fall appeared as the main cause of the first dislocation. No higher recurrence rate occurred among athletes. Arm dominance and length of immobilization played no role in the recurrences. A fracture of the greater tuberosity or the presence of a Hill-Sachs lesion did not influence the recurrence rate.

Conclusions.—Although sports activity has been linked with recur-rence of dislocation, these results do not support this observation. Physi-cians should be cautioned against using primary operative treatment as prophylaxis for young patients with this type of injury.

► This article emphasizes that recurrence of anterior shoulder dislocation is not so common as the classic articles would suggest. We also found this to be true in a review of dislocations occurring in the Olmstead County (Minnesota) pop-ulation. These authors conclude that athletics had no effect on recurrence of dislocation. They, however, have analyzed their material related to the cause of the initial dislocation and have not analyzed it relative to time of return to the sporting activity in which the dislocation initially occurred. These authors do ad-dress immobilization quite nicely. There is not very much comment, though, on rehabilitation. The authors seem quite correct in their conclusion. Operative treatment for the acute dislocation would seem excessive. There are many ex-periencing this injury who will not need significant further treatment.—R.H. Cofield, M.D.

Anterior Capsulolabral Reconstruction of the Shoulder in Athletes in Overhand Sports

Jobe FW, Giangarra CE, Kvitne RS, Glousman RE (Kerlin-Jobe Orthopaedic Clinic, Inglewood, Calif; Orthopedic Hand and Sports Specialists, Camarillo, Calif)

Am J Sports Med 19:428–434, 1991   2–15

Introduction.—Surgical procedures can correct anterior glenohumeral instability in athletes participating in sports that require overhand throwing, but many of these patients do not regain their previous level of throwing skill. A modified anterior capsulolabral reconstruction (ACLR) was developed that often can restore the preinjury level of function.

Patients.—Twenty-five athletes, 13 of whom competed at the professional level, were included. All had documented anterior shoulder instability and shoulder pain that failed to improve with conservative therapy. Twenty athletes competed in baseball, 2 in football, 1 in basketball, 1 in softball, and 1 in water polo. Their average age at time of operation was 21 years. All underwent ACLR and a formal program of rehabilitation exercises.

Results.—The exercise program was continued for at least 1 year. By 2½ months, full range of motion was achieved, and most patients were free of pain. Results at follow-up were rated excellent in 68% of the athletes, good in 24%, fair in 4%, and poor in 4%. All patients had negative impingement signs. Eighteen athletes were able to return to their previous level of competition for at least 1 complete season. The 7 remaining players were satisfied with the stability, almost full range of motion, and freedom from pain resulting from the procedure and rehabilitation program.

Conclusion.—Most athletes with anterior glenohumeral instability associated with repetitive throwing respond to nonoperative treatment. The ACLR procedure offers excellent results for many of those who require surgery and is a significant improvement compared with previous methods.

▶ This article is of great importance. There is now hope for athletes with shoulder subluxation in the anterior direction. If their problem does not respond to the usual nonoperative treatment methods, surgery may be an option, and, certainly, the results reported are very reasonable. The only criticism one might have of the structure of this article is in the description of the patient characteristics and their pathology. The first could certainly be more ample to help us all understand the patient population somewhat better. In addressing the second, the authors state that the presence of anterior instability was confirmed by examination under anesthesia and at arthroscopy. However, none of those findings are reported in the article. So, unfortunately, readers are somewhat uncertain about the population being treated.—R.H. Cofield, M.D.

Results of the Putti-Platt Operation for Recurrent Anterior Dislocation of the Shoulder

Fredriksson A-S, Tegner Y (Central Hospital, Boden, Sweden)

Int Orthop 15:185–188, 1991

2–16

Background.—The goal of the Putti-Platt repair of recurrent anterior shoulder dislocation is to prevent recurrent dislocation by limiting external rotation. Reported recurrence rates range from 0% to 36%, but many investigations have involved only short follow-ups.

Methods.—Of 101 patients undergoing a Putti-Platt repair for recurrent shoulder dislocation between 1973 and 1981, 89 were followed and 43 were examined clinically (23 with a dynamometer). The mean follow-up was 8 years. Most of the dislocations had occurred during normal activity, but 38% of patients were engaged in athletic activity at the time of injury.

Findings.—Eighteen patients (20%) had recurrent dislocation, but 8 had fewer than 4 redislocations. Older patients had a relatively low recurrence rate; there was no difference between patients injured during athletic activity and other patients. Only 2 patients had a full range of motion. Reduced strength and power were found in the injured shoulders.

Conclusions.—Recurrent shoulder dislocation is relatively frequent in younger patients having the Putti-Platt operation. One should hesitate to recommend this procedure for young persons who are active.

▶ Amen! If stretching of the anterior capsule and subscapularis is a major or the only abnormal finding at the time of surgery, shortening these structures certainly is reasonable. However, if the capsule is torn from the edge of the glenoid (as is the rule), addressing this abnormality by shortening the capsule and subscapularis, although reasonable in the past, is recognized to have its limitations. As is so nicely illustrated in this article, the recurrence rate is higher, and the loss of movement is greater.—R.H. Cofield, M.D.

Alvik's Glenoplasty for Humeroscapular Dislocations: 6-Year Follow-Up of 52 Shoulders

Niskanen RO, Lehtonen JY, Kaukonen J-P (Päijät-Häme Central Hosp, Lahti, Finland)

Acta Orthop Scand 62:279–283, 1991

2–17

Background.—The Eden-Hybbinette operation for anterior recurrent dislocation of the shoulder, modified by Alvik 40 years ago, has been used successfully in Scandinavia. In Alvik's modification, an iliac-crest, bone graft is inserted into a groove in the glenoid rim of the scapula (Fig 2–4). The results of this procedure, the incidence of redislocations, the development and significance of arthrosis, and the future of the bone transplant were examined retrospectively.

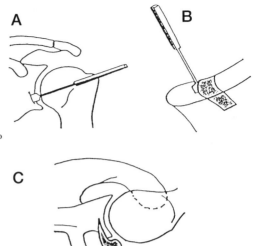

Fig 2–4.—A groove is made with an osteotome through the capsule into the anteroinferior aspect of the scapular neck (**A**), an iliac-crest bone graft (**B**) is jammed into the groove without any fixation. Inferosuperior view (**C**). (Courtesy of Niskanen RO, Lehtonen JY, Kaukonen J-P: *Acta Orthop Scand* 62:279–283, 1991.)

Patients.—Fifty-two shoulders in 46 patients were surgically treated using the modified Alvik method. At the time of surgery, patients had a mean age of 32 years. Average follow-up was 6 years.

Results.—No operative complications occurred. Two thirds of the patients were satisfied with the operation. After surgery, spontaneous redislocation occurred in only 1 patient. There were also 10 traumatic redislocations. Nine shoulders showed signs of postoperative arthrosis. Arthrosis correlated more strongly with the patient's age at surgery than with length of follow-up. Bony healing of the transplant was noted in 41 shoulders.

Conclusions.—One fifth of patients had postoperative redislocations or subluxations. However, there was relevant trauma in 10 of 11 patients, indicating only 1 real failure. Alvik's glenoplasty is recommended as 1 of the methods, for treating habitual anterior humeroscapular dislocation and subluxation.

▶ This very useful article points out, as we have come to learn, that the Eden-Hybbinette operation is relatively effective. The recurrence rate may be higher than we have come to expect with the soft tissue repairs (about 20% in this series). Most importantly though, placing a bone graft where it might come in contact with cartilage has the potential to create glenohumeral arthritis. In this patient series, 9 shoulders had moderate or severe arthritis, and 18 additional shoulders had "incipient" arthritis. With soft tissue repairs being so effective, one would believe that many surgeons would not elect to perform this type of procedure, not only because the recurrence rate is somewhat higher than the soft tissue procedures but also because the opportunity for arthritis to develop is distinctly greater.—R.H. Cofield, M.D.

Complications of a Failed Bristow Procedure and Their Management

Young DC, Rockwood CA Jr (Univ of Texas, San Antonio)
J Bone Joint Surg 73-A:969–981, 1991   2–18

Background.—When the Bristow procedure for reconstruction of the shoulder fails, the subsequent management can be difficult. Forty such cases were reviewed to identify the complications, define the processes leading to failure, and assess the results of the subsequent treatment.

Patients.—Thirty-nine patients who underwent 40 failed procedures were treated during a 10-year period. The average follow-up was 4.4 years. The mean age at presentation was 30 years. In addition to the Bristow procedure, patients had undergone 36 previous operations, including 23 anterior reconstructions in 17 patients. The initial complaint was chronic painful anterior instability in 28 shoulders, pain with no subjective instability in 6 shoulders, and posterior instability in 4 shoulders; 2 patients had no pain and no instability.

Findings.—All patients were started on a shoulder rehabilitation program. Those who had continued signs or symptoms had surgery; this was done in 31 of the 40 shoulders (78%). A special anterior capsular shift was done in 16 shoulders, 4 had capsular release, 4 had total shoulder arthroplasty, and other procedures were done in the remaining 7 shoulders. Complications of the initial procedure included recurrent painful anterior instability, injury to the articular cartilage, nonunion of the coracoid bone-block and the glenoid, loosening of the screw, neurovascular injury, and posterior instability. The main cause of failure was excessive laxity of the capsule, which occurred in 80% of shoulders and caused chronic, painful anterior or posterior instability. The remaining 20% had an untreated Perthes-Bankart lesion. Outcome was judged good or excellent in only 50% of patients.

Conclusions.—These findings suggest that the Bristow procedure should not be used for primary treatment of the shoulder with symptomatic anterior instability. The anterior reconstruction described is a difficult procedure that requires meticulous technique. The Bristow procedure carries no better rate of success than other standard operations, and it causes a wide range of minor and serious complications.

▶ As with the Putti-Platt and the Eden-Hybbinette procedures described in reports above, the Bristow procedure can also lead to a significant number of poor results or complications. Certainly, this procedure has been shown to be effective for a number of individuals. However, it will not necessarily create a situation that will lead to healing of a Bankart lesion or to capsular tightening. Failure to address these 2 pathologic changes renders the security of an operation much less certain. In addition, one is then left with a situation of possible bone or metal contact against cartilage, neurovascular injury, or other metal problems. As can easily be gleaned from the 3 previous articles, evidence is mounting indicating that, for shoulder instability, the treatment should be either repair of the torn capsular ligaments when they are disrupted (usually at the glenoid rim) or tightening of a stretched capsule. This is conceptually very direct, complications are minimized, and the results are optimized.— R.H. Cofield, M.D.

Concurrent Rotator-Cuff Tear and Brachial Plexus Palsy Associated With Anterior Dislocation of the Shoulder: A Report of Two Cases
Gonzalez D, Lopez RA (Albert Einstein College of Medicine, New York)
J Bone Joint Surg 73-A:620–621, 1991   2–19

Background.— In middle-aged patients, acute tears of the rotator cuff associated with anterior dislocation of the shoulder may be misdiagnosed initially, especially when a concurrent brachial-plexus palsy also exists. Two patients with all 3 of these lesions were treated.

Case Report.— Woman, 57, came to the emergency room with pain and swelling of the shoulder after an assault. Other symptoms included paresthesias in the right arm and weakness of flexion of the elbow. The weakness and paresthesias persisted after a closed reduction of the anterior dislocation. There was no radiographic evidence of fracture. When the patient's symptoms persisted at 1-week follow-up, additional studies were undertaken. An arthrogram showed a complete tear of the rotator cuff. At surgery, a full-thickness, 6-cm wide tear was found and primarily repaired. The patient was given standard postoperative rehabilitation. She remains free of pain and enjoys normal function at 2-year follow-up.

Conclusions.— Patients who have sustained an anterior dislocation of the shoulder, especially older patients whose injury was caused by severe trauma, should be evaluated carefully for additional injury to the rotator cuff and brachial plexus. Early diagnosis and treatment is important in obtaining an optimal functional outcome.

▶ It is known that rotator cuff tearing or nerve injury may occur in association with shoulder dislocation. It is important to recall that both may occur. Arthrography or MRI plus electromyographic testing may be necessary in a patient with shoulder dislocation that does not rapidly recover active movement.— R.H. Cofield, M.D.

The Effect of Capsular Venting on Glenohumeral Laxity
Gibb TD, Sidles JA, Harryman DT II, McQuade KJ, Matsen FA III (Univ of Washington, Seattle)
Clin Orthop 268:120–127, 1991   2–20

Background.— Although the shoulder muscles are inactive and do not contribute to stability, anesthetized shoulders often are stable against forces applied during drawer and sulcus tests. The glenohumeral joints of anatomical specimens also exhibit this passive stability.

Methods.— The effect of capsular venting on glenohumeral laxity was investigated in 8 fresh cadaver shoulders from persons aged 57–87 years, including 6 contralateral pairs. A 6-degrees-of-freedom force transducer and a 6-degrees-of-freedom spatial tracker were used. Air was admitted ad libitum through an 18-gauge needle to provide capsule ventilation.

Results.—Venting decreased the force needed to translate the humeral head with respect to the glenoid fossa by a mean of 15.3N (55%) for anterior forces; 10.8N (43%) for posterior forces; and 19N (57%) for inferior forces.

Conclusion.—Laxity was substantially increased when air was admitted to the capsules. Passive stability is likely to be diminished by a similar mechanism in patients with intact but excessively lax capsules. Clinicians should consider this principle when evaluating glenohumeral stability.

ELBOW

Posterolateral Rotatory Instability of the Elbow

O'Driscoll SW, Bell DF, Morrey BF (St Michael's Hosp; The Hospital for Sick Children, Toronto; Mayo Clinic and Found, Rochester, Minn)
J Bone Joint Toronto Surg 73-A:440–446, 1991   2–21

Background.—Recurrent posterolateral rotatory instability of the elbow is hard to diagnose. A new test was developed to diagnose posterolateral rotatory instability of the elbow.

Patients.—Five patients aged 5–46 years were treated. The age at injury ranged from 3 to 42 years. Two patients had more than 100 recurrences. Operative findings were avulsion in 2 patients and laxity in 3.

Technique.—The instability in these patients could be demonstrated only by the posterolateral rotatory instability test. It consists of supination of the forearm and application of a valgus moment and axial compression force to the elbow while it is flexed from full extension. The elbow is reduced in full extension and subluxation during flexion to obtain a positive test result. Further flexion (more than 40 degrees) produces a sudden palpable, visible reduction of the radiohumeral joint (Fig 2–5).

Conclusions.—The cause of this condition is believed to be laxity of the ulnar part of the lateral collateral ligament. This laxity allows a transient rotatory subluxation of the ulnohumeral joint and an associated dislocation of the radiohumeral joint. The annular ligament is intact, preventing the radioulnar joint from dislocating. Surgical repair of the lax ulnar part of the collateral ligament will eliminate the posterolateral rotatory instability.

▶ Perhaps this has been hard to delineate in the past because diagnosis is so physician-dependent rather than test-dependent. The authors have nicely described the clinical evaluation needed to make the diagnosis. Because the number of patients seen with this problem is small, treatment recommendations cannot be presented forcefully. The authors, though, have suggested a quite

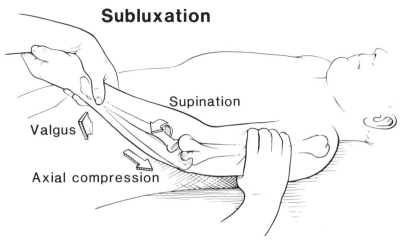

Fig 2–5.—Test for posterolateral rotary instability of the elbow. With the arm at the side and the forearm in supination, supination and valgus moments, as well as axial forces, are applied to the elbow, which is flexed approximately 20 to 30 degrees. The posterolateral subluxation is visibly and palpably reduced when the elbow is flexed farther. (Courtesy of O'Driscoll SW, Bell DF, Morrey BF: *J Bone Joint Surg* 73-A:440–446, 1991.)

reasonable approach to ligament repair for this type of instability.—R.H. Cofield, M.D.

Chronic Posterior Subluxation and Dislocation of the Radial Head
Bell SN, Morrey BF, Bianco AJ Jr (Mayo Clinic and Found, Rochester, Minn)
J Bone Joint Surg 73-A:392–396, 1991   2–22

Background.—Congenital posterior displacement of the radial head is usually associated with other anomalies or systemic conditions but can occur in otherwise normal people. The latter situation, which is relatively rare, was investigated.

Patients.—From 1965 to 1985, 27 of 79 patients with a diagnosis of chronic posterior displacement of the radial head had no other musculoskeletal anomalies or history of trauma to the elbow. The mean age of the 27 patients was 7.8 years. Three characteristic radiographic types were noted: subluxation (type I), posterior dislocation with minimum displacement (type II), and posterior dislocation with substantial proximal migration of the radius (type III). Eighteen patients (21 elbows) were available for follow-up 2.5–13.5 years after initial examination.

Results.—The most common initial problems were pain, loss of motion of the elbow, and deformity. Ten patients were treated with excision of the radial head, and 8 were not treated. Only 1 patient with an untreated elbow noted an increase in pain, about 5 years after the initial assessment. A slight loss of extension was noted in patients with a type II dislocation, but in only 1 with a type III dislocation. All untreated patients had a normal range of flexion initially and at follow-up. Postoperatively, 5 treated patients were relieved of all pain, and 2 had less pain. Cosmetic deformity was mild at follow-up in all but 1 of the treated patients. Range of motion was significantly improved in 1 patient.

Conclusions.—Classification according to radiographic type correlated well with the indications for surgery and prognosis. Type I dislocation caused pain and clicking and was associated with later degenerative arthritis. Type II resulted in less severe pain than type I and only moderately impaired the arc of motion. Cosmetic deformity was a problem in type III elbows.

Tendon Injury and Disease

Shoulder Disorders in the Elderly: A Community Survey

Chard MD, Hazleman R, Hazleman BL, King RH, Reiss BB (Addenbrooke's Hosp, East Barnwell Health Ctr, Cambridge, England)
Arthritis Rheum 34:766–769, 1991   2–23

Background.—Hospital-based studies indicate that nontraumatic symptomatic shoulder disorders, which are common in middle-aged individuals, are relatively rare in the elderly. However, pathologic studies suggest that there is a progressive degeneration of the rotator cuff with age. A community-based prevalence study investigated the prevalence of symptomatic shoulder disorders in the elderly.

Methods.—A community sample of 644 individuals older than 70 years of age was surveyed. The sample consisted of 318 men and 326 women.

Results.—The prevalence of symptomatic shoulder disorders was 21%. These disorders were reported by 25% of the women and 17% of the men. Approximately 70% of those with shoulder pain had rotator cuff involvement. Fewer than 40% of the individuals surveyed sought medical attention for their complaints.

Conclusions.—Symptomatic shoulder disorders are common among the elderly. They occurred in 1 of 5 individuals of this group. Because elderly individuals often do not volunteer information about shoulder pain, increased medical awareness is needed.

▶ This nice study helps to dispel some of the incorrect implications in the literature. Soft tissue problems in the shoulder are very common in the elderly. As a corollary to this, it is reasonable to conclude that the large number of lesions identified in cadavers were in fact not asymptomatic. Probably many were symptomatic but not to the extent that surgery would have been required in a population group with lower physical demands.—R.H. Cofield, M.D.

Bicipital Groove Dysplasia and Medial Dislocation of the Biceps Brachii Tendon

Levinsohn EM, Santelli ED (State Univ of New York, Syracuse)
Skeletal Radiol 20:419–423, 1991   2–24

Background.—The long head of the biceps brachii tendon is a recognized source of shoulder pain. If the bicipital groove is shallow, the tendon may tend to sublux medially or dislocate. If the groove is deficient, unroofing by avulsion of the subscapularis tendon may facilitate subluxation or dislocation of the tendon medially. The plain film finding of dysplasia of the lesser tubercle of the humerus and its relationship to medial dislocation of the biceps brachii was examined.

Methods.—Fifty-five patients were referred for arthrography because of shoulder pain. Plain films included the anteroposterior view with internal rotation, Grashey view, axillary view, and bicipital groove view, taken both before and after injection of contrast. The bicipital groove was measured by the method of Cone et al. (Fig 2–6).

Results.—Mean medial wall angle was 41 degrees. Twelve patients had a medial wall angle of 30 degrees or less, 7 of whom had concurrent medial dislocation of the biceps tendon; 3 of the latter had a rotator cuff tear. None of the patients whose medial wall angle measured greater than 30 degrees had a dislocated bicipital tendon, and only 3 had a rotator cuff tear.

Conclusions.—Radiographic examination of the bicipital groove appears to be an important adjunct in the evaluation of patients with possible abnormalities of the biceps tendon. The diagnosis of medial dislocation of the biceps tendon can be made by arthrography, with or without CT. On arthrography the tendon lies medial to the lesser tubercle of the humerus.

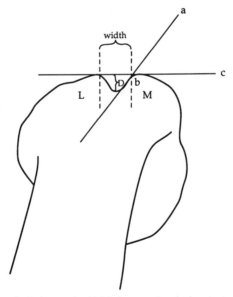

Fig 2–6.—Cone's method of measuring bicipital groove. Standard projection is taken with cassette at right angle to long axis of humerus. Patient is supine with humerus in maximal external rotation. Cranially directed central beam is projected medially 15 degrees and as parallel as possible to long axis of humerus. *a, b, c,* medial wall angle of lesser tubercle; *dotted lines,* width of groove, *D,* depth of groove; *L,* greater tubercle; *M,* lesser tubercle. (Courtesy of Levinsohn EM, Santelli ED: *Skeletal Radiol* 20:419–423, 1991.)

▶ It is an interesting observation that shallow medial wall angles correlate not only with biceps tendon dislocation but also with rotator cuff tearing. This finding may or may not be confirmed by subsequent investigators. An important implication is that the shape of the humeral head may play a role in the propensity to develop rotator cuff disease with tearing. The acromion certainly has been implicated, but perhaps we should not neglect considering the importance of structural variations in the humeral head.—R.H. Cofield, M.D.

Shoulder Strength Analysis Using the Cybex II Isokinetic Dynamometer
Cahalan TD, Johnson ME, Chao EYS (Mayo Clinic and Found, Rochester, Minn)
Clin Orthop 271:249–257, 1991   2–25

Introduction.—In the past, shoulder strength was assessed by subjective manual muscle testing. This method is of limited usefulness because of problems with interrater reliability and because muscle strength cannot be tested under dynamic conditions. Both problems have been eliminated with the new isokinetic devices. A clinically useful method of isokinetic shoulder strength assessment was developed to create a database of normal shoulder muscle strength values under isometric and multiple isokinetic conditions.

Methods.—Fifty healthy volunteers aged 21–40 years with normal active shoulder motion and no history of upper extremity symptoms were included. A Cybex II isokinetic dynamometer was modified to allow a wide range of placements of the dynamometer head. Isokinetic testing was performed at speeds of 0, 60, 180, and 200 degrees per second. Each person was allowed 5 or 6 submaximal repetitions at 60 degrees per second before testing in a new plane, and 2 or 3 repetitions before testing at each speed. All tests consisted of 5 maximal and reciprocal contractions. The best 3 contractions were used for data analysis.

Results.—Mean peak torque values generally decreased as contraction speed increased. Shoulder extension torque was greatest, followed by adduction, flexion, internal rotation, abduction, and external rotation. Men were significantly stronger than women for all motions and at all speeds tested. Torque values for the dominant extremity were significantly greater than for the nondominant extremity.

Conclusions.—Shoulder strength is variable, even within the healthy young adult population. The normal shoulder strength data obtained in this study can be used for comparison when assessing disability of the upper extremity.

▶ We really do need more accurate methods of measuring shoulder strength and methods that would be practical in a clinical setting. In this study, the investigators attempt to isolate the shoulder muscles as much as possible. The study has evidently been very carefully done, and in certain measurements there are distinct differences between the dominant and nondominant extremity. This has been inconsistently demonstrated in the past. In the clinical setting, many patients with shoulder injury or disease are middle-aged or older and have compromised musculotendinous units. It would be wonderful to have a more precise method of measuring these deficiencies. Unfortunately, isokinetic testing has seemed to be quite rigorous for these individuals and has not offered as much useful information as one would like relative to the difficulties associated with the testing.—R.H. Cofield, M.D.

Arthroscopic Distension in the Management of Frozen Shoulder
Hsu SYC, Chan KM (The Chinese University of Hong Kong, Shatin)
Int Orthop 15:79–83, 1991   2–26

Background.—Frozen shoulder is a common problem in Hong Kong. When patients are treated early, physiotherapy and anti-inflammatory drugs often relieve the pain and improve stiffness; those treated later may be resistant to such treatment. A prospective study was done to compare manipulation and physiotherapy, physiotherapy alone, and arthroscopic distention in patients with frozen shoulder.

Methods.—Between 1985 and 1987 75 patients with a history of symptoms for longer than 3 months and abduction restricted to 90 degrees or less were treated. The 25 patients in group 1 were treated by manipulation and physiotherapy in a standard fashion. The 25 patients in group 2 were treated with arthroscopic distention and standard physiotherapy. The 25 patients in group 3 had standard physiotherapy alone. All patients were assessed at weeks 1, 2, 3, 5, 8, and 12.

Results.—Pain relief was greater in the first 2 groups. Patients in group 1 had greater relief than those in group 2 for the first 3 weeks, but the difference was insignificant thereafter. The degree of pain relief increased with time regardless of the treatment used and was most dramatic in the first 4–5 weeks. Group 1 had more shoulder flexion than group 2 in the first 5 weeks, a difference that decreased beyond week 5. Group 1 had better flexion than group 3 throughout the trial period. After 5 weeks group 2 had significantly greater flexion than group 3. Shoulder abduction range was significantly greater in group 1 than in group 2 at weeks 2, 3, and 8. Abduction strength did not differ between groups 1 and 2. After 3 and 5 weeks, respectively, patients in group 3 were weaker than those in groups 1 and 2. After 3 weeks, groups 1 and 2 had a significantly higher mean functional score than group 3. Functional scores were not significantly different in groups 1 and 2 throughout the 12 weeks.

Conclusion.—Treatment with manipulation and physiotherapy and with arthroscopic distention and physiotherapy are better than treatment with physiotherapy alone. Arthroscopic distention is a good alternative to manipulation, as it is more controllable and provides important information about the pathologic lesions in the joint.

▶ This study details the results (short-term follow-up) of patients treated for frozen shoulder. With more aggressive treatment, including manipulation or arthroscopy, improvement seems to occur sooner. However, the study does not address the final outcome, which occurs for many patients beyond 12 weeks. It is important to recall that arthroscopy may be of help in diagnosis; however, arthrography in this setting may be just as useful by excluding a significant intra-articular synovitis and the presence of rotator cuff tearing.—R.H. Cofield, M.D.

Surgical Treatment of Medial Epicondylitis: Results in 35 Elbows
Vangsness CT Jr, Jobe FW (Univ of Southern California)
J Bone Joint Surg 73-B:409–411, 1991   2–27

Background.—Medial epicondylitis at the elbow, a relatively uncommon condition, usually responds to conservative treatment. However, when such treatment fails and when pain persists after 6–12 months, surgery may be considered (Fig 2–7). Reports on the surgical treatment of medial epicondylitis have not been published in the past.

Patients.—Between 1974 and 1984, 38 patients at 1 center required surgery for medial epicondylitis after conservative treatment failed. Thirty-five of these patients were reviewed. The mean age was 43 years, and the mean follow-up was 85 months.

Results.—At surgery the residual tears with incomplete healing were consistently found in the flexor origin at the medial epicondyle. Microscopy showed reactive fibrous connective tissues with various degrees of inflammation. The mean subjective estimate of elbow function improved from 38% to 98% after surgery. Isokinetic and grip strength testing after surgery in 16 patients showed strength equivalent to the healthy limb. The results were classified as excellent in 25 patients, good in 9, and fair in 1. Eighty-six percent of the patients had no limitation in elbow use.

Conclusions.—Surgery for medial epicondylitis after the failure of conservative treatment is predictably effective. It relieves pain, restores strength, and allows patients to return to their previous levels of daily activity and sports participation after surgery.

▶ The authors present a simple and, as they demonstrate, effective treatment method for symptomatic, incomplete tearing and reactive changes at the me-

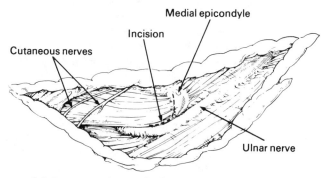

Fig 2–7.—Medial skin incision, showing the deep strictures. (Courtesy of Vangsness CT Jr, Jobe FW: *J Bone Joint Surg* 73-B:409–411, 1991.)

dial humeral epicondyle. Fortunately, surgery is seldom necessary in this condition, but, should it prove to be necessary, a simple, sound, and effective solution is possible.—R.H. Cofield, M.D.

SHOULDER IMPINGEMENT

Arthroscopic Subacromial Decompression for Chronic Impingement: Two- to Five-Year Results
Ellman H, Kay SP (Univ of California, Los Angeles)
J Bone Joint Surg 73-B:395–398, 1991   2–28

Background.—Preliminary research and a short-term follow-up study have suggested that arthroscopic subacromial decompression (ASD) is an effective alternative to open acromioplasty for patients with chronic impingement syndrome in the shoulder. The longer term results of ASD in patients without evidence of full thickness rotator cuff tears were analyzed.

Patients.—Ninety ASDs were done between 1983 and 1986. Eighty-two of these patients were available for a minimum 2-year follow-up; the longest follow-up was 5 years. Seventeen of the 82 patients had full thickness rotator cuff tears and were excluded. The remaining 65 patients were 34 women and 31 men (average age, 45 years). The mean duration of symptoms before surgery was slightly more than 2 years.

Results.—Eighty-nine percent of the patients had a satisfactory result according to the University of California, Los Angeles shoulder rating scale. Thirty-two patients were classified as excellent. The results were fair in 4 patients and poor in 3. The most dramatic benefit was pain relief, but function improved as well. The mean pain rating improved from 2.8 to 8.2, indicating slight discomfort and occasional pain. In addition, 55% of the shoulders became completely pain free.

Conclusions.—These outcomes compare favorably with those of open acromioplasty. The arthroscopic procedure is technically demanding, however, when it is done properly in appropriately selected patients, hos pitalization is brief, the return to activities is rapid, the risk of deltoid muscle complications is minimal, and the results are lasting.

▶ This nicely performed patient series demonstrates that, using contemporary clinical diagnostic means, arthroscopic acromioplasty is effective for patients with the impingement syndrome in the absence of full-thickness rotator cuff tearing. We now have in hand MRI, which offers the opportunity to assess carefully rotator cuff tendon pathology. With this more precise diagnostic tool, perhaps it will become increasingly apparent who should and who should not be considered for this treatment option.—R.H. Cofield, M.D.

Total Acromionectomy: A Twenty-Year Review
Bosley RC (Boulder Orthopedics, Colo)
J Bone Joint Surg 73-A:961–968, 1991   2–29

Background.—Impingement of the rotator cuff can cause chronic and disabling pain in the shoulders. Conservative treatment is often effective, but some patients require surgical intervention. Good results after total acromionectomy initially were reported in 1949 and in some trials thereafter, but poor results reported in recent years led to a recommendation against its use.

Patients.—Between 1969 and 1991, 40 patients underwent total acromionectomy on 45 shoulders. Thirty-one patients (aged 31–70 years) who underwent operation on 34 shoulders were available for examination and interview. The duration of follow-up ranged from 2 to 20 years. Total acromionectomy was performed on 27 dominant shoulders and on 7 nondominant shoulders. Three patients had bilateral procedures. All patients had disabling shoulder pain that often radiated to the midpoint of the arm. Nineteen shoulders had a tear of the rotator cuff, of which 8 were small and 11 were massive. Six shoulders had degenerative lesions of the rotator cuff accompanied by a large calcific deposit. The remaining shoulders had a degenerative lesion with chronic subdeltoid bursitis. All patients had chronic impingement syndrome. All patients completed a questionnaire to rate their overall level of satisfaction. In addition, shoulders were examined for strength, range of motion, presence of crepitus or atrophy, and symmetry of appearance.

Results.—The clinical results were excellent for 25 shoulders, good for 4, fair for 4, and poor for 1. Twenty-eight patients stated that they were very satisfied with the outcome and would certainly have the operation again. The remaining 3 patients were satisfied and likely to have the operation again, if needed. The 4 least satisfactory results were obtained in patients who had a long-standing massive tear of the rotator cuff. Retraction of the deltoid, considered the major drawback of total acromionectomy, did not occur in any of the patients.

Conclusions.—The unsatisfactory results attributed to total acromionectomy are likely the result of an avoidable complication rather than of the procedure itself. Failure to repair the deltoid adequately results in the muscle's retraction, which has given the procedure an unfavorable reputation.

▶ The author has very nicely documented that, given exacting technique and adequate postoperative support, deltoid retraction after total acromionectomy can be prevented. Eleven of 40 shoulders had more than a small amount of rotator cuff tearing. The least satisfactory results were in this patient group. One might reasonably comment that for lesser degrees of involvement of the rotator cuff an operation as substantial as total acromionectomy is not necessary, while for patients with larger rotator cuff tears it is not desirable. These would be the points of a devil's advocate and perhaps represent the majority opinion among orthopedic surgeons today.—R.H. Cofield, M.D.

Superior Humeral Dislocation: A Complication Following Decompression and Debridement for Rotator Cuff Tears
Wiley AM (Toronto Western Hosp)
Clin Orthop 263:135–141, 1991   2–30

Introduction.—Bursal decompression and débridement of the edges of the rotator cuff are used to treat irreparable rotator cuff tears. Superior migration of the humeral head was seen in 4 patients who had undergone decompression and débridement of the rotator cuff.

Patients.—To correct impingement and improve access for rotator cuff repair, subacromial decompression was performed in 4 patients while attempts were made to repair the rotator cuff. Healing of the repairs did not occur. In 2 patients who required humeral head replacement, the prosthesis dislocated superiorly. In 2 patients, migration of the humeral head was treated successfully by reestablishing the roof of the bursa with a bone graft. The treatment resulted in significant or complete pain relief; however, long-term follow-up was not possible. In 1 patient, 40 degrees of forward flexion and 40 degrees of abduction resulted; in the other, abduction and forward flexion were impossible.

Conclusions.—Decompression and débridement should rarely be performed in the treatment of large irreparable rotator cuff tears. Where migration of the humeral head has occurred, re-establishment of the coracoacromial arch by bone grafting, together with a capsular release, may be an effective procedure.

▶ Anterior acromioplasty is performed to prevent injury to the rotator cuff while it is healing after an operative procedure. It is also performed to prevent further damage to the rotator cuff. In these situations, pain relief is a most fortunate accompanying feature. Some have extended this concept to conclude that pain is treatable by anterior acromioplasty even in the absence of a rotator cuff. In some situations, this may prove to be true; however, in others, as is so nicely illustrated in this article, significant instability may result, causing harm to the patient.—R.H. Cofield, M.D.

ROTATOR CUFF TEARING

Repairs of the Rotator Cuff: Correlation of Functional Results With Integrity of the Cuff
Harryman DT, Mack LA, Wang KY, Jackins SE, Richardson ML, Matsen FA III (Univ of Washington, Seattle)
J Bone Joint Surg 73 A:982–989, 1991   2–31

Background.—In some cases patients with untreated rotator cuff tears have relatively good function and comfort, and function may be good even when there is a defect after operation. The functional results after operation were correlated with the integrity of the cuff using ultrasonography.

Methods.—Included were 89 patients who had undergone repair of 105 chronic tears of the rotator cuff. All operations included anteroinferior acromioplasty. Average patient age was 60 years at the time of repair. Patients were assessed by ultrasonography an average of 5 years after operation.

Results.—When tears involved the supraspinatus tendon only, 80% of cuffs were found to be intact. When other parts were also involved, more than 50% had a recurrent defect. Prevalence of recurrent defects was greater in older patients and in those who had a larger tear. Most patients, even those with sonographic signs of a recurrent defect, were satisfied with their results. Function during activities of daily living was better in shoulders with an intact cuff at follow-up than in those with a large recurrent defect. Range of active flexion was also better, 129 degrees in the intact group compared to 71 degrees in the recurrent defect group. Range of active external and internal rotation and strength of flexion, abduction, and internal rotation showed similar correlations. The degree of functional loss was related to the size of the defect when the cuff was not intact.

Conclusions.—In rotator cuff tears the integrity of the cuff at follow-up, rather than the size of the tear at operation, is the major determinant of outcome. In a patient who undergoes repair of a secondary tear the result is comparable to that of a repaired primary tear if the cuff remains intact. Age or disuse may lessen the quality of the cuff tissue, its attachment to bone, and the chance for a durable repair.

▶ Ultrasonography as a measuring method has allowed us to know that patients do better after rotator cuff surgery when the rotator cuff is repaired and remains intact. The chances of the repair remaining intact and the quality of the outcome after surgery are determined by the extent of the tearing. However, as the authors so nicely demonstrate, even quite large tears that undergo repair do well if the repair heals satisfactorily.—R.H. Cofield, M.D.

Shoulder Surgery for Rotator Cuff Tears: Ultrasonographic 3-Year Follow-Up of 97 Cases

Wülker N, Melzer C, Wirth CJ (Hannover Med School; Justus-Liebig-Univ, Giessen, Germany)
Acta Orthop Scand 62:142–147, 1991   2–32

Background.—Satisfactory clinical results are usually reported after surgical closure of rotator cuff tears, but those reports do not address the anatomical integrity of the rotator cuff. Ultrasonography was used to evaluate shoulders after surgical treatment of rotator cuff tears.

Methods.—Ninety-seven of 116 shoulders were available for clinical reexamination and ultrasonography a mean of 37 months postoperatively. All shoulders had been operated on because of persistent pain on movement accompanied by significant loss of function, usually after unsuccessful nonsurgical treatment. Surgery included the saber-incision approach, with removal of the deltoid attachments as required for exposure, and resection of the subacromial bursa. In 48 shoulders, additional anterior acromioplasties with resection of the coracoacromial ligament were performed; in other cases, resection of the coracoacromial ligament alone, resection of reattachment of the long biceps tendon, synovectomies, or mere débridements provided treatment.

Results.—Good or excellent clinical results occurred in 70% of patients, with poor results in 14%. Ultrasonography showed a normal rotator cuff in 37 shoulders; loss of thickness or hyperdensity, or both, of the rotator cuff in 31 shoulders; and complete rupture in 29 shoulders. Almost one fifth of the contralateral shoulders had clinical abnormalities, and one third had ultrasonographic abnormalities. Good clinical outcomes were associated with decreasing age and concomitant anterior acromioplasties. Ultrasonographic follow-up in general did correlate with clinical results. However, a patient with on intact tendon might have a poor result and vice versa.

Conclusions.—Because the anatomical integrity of the rotator cuff does not necessarily yield results that satisfy the patient, tears should be closed only if this can be achieved without undue tension. For large defects, the lesion should be débrided and left open. When surgery is indicated, an anterior acromioplasty with division of the coracoacromial ligament and excision of the subacromial bursa should always be performed.

▶ The details of the physical examination in these patients are not recorded in the manuscript such that readers can easily interpret the results. The authors did demonstrate that clinical scores were best in patients with normal ultrasonographic findings, were intermediate in the group with thinning or nonhomogeneous echo patterns, and were lowest in the group with recurrent defects of the rotator cuff. These differences were statistically significant. So, it would seem difficult to justify the conclusions reached by these authors—at least based on the information included in the article. The above 2 articles (Abstracts 2–31 and 2–32) do illustrate the usefulness of ultrasonographic evaluation in the postoperative patient. However, particularly as emphasized in the second article, the ultrasonographic evaluation alone will not dictate with assurance whether or not a patient has a good or poor result.—R.H. Cofield, M.D.

Discussion and Validation of Several Methods of Evaluation of the Results of Surgery for the Rotator Cuff: A Plea for Uniformity
Urvoy P, Boileau G, Berger M, Vanveicenaher J, Schmidt D, Herlant M, Mestdagh H (Centre Hospitalier de Lille, France; Centre de Rééducation fonctionelle l'Espoir, Hellemes, France)
Rev Chir Orthop 77:171–178, 1991   2–33

Introduction.—There is controversy whether conservative treatment or surgery is the optimal treatment for lesions of the rotator cuff. The resolution of this controversy requires objective evaluation of outcomes, but there is no standard method for evaluating treatment outcomes. Three different methods for evaluating the outcomes of surgical treatment for rotator cuff lesions were compared.

Methods.—Between 1986 and 1988, 21 patients were operated on for an extensive rupture of the rotator cuff. The same surgical technique was used in all patients. The functional results were evaluated and scored on the forms proposed by Patte, Kénési, and Constant. In addition, 2 other simple tests were used: the measurement of the triple point distance described by Kapandji and the carrying of a series of weights ranging from .5 kg to 11 kg for at least 5 seconds in the position known as the "barman" position.

Results.—There was good correlation between the 3 evaluation methods. Correlation between the forms of Patte and Constant was excellent. The mean triple point measurement was 26.7 cm, and the mean weight lifted was 3.65 kg. However, the measurement of the triple point and the weight lifted had only a fair correlation with the Patte form. The method proposed by Constant combined with the triple point measurement appears to be the simplest and most complete for routine use. The Patte form is more extensive and can be reserved for more detailed evaluation in scientific studies. The use of any of these forms does not eliminate the need for assessment of specific clinical signs nor for radiographic evaluation.

Conclusions.—All 3 forms are reliable for evaluating the functional postoperative results after rotator cuff repair. The modified Constant form combined with the triple point measurement is the most suitable for routine use.

▶ There are a number of things that can be evaluated to assess the result of treatment for rotator cuff disease. These authors nicely demonstrate that some complex evaluations or simple evaluations assessing motion or strength often seem to correlate quite well. One should probably not be too surprised, because the rotator cuff is intimately involved with the shoulder capsule in providing stability and is also, of course, a muscular structure that contributes significantly to both movement and strength. As the previous articles on ultrasonography have indicated, when the rotator cuff repair heals well the subjective clinical parameters also improve. Thus, measuring various parameters is a check, one against the other. Patients who feel they have done well after surgery not only will generally have good pain relief and functional capabilities but also will have better movement and greater strength.—R.H. Cofield, M.D.

Isolated Rupture of the Tendon of the Subscapularis Muscle: Clinical Features in 16 Cases
Gerber C, Krushell RJ (University of Berne, Switzerland)
J Bone Joint Surg 73-B:389–394, 1991
2–34

Background.—Few cases of isolated subscapularis tendon rupture have been reported. Sixteen patients with a characteristic clinical syndrome that had not been described previously were assessed.

Patients.—The patients were 16 men aged 25–64 years. Traumatic rupture of the tendon of the subscapularis muscle was documented as an isolated lesion in the shoulder. The injury was caused by forceful hyperextension or external rotation of the adducted arm. The men complained of anterior shoulder pain and weakness of the arm when used above and below the shoulder level. None of the men had shoulder instability. The injured shoulders displayed increased external rotation and decreased strength of internal rotation. The lift-off test, a simple clinical maneuver, reliably diagnosed or clinically excluded relevant subscapularis tendon rupture. The clinical diagnosis was best confirmed by either ultrasonography or MRI; however, arthrography and CT arthrography also were useful. In each patient, surgical exploration confirmed the diagnosis. Ruptured tendon repair was technically demanding and required good exposure to identify and protect the axillary nerve (Fig 2–8).

Conclusions.—The most important and consistent clinical findings in these 16 patients were an increased range of external rotation, loss of internal rotation strength, and an abnormal lift-off test result. All of the imaging studies also were helpful in establishing the diagnosis. A deltopectoral surgical approach should be used because the dissection is nearly impossible through the superolateral approach.

▶ This article suggests several things: first, that tearing of the tendon of the subscapularis muscle is perhaps somewhat more common than has been appreciated to date; second, that ample diagnostic means are readily available; and, third, that all patients who have this problem do not necessarily do well

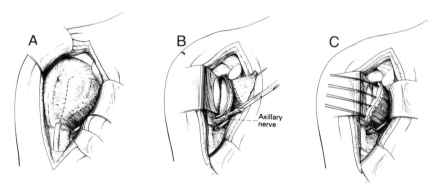

Fig 2–8.—Diagrams of a right shoulder with ruptured subscapularis tendon. **A,** the humeral head is covered with thin scar tissue that can be mistaken for intact tendon. The biceps tendon may be dislocated medially into the joint. The scar that has replaced the subscapularis tendon is incised vertically *(dotted line).* **B,** the lesser tuberosity is found to be bald. Scar tissue is excised to reveal the tendon *(dotted line),* the axillary nerve being carefully protected. **C,** the subscapularis tendon is transfixed with heavy sutures and the musculotendinous unit is mobilized and prepared for reinsertion. (Courtesy of Gerber C, Krushell RJ: *J Bone Joint Surg* 73-B:389–394, 1991.)

with nonoperative treatment. The reader is well advised to remember that this tendon tearing may be a part of the impingement process with involvement of the supraspinatus and the subscapularis. So, on approach through the deltopectoral interval, one must also consider thorough evaluation of the coracoacromial arch and assessment of the supraspinatus tendon and must strongly consider anterior-inferior acromioplasty as an adjunct to the repair.—R.H. Cofield, M.D.

The Effect of Arm Position and Capsular Release on Rotator Cuff Repair: A Biomechanical Study
Zuckerman JD, LeBlanc J-M, Choueka J, Kummer F (Hosp for Joint Diseases, New York)
J Bone Joint Surg 73-B:402–405, 1991   2–35

Background.—Clinicians need to understand the effect of arm position and capsular release on the tension in a rotator cuff repair for proper postoperative management. The goal of rotator cuff tear surgical repair is the restoration of integrity under minimal tension. Because the optimal method and position of postoperative immobilization is widely debated, a cadaver was examined to assess the effect of arm position and capsular release on rotator cuff repair.

Methods.—Artificial defects in the rotator cuff were created to include the supraspinatus only or both the supraspinatus and the infraspinatus. The defects were then repaired in a standard fashion, with shoulders abducted 30 degrees at the glenohumeral joint. Strain gauges were placed on the lateral cortex of the greater tuberosity, and measurements were obtained in 36 combinations of abduction, flexion/extension, and medial/lateral rotation both before and after capsular release.

Results.—With small tears, tension in the repair increased significantly with movement from 30 degrees to 15 degrees of abduction. However, it was minimally affected by flexion or rotation changes. Capsular release significantly decreased the force at 0 abduction and 15 degrees of abduction. For large tears, abduction of at least 30 degrees with lateral rotation and extension consistently produced the lowest values. Thirty percent less force at 0 abduction resulted from capsular release.

Conclusions.—These findings provide some relevant information about postoperative positioning after rotator cuff repair. Repair should be done at or near the abduction position to be held after surgery. The position of abduction has a much more important effect on repair tension than either rotation or flexion/extension. Capsular attachment release at the glenoid rim significantly decreases the tension on the supraspinatus repair, particularly for large defects. When clinicians test the security of a repair intraoperatively, they should examine the anterior part of the supraspinatus carefully because this is the most common site of failure.

▶ This laboratory study reinforces the importance of the position of the arm at the time of rotator cuff repair and informs us in a scientific fashion that release of the shoulder capsule is a useful adjunct to eliminating tension at the repair site. The position of abduction is the most important position to determine when performing the rotator cuff repair. As demonstrated by these authors, flexion and extension or rotational positioning is not nearly so important for tears involving the supraspinatus or the supraspinatus and infraspinatus tendons.—R.H. Cofield, M.D.

Arthroplasty and Arthrodesis

SHOULDER

Shoulder Arthroplasty in Complex Acute and Chronic Proximal Humeral Fractures

Frich LH, Søjbjerg JO, Sneppen O (Orthopaedic Hospital, Aarhus, Denmark)
Orthopedics 14:949–954, 1991   2–36

Background.—There is disagreement as to the treatment of comminuted or displaced fractures of the proximal humerus. The results of shoulder arthroplasty were in examined patients with complex acute and chronic fractures of the humeral head.

Patients.—During a 6 year period, 42 patients underwent prosthetic replacement. Fifteen patients had acute fractures, all of them 4-part. Median postfracture delay in this acute group was 13 days. A second group of 27 patients had chronic fractures; 11 of these were 4-part, 9 were 3-part, and 7 were 2-part. Median postfracture delay in this chronic group was 14 months. For all patients follow-up was approximately 2 years.

Results.—The acute group had satisfactory pain relief, but pain relief was unpredictable in the chronic group. There were no significant differences between the 2 groups in active elevation, external rotation, and function score. Active elevation and function score were correlated, but pain decreased the final result in the chronic group. In the acute group results were excellent in 20% of patients and good in 40%; in the chronic group only 22% had a good result. A poor result occurred in only 13% of the acute group and in 40% of the chronic group. No differences were noted in the chronic group among patients with 2-, 3-, and 4-part fractures. Five patients who were previously treated with osteosynthesis had persistent instability, and 2 of them had an infection.

Conclusions.—Prosthetic replacement offers good results in patients with acute proximal humeral fractures. The possibility of a good result with revision arthroplasty is reduced by failed primary treatment.

▶ This paper again demonstrates that these fractures can be very difficult to treat effectively, and some patients seem to obtain a less than satisfactory result in spite of excellent care. It again demonstrates that the likelihood of treatment success is better if definitive care is given in the acute setting. It also again reiterates to us that the results of revision surgery are less satisfactory than a primary procedure.—R.H. Cofield, M.D.

Total Shoulder Arthroplasty Versus Hemiarthroplasty: Indications for Glenoid Resurfacing
Boyd AD Jr, Thomas WH, Scott RD, Sledge CB, Thornhill TS (Brigham and Women's Hosp, Boston)
J Arthroplasty 5:329–336, 1990   2–37

Background.—Shoulder hemiarthroplasty (HEMI) and total shoulder arthroplasty (TSA) have both had good results in 80% to 94% of patients. The decision to resurface the glenoid is usually based on radiographic evidence of joint destruction, but previous reports have demonstrated a need to define the indications for this procedure more clearly. Records of 134 patients were reviewed to compare the results of HEMI and TSA.

Patients.—Criteria for inclusion were met by 64 HEMI procedures in 59 patients and 146 TSA procedures in 134 patients. The primary indication for surgery in these patients was pain unresponsive to conservative management; loss of function was a secondary consideration. Average follow-up was 43 months for the HEMI group and 45 months for the TSA group. The average age for the HEMI group (58 years) was similar to that of the TSA group (60 years). Rheumatoid arthritis accounted for 71% of the diagnoses in the TSA group and 46% in the HEMI group.

Results.—Complete pain relief was achieved in 55% of shoulders in the TSA group and 47% in the HEMI group. In most of the remaining shoulders, only slight or moderate pain was reported with activity. Thus, good results were obtained in 93% of shoulders treated with TSA and 92% of shoulders treated with HEMI. Patients with rheumatoid arthritis had a higher rate of complete pain relief with TSA (49%) than with HEMI (29%).

Conclusions.—Based on these findings, TSA is recommended for patients with inflammatory arthropathies and HEMI for patients with osteoarthritis, avascular necrosis, and 4-part fractures with preservation of glenoid congruity and absent synovitis. Although progressive glenoid loosening was noted in 12% of TSAs, this finding did not correlate with pain relief or range of motion.

▶ These authors' results are certainly clear and well accepted for the diagnoses of osteonecrosis and 4-part fractures. In their patients with rheumatoid arthritis, the results were better with TSA. In the article, osteoarthritis and osteonecrosis are evaluated as a single group, so it is difficult to know exactly the outcome in osteoarthritis relative to the use of HEMI or TSA. The authors recommend HEMI for patients with osteoarthritis, avascular necrosis, and 4-part fractures with preservation of glenoid congruity and in the absence of synovitis. However, it is difficult to have a great deal of certainty about thisfinal conclusion because of the way the data have been grouped for presentation.—R.H. Cofield, M.D.

Rigid Internal Fixation for Shoulder Arthrodesis

Stark DM, Bennett JB, Tullos HS (Baylor College of Medicine, Houston)
Orthopedics 14:849–855, 1991   2–38

Background.—There are several indications for shoulder arthrodesis. The rate of successful shoulder arthrodesis was assessed using dynamic compression plates for internal fixation with limited postoperative immobilization.

Patients.—Fifteen of 16 patients treated in 1984–1985 were available for chart and radiographic review. At the time of surgery, the patients' age ranged from 7 to 77 years; follow-up ranged from 3 to 32 months. In each patient, the position of the extremity relative to the scapula and trunk was noted just after surgery, at regular intervals until fusion, and at follow-up examinations.

Results.—In 13 shoulders, fusion occurred without change of intraoperative position after a mean of 4 months. The shoulder position was lost in 1 patient just after surgery because of inadequate fixation; subsequently, this shoulder fused. A bone graft was performed in another patient who had persistent nonunion for 2½ years. Of 4 patients who complained of residual symptomatic hardware, 2 required surgical removal of the plate and screws. Only 1 patient was dissatisfied with the clinical result at follow-up. Two patients were within 5 degrees of the preoperatively determined position of 30 degrees abduction, 30 degrees forward flexion, and 30 degrees internal rotation. Almost all patients could function satisfactorily (Fig 2–9).

Conclusions.—Shoulder arthrodesis using rigid internal fixation without postoperative cast or brace immobilization maximizes patient comfort without compromising arthrodesis success. However, arm position control remains inexact. Additional modifications are needed to assure fusion position and minimize disability.

▶ Internal fixation for shoulder arthrodesis has improved dramatically during the past decade. Fusion rates are indeed quite high using contemporary techniques.—R.H. Cofield, M.D.

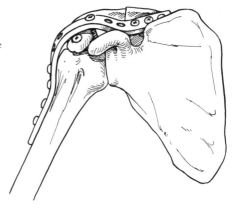

Fig 2–9.—Shoulder arthrodesis technique emphasizing plate and screw position. (Courtesy of Stark DM, Bennett JB, Tullos HS: *Orthopedics* 14:849–855, 1991.)

ELBOW

Total Replacement for Post-Traumatic Arthritis of the Elbow
Morrey BF, Adams RA, Bryan RS (Mayo Clinic and Found, Rochester, Minn)
J Bone Joint Surg [Br] 73-B:607–612, 1991   2–39

Background.—There have been no reports exclusively on the treatment of posttraumatic arthritis.

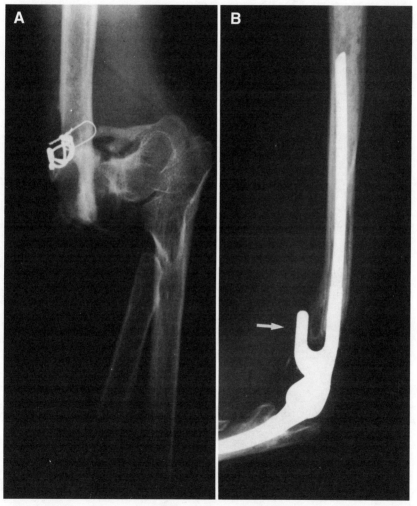

Fig 2–10.—**A,** an ununited supracondylar fracture in a 67-year-old woman. **B,** there is an intact bone-cement interface and incorporation of the bone graft behind the flange *(arrow)* 5 years after arthroplasty with a type III implant. (Courtesy of Morrey BF, Adams RA, Bryan RS: *J Bone Joint Surg* 73-B:607–612, 1991.)

Methods.—Data on 55 surgical procedures using the original Coonrad implant or 1 of its 2 modifications performed on 54 patients in 1973–1985 were reviewed. The 53 elbow replacements were followed-up for at least 2 years (mean, 6.3 years). The treatment of these patients was difficult because the patients had an average of 2 previous operations per joint. There had been previous complications in 22 joints; 18 had less than 50 degrees of flexion, and 6 were flail.

Results.—During follow-up 10 patients needed 14 revision procedures for aseptic loosening. At last follow-up 38 elbows were without progressive radiolucent lines. In 2 patients, the elbow had to be resected, 1 for deep infection and 1 for bone resorption after a foreign-body reaction to titanium (Fig 2–10).

Conclusions.—The Coonrad prosthesis offers a reliable option for the treatment of patients with posttraumatic arthritis. However, prosthetic replacement for posttraumatic arthritis should not be performed in persons younger than 60 years of age. Careful selection of patients older than 60 years of age is necessary.

Capitellocondylar Total Elbow Replacement for Rheumatoid Arthritis
Hodgson SP, Parkinson RW, Noble J (Univ of Manchester, Salford, England)
J R Coll Surg Edinb 36:133–135, 1991   2–40

Background.—The capitellocondylar elbow, first used in 1974, has yielded encouraging results. However, problems of postoperative dislocation and ulnar nerve palsy have not been eliminated completely, despite changes in prosthesis design and the use of a lateral approach. Results of a series of capitellocondylar total elbow replacements were reported.

Patients.—Twenty-three replacements were done in 18 patients with rheumatoid arthritis. The patients were 16 women and 2 men aged 54–77 years at the time of operation. Follow-up ranged from 1.5 years to 5 years (mean, 3 years).

Results.—All patients had relief of pain after surgery. Postoperative range of movement was improved in all directions. There was no evidence of radiologic loosening. Complications included transient ulnar nerve palsy in 15 elbows (65%) and a permanent ulnar nerve palsy in 1 elbow (4%). Wound healing was delayed in 2 elbows.

Conclusions.—Capitellocondylar total elbow replacement for rheumatoid arthritis is rewarding in the short term. The ulnar nerve problem is usually transient. Although this complication is common, this prosthesis has greatly improved the outcome of elbow replacement.

▶ The patients and the results presented in the preceding 2 articles (Abstracts 2–39 and 2–40) suggest that total elbow replacement is indeed becoming much more reliable as an operation. However, patient selection and surgical technique continue to be critical, suggesting that this operation is indeed somewhat more marginal than many of those done in orthopedic surgery.—R.H. Cofield, M.D.

Results of Elbow Synovectomy in Rheumatoid Arthritis

Vahvanen V, Eskola A, Peltonen J (Orthopaedic Hosp of the Invalid Found, Helsinki, Finland)
Arch Orthop Trauma Surg 110:151–154, 1991   2–41

Background.—The benefit of elbow synovectomy in rheumatoid arthritis is debated. The long-term effects of elbow synovectomy, as assessed by clinical criteria and radiographic findings, were investigated.

Patients.—Between 1966 and 1986, 46 women and 8 men had synovectomies on 70 elbows. In all patients, the indication for surgery was rheumatoid arthritis. Mean follow-up was 7.5 years (range, 1.5–22 years).

Outcomes.—Clinical assessment revealed marked pain relief in 28 elbows, (40%). In 38.5% the pain was moderate but still better than it had been before surgery. Pain was severe in 21.5%. Mean flexion arc was 114.5 degrees, and mean rotation arc was 134.5 degrees. Latitudinal instability of as much as 5 degrees was noted in 47% of elbows, of as much as 10 degrees in 28.5%, of as much as 15 degrees in 8.5%, and of more than 15 degrees in 16%. The mean carrying angle in valgus was 10 degrees. Measures of strength in flexion and extension in these patients showed a reduction of approximately 50% those of age-matched, healthy controls. Reoperation was needed in 10 elbows (14%). The period between the primary synovectomy and second operation in these patients averaged 8 years.

Conclusion.—Although the results of elbow synovectomy deteriorate in the long term, it is still suggested that this operation can be done successfully, even in grade 3 elbows (as defined by Larsen).

Varied Topics

One Hundred Percent Incidence of Hemidiaphragmatic Paresis Associated With Interscalene Brachial Plexus Anesthesia as Diagnosed by Ultrasonography

Urmey WF, Talts KH, Sharrock NE (Cornell Univ)
Anesth Analg 72:498–503, 1991   2–42

Background.—Sensory anesthesia of the fourth and fifth cervical nerves is a routine part of interscalene brachial plexus anesthesia for shoulder surgery. Interscalene blocks that produce surgical C3-C5 sensory anesthesia should cause some degree of diaphragmatic paralysis. The incidence of ipsilateral hemidiaphragmatic paresis during routine interscalene block was assessed by ultrasonography.

Methods.—Thirteen healthy patients who were scheduled for elective upper extremity surgery with interscalene blocks were evaluated. Brachial plexus block was achieved with an injection of 34–52 mL of 1.5% mepivacaine with 5 μg/mL of epinephrine and .05 mEq/mL of sodium bicarbonate. All of the patients had cervical sensory anesthesia. Ultrasonography measurements were made 2, 5, and 10 minutes after injection and hourly after surgery in 11 patients.

Results.—Within 5 minutes all of the patients showed a change from normal to paradoxical motion of the ipsilateral hemidiaphragm during sniff and Mueller maneuvers. Eleven of the patients showed this change at 2 minutes. Between 3 and 4 hours after injection, 10 of the 11 patients returned to normal diaphragmatic motion; in the remaining patient, the return to normal took place by the fifth hour after injection. Despite the fact that all of the patients were unsedated, only 5 of 13 noticed any change in breathing.

Conclusions.—Interscalene brachial plexus block anesthesia for shoulder surgery appears to result inevitably in diaphragmatic paresis. Although this may occur without symptoms, more marked changes in ventilation may occur in patients with preexisting respiratory system pathology.

▶ It seems apparent from this article that ipsilateral diaphragmatic paralysis is an expected part of interscalene brachial plexus anesthesia. It should not be considered a complication. It is interesting how short-lived the paralysis was, as the sensory blockade may extend much longer than a 4–5-hour time period.—R.H. Cofield, M.D.

The Shoulder in Multiple Epiphyseal Dysplasia
Ingram RR (Royal Infirmary, Glasgow)
J Bone Joint Surg 73-B:277–279, 1991   2–43

Background.—Multiple epiphyseal dysplasia results in abnormal limb epiphyses. At approximately age 7 years, short-limbed dwarfism and painful joints may develop in individuals with this autosomal dominant disorder.

Methods.—To define the frequency with which this condition affects the shoulder joint and to outline its radiologic characteristics, 23 females and 27 males, aged 4–67 years, (mean age, 30 years) were examined. Only those shoulders that exhibited symptoms underwent consistent radiographic examinations to avoid overexposure in the patients.

Results.—Of the 100 shoulders evaluated, 16 patients had 31 symptomatic joints. All patients with symptomatic shoulders were classified as having severe multiple epiphyseal dysplasia accompanied by stubby digits, serious lower limb joint abnormalities, and short-limbed dwarfism. Radiographic examinations were performed on 32 symptomatic and 22 asymptomatic shoulders. The 8 patients with restricted joint movement tended to be younger (mean age, 26.5 years) than the overall population. Patients classified as osteoarthritic were usually older, and all had symptoms. In 20 shoulders, there was a hatchet head formation on the radiographs; all these patients had symptoms of the condition. In each of these patients, the glenoid fossa was poorly formed, and its inferior portion merged into the lateral border of the blade of the scapula. The individuals with hatchet head shoulders experienced pain, usually in the fifth and sixth decades of life. One third of the patients had bilateral symptoms.

Conclusions.—Although knee and hip complications predominate in patients with multiple epiphyseal dysplasia, many patients have shoulder abnormalities as well. There are 2 distinct radiologic groups: the hatchet-head group, which lacks significant glenohumeral movement early, and the minor epiphyseal abnormality group.

▶ This study nicely defines changes in the shoulder in multiple epiphyseal dysplasia. The condition is rather rare; therefore, little is known about the effectiveness of surgical treatment for this problem.—R.H. Cofield, M.D.

Pustular Osteoarthropathy and Its Differential Diagnosis
Wetzel R, Gondolph-Zink B, Puhl W (Universität Ulm, Germany)
Int Orthop 15:101–104, 1991   2–44

Introduction.—Pustular osteoarthropathy consists of a combination of costosternoclavicular hyperostosis and palmoplantar pustulosis, some times with hyperostotic spondylosis and spondylarthritis. Only 40 patients with this disease have been reported in the Western hemisphere; the condition is more common in the Far East. Data on 4 women and 1 man with pustular osteoarthropathy were reviewed.

Patients.—All of the patients had pustolosis, hyperostosis, and sternoclavicular arthritis. There was spondylosis in 2 patients. All 11 patients were negative for HLA-Bw27. In the 2 patients, anti-inflammatory drugs and tetracycline reduced pain and swelling; in 1 patient, the symptoms recurred when the anti-inflammatory medication was discontinued.

Conclusion.—The diagnosis of pustular osteoarthropathy is difficult, because the skin lesions can develop before the costosternoclavicular hyperostoses. Radiographically, pustular osteoarthropathy is characterized by hyperostosis, sclerosis, and erosions of the clavicle and adjacent parts of the manubrium. It appears to be an enthesopathy, and the paloplantar pustulosis is interpreted as a form of psoriasis.

▶ If this syndrome is recognized, unnecessary surgical biopsy or other forms of interventional treatment may be avoided.—R.H. Cofield, M.D.

3 General Adult Reconstruction

Introduction

It has been said that there are no new conditions in orthopedic surgery, most having been described by Hippocrates, yet we know the natural history of very few of these conditions. Although there is some truth to that statement, several papers this year have studied the natural history of some of the conditions with which we deal: osteochondritis dissecans is one example. The paper by Twyman, Desai, and Aichroth points out that lesions in the lateral condyle have a poorer prognosis than do similar lesions located on the medial femoral condyle. Another paper suggests that the treatment of osteonecrosis of the knee in elderly patients has been variable because of the lack of information regarding the natural history of this process. The recent availability of MRI as well as radioisotope scintigraphy has led to a greater understanding of the natural history of the condition and an appreciation of the appropriate application of treatment modalities such as tibial osteotomy. Studies of the natural history of conditions diagnosed by MRI raise the issue of diagnostic specificity; does everything presenting as a signal abnormality on MRI really relate to an anatomical lesion of bone? There is at least the possibility that MRI overreads lesions of the marrow that would heal spontaneously without treatment. The same question is raised by another paper, which examines the natural history of "lesions" seen as signal changes within the body of the meniscus. Similarly, we know that some signal abnormalities seen in the contralateral hip of patients with clinically unilateral osteonecrosis never develop into a clinically recognizable condition. What do those changes represent—"bone bruises," abnormalities of marrow metabolism, or the subchondral response to changes in the overlying cartilage? Only careful documentation of these conditions and long-term follow-up studies will help decide which lesions need treatment and which are transient signal changes that do not progress to lesions of consequence.

Another paper in this section traces the natural history of medial arthritis of the knee. The study demonstrates quite conclusively that medial compartment osteoarthritis is slowly but uniformly progressive and that the vast majority of the patients will eventually require surgical treatment. Another important and related paper demonstrates that acetaminophen may be as effective as nonsteroidal and inflammatory agents in the management of osteoarthritis of the knee, with obvious implications in cost-effectiveness and frequency of side effects. Arthroscopic débridement for osteoarthritis of the knee, especially that localized to the medial compartment, is a frequently performed procedure. A careful study by

McLaren, et al. demonstrates the transient nature of relief after such débridement.

There are a number of important papers on the technique of total knee arthroplasty (TKA) included in the section this year. The subvastus approach is suggested as a useful routine incision for arthroplasty of the knee. In my experience, however, this approach is most useful for certain revision situations rather than as a routine. Other papers address the importance of coronal alignment in TKA, methods to augment deficient bone stock, the importance of joint-line position and its relation to function after arthroplasty, studies of the time and quantity of blood loss after TKA, and the usefulness of reinfusion of the blood collected from suction drains.

A number of papers address the usefulness of unicompartmental arthroplasty of the knee and arrive at the conclusion that this procedure is extremely useful in a small subset of patients who have something important to gain from the increased motion and proprioception usually seen in patients who have unicompartmental replacement as compared to those who have tricompartmental replacement. The 10-year survivorship of tricompartmental replacements is so good, however, that most patients are probably better off having tricompartmental replacement rather than unicompartmental replacement, with its greater annual failure rate. An elderly patient with multiple joint restrictions in whom the achievement of nearly normal postoperative knee motion would be functionally important and whose disease is located exclusively in the medial or lateral compartment might be a suitable candidate for unicompartmental replacement.

There are also a number of papers on the results of TKA, including papers that demonstrate the predictable high success rate at 10 years after TKA using current design concepts and techniques. These papers provide strong evidence to support the contention that knee arthroplasty today is as predictably successful as is total hip arthroplasty. Whether polyethylene wear in the second decade after the arthroplasty will increase failure rates to levels higher than are seen after hip arthroplasty remains to be seen. It is becoming evident, however, that polyethylene wear is the limiting factor in both hip and knee arthroplasty, and better methods to address this problem will have to be discovered if the longevity of arthroplasties is to be increased. It appears to me, at least, that fixation of implant devices into the skeleton has largely been solved, as have the design features necessary to produce nearly normal function. If those statements are true, wear of the articulating surface will be the predominant mode of late failure. The next few years should see an enormous increase in our efforts to improve the wear characteristics of polyethylene, to improve the composition of polyethylene, or to find substitute materials, including the possibility of metal-on-metal articulations.

Clement B. Sledge, M.D.

Diagnosis and Management of Knee Injuries

Clinical Course and Roentgenographic Changes of Osteonecrosis in the Femoral Condyle Under Conservative Treatment
Motohashi M, Morii T, Koshino T (Yokohama City Univ, Japan)
Clin Orthop 266:156–161, 1991   3–1

Background.—Spontaneous osteonecrosis of the femoral condyle may be 1 of the few clinical conditions characteristic of old age. Its natural history has not been examined. The clinical course and radiographic changes of 14 patients with osteonecrosis of the femoral condyle undergoing conservative treatment were examined.

Methods.—Fifteen knees in 9 women and 5 men (average age, 62.8 years) were examined. Follow-up averaged 4.9 years. The condition was spontaneous in 12 knees in 11 patients and was steroid-induced in 3 patients; the medial femoral condyle was affected in 13 knees. Conservative treatment consisted of quadriceps exercise, analgesics, crutches or braces, and weight control. Each patient underwent measurement of the maximum width of the lesion on anteroposterior radiographs; lesions of less than 10 mm were considered small.

Results.—At follow-up 5 patients could walk 1 km with no pain, 4 patients had occasional pain, and 1 had mild pain while walking. Full range of motion was preserved in 12 knees. At the first visit average lesion size was 2.1 cm^2, with 5 lesions measuring less than 1.5 cm^2, and 3 measuring more than 3.5 cm^2. At follow-up average size was 3 cm^2, with size increasing by more than 18% in 8 knees. Five lesions were considered small at the first visit, and 10 were considered large; at follow-up only 2 lesions were still small. No changes in staging or limb alignment were seen in knees with small lesions. The steroid-induced lesions were significantly larger than the spontaneous lesions.

Conclusions.—The natural history of osteonecrosis of the femoral condyle is examined. Lesions increase in size gradually, especially in the early stages. Operation may be indicated even for knees with small lesions; conservative treatment should be reserved for patients with only mild pain and no malalignment of the limb.

▶ Spontaneous osteonecrosis of the elderly knee is usually readily diagnosed but difficult to manage because of the age of the involved patients and uncertainty regarding the natural history. In this study, radiographic progression is well documented in the 15 lesions followed for an average of nearly 5 years. Most lesions increased in size, especially those related to steroid use. The lesion did not disappear in any of the 15 knees, although pain diminished in 11. The authors recommend tibial osteotomy for patients with knee pain and malalignment. It would appear that patients can be followed safely until their symptoms are sufficient to justify surgery. Early intervention, except for the small lesions in young patients in whom tibial osteotomy would be appropriate, does not seem justified.—C.B. Sledge, M.D.

Osteonecrosis of the Knee Detected Only by Magnetic Resonance Imaging

Healy WL (Lahey Clinic Med Ctr, Burlington, Mass)
Orthopedics 14:703–704, 1991   3–2

Introduction.—Biopsy-proved osteonecrosis was diagnosed by MRI only in a patient who was seen with chronic, disabling knee pain.

Case Report.—Man, 39, had pain in both knees and legs for 3 years after brief, high-dose steroid treatment for asthma. The patient described a constant ache that began in the distal thigh but did not extend below the ankle. The ache increased on weight-bearing. The knees were stable and had a full range of motion. Both conventional radiography and bone scanning were negative; however, MRI showed osteonecrosis of both femoral heads, the distal segments of both femurs, and the proximal segments of both tibias. Core decompression was performed, and biopsy specimens confirmed osteonecrosis.

Discussion.—Plain roentgenograms failed to demonstrate a loss of structural integrity in the patient's knee. Although a normal bone scan seemed to rule out avascular necrosis, an MRI study showed widespread osteonecrosis.

▶ The usefulness of MRI in the diagnosis of osteonecrosis in several sites is becoming evident. This case report demonstrates that MRI can show distinctive abnormality, even though the bone scan is normal. However, until large numbers of patients are followed for several years to reveal the natural history of lesions demonstrated by MRI only, it is possible that the sensitivity of the study is such that it will detect lesions that may not be progressive.—C.B. Sledge, M.D.

Fresh Osteochondral Allografting of the Femoral Condyle

Convery FR, Meyers MH, Akeson WH (Univ of California, San Diego)
Clin Orthop 273:139–145, 1991   3–3

Introduction.—Fresh osteochondral shell autografting of the femoral condyle is an alternative to hemiarthroplasty or total arthroplasty in young patients with localized osteochondral defects. The results were reviewed in 36 patients who underwent 37 such operations. The indication was traumatic osteochondral defect in 23 patients, osteochondritis dissecans in 8, and steroid-related avascular necrosis of the femoral condyle in 6.

Management.—A total of 25 patients had allografting of the femoral condyle only. Eleven patients had additional sites in the same knee allografted. The allografts ranged from 1 × 1 to 2 × 6 cm in size. The thickness of the subchondral bone was kept to within 5 mm. Before June 1989, the allografts were press-fitted into the surgically prepared site, and they were sometimes supplemented with screws. More recently they have been press-fitted and further secured with orthosorb biodegradable polydioxanon pins.

Results.—Of the 9 evaluable knees operated on more than 5 years ago, 8 were rated good or excellent. The 1 poor result appeared to reflect a technical deficiency. Three procedures subsequently failed in young females with traumatic osteochondral defects who lacked an anterior cruciate ligament. Five of the 8 knees operated on 2–5 years ago had a good or excellent outcome. Of the 17 knees treated in the past 2 years, 5 had problems. No wound infections occurred, and no patient had evidence of an immune response. All of the failures appeared to be mechanical in origin.

Conclusions.—Technical proficiency is especially important when performing fresh osteochondral shell allograft surgery. A perfect press fit is critical. Any ligamentous deficiency should be corrected before or at the time of allografting.

▶ The authors report on their extensive experience with the use of fresh osteochondral shell allografts in a variety of cartilage defects involving the femoral condyle. The report suggests that most, if not all, of the failures were related to technical problems. They leave us with the optimistic impression that if ligament injuries are corrected to restore normal knee kinematics and if technical problems of fixing the grafts securely are overcome this technique should offer promise for patients with localized defects in the articular cartilage of the knee.—C.B. Sledge, M.D.

Stability of Osteochondral Fragments of the Femoral Condyle: Magnetic Resonance Imaging With Histopathologic Correlation in an Animal Model
Adam G, Bühne M, Prescher A, Nolte-Ernsting C, Bohndorf K, Günther RW (Univ of Technology, Aachen, Germany)
Skeletal Radiol 20:601–606, 1991

3–4

Background.—Magnetic resonance imaging might be useful in assessing the stability of osteochondral fragments in osteochondritis dissecans or after osteochondral transplantation. However, reports correlating MRI scans with histologic findings have been lacking.

Methods.—Osteochondral fragments of the femoral condyle were created in 7 adult dogs. Fragment stability was assessed every 1–4 weeks using T1- and T2-weighted spin echo sequences and contrast-enhanced T1-weighted spin-echo sequences. The dogs were killed between the 34th and 196th days postoperatively, and the MRI and histopathologic findings were compared.

Results.—Contrast-enhanced MRI studies revealed 2 loose and 5 stable fragments, with the loose fragments having a well-defined high-signal intensity line between the fragment and the epiphysis (Fig 3–1). Histologically, this interface showed vascularized granulation tissue. A similar line was seen on plain sequences, but it was irregularly defined and not enhanced on contrast studies. No granulation tissue was seen at the inter-

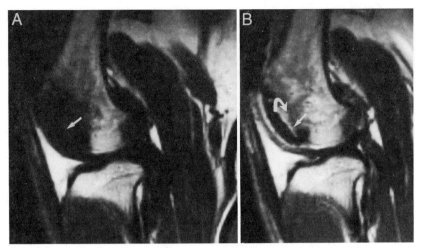

Fig 3–1.—Dog 64 days after surgery, loose fragment. **A,** T1-weighted (SE 500)/15); **B,** T1-weighted after gadopentetate dimeglumine. (Courtesy of Adam G, Bühne M, Prescher A, et al: *Skeletal Radiol* 20:601–606, 1991.)

face in those fragments, but the fracture was repaired completely with intact bone trabeculae. On the articular cartilage surface, areas of fibrocartilaginous repair also were enhanced.

Conclusions.—In experiments in dogs, contrast-enhanced MRI precisely delineates a line separating unstable osteochondral fragments that can be differentiated from a similar line in stable fragments. In stable fragments, the histologic basis of this line is unexplained; it may reflect differences in binding or proton distribution in healing fragments.

▶ A major component of the decision to operate on a patient with osteochondral fragment of the femoral condyle is whether or not the fragment is "stable" or "loose." The rationale is that stable fragments will heal if protected, whereas loose fragments are likely to drop out of their beds, become loose bodies, and leave behind a large defect that will heal only with inadequate fibrocartilage. The authors of this paper, therefore, undertook a study of the usefulness of MRI in assessing the stability of osteochondral fragments in experimental animals. With Gd enhancement, they were able to demonstrate clear differences between fixed and loose fragments. If confirmed in a human clinical series, this imaging technique will provide useful guidance in the management of patients with osteochondritis dissecans.— C.B. Sledge, M.D.

MR of the Knee: The Significance of High Signal in the Meniscus That Does Not Clearly Extend to the Surface
Kaplan PA, Nelson NL, Garvin KL, Brown DE (Univ of Nebraska, Omaha)
AJR 156:333–336, 1991   3–5

Background.—A meniscal tear is characterized by increased signal intensity within the structure on MRI; however, it is not always possible to know whether a focus of high signal is confined to the substance of the meniscus or whether it extends to the surface.

Methods.—Magnetic resonance studies of the knee in 142 consecutive patients were examined prospectively by 2 experienced radiologists. All patients were referred with suspected internal derangements of the knee. Arthroscopic findings were available for 92 of the patients.

Observations.—Evidence of a meniscal tear was equivocal in 20 knees (14% of those examined). The signal was horizontal in the midportion of the meniscus, and it extended almost to the inferior meniscal surface. The posterior horn of the lateral meniscus was the site of involvement in 17 of the 20 knees. None of the tears found at arthroscopy were considered equivocal on MRI. Examination of 1 meniscus that was removed showed degenerative changes but no tear. The equivocal tears were best seen on sagittal views, and they were detected on T1-weighted, proton-density, and gradient-echo sequences, but not on T2-weighted images.

Conclusion.—A meniscal tear is unlikely to be present when MR scans show a high-signal focus that does not unequivocally extend to involve the meniscal surface.

▶ Magnetic resonance imaging is now well established in the diagnosis of meniscal pathology, but there remains a group of patients with ambiguous MRI findings, especially those with increased signal intensity within the structure of the meniscus though without extension to the periphery. The authors conclude that such findings do not predict a meniscal tear.—C.B. Sledge, M.D.

Analgesic Effect of Intraarticular Morphine After Arthroscopic Knee Surgery

Stein C, Comisel K, Haimer E, Yassouridis A, Lehrberger K, Herz A, Peter K (Ludwig-Maximilians-Universität München, Germany)
N Engl J Med 325:1123–1126, 1991   3–6

Background.—Recent animal studies have demonstrated that both exogenous and endogenous opioid agonists have peripheral antinociceptive effects in inflamed tissue. The analgesic effect on postoperative pain of low doses of morphine administered intra-articularly in patients undergoing arthroscopic knee procedures was evaluated.

Methods.—At the end of the operation and before the arthroscope was removed, a total of 52 patients received simultaneous injections: 18 patients (group 1) received 1 mg of morphine hydrochloride in 40 mL of normal saline intra-articularly and 1 mL of normal saline intravenously; 15 controls (group 2) received 40 mL of saline intra-articularly and 1 mg of morphine intravenously; 10 (group 3) received .5 mg of morphine in 40 mL of saline intra-articularly and 1 mL of saline intravenously; and 9 (group 4) received 1 mL of morphine plus .1 mg of naloxone in 40 mL of saline intra-articularly and 1 mL of saline intravenously. These solutions were prepared in coded syringes to blind their administration. Postoperative pain assessment used the 100-mm visual analog scale, a numerical rating scale, and a German adaptation of the McGill pain questionnaire.

Results.—The patient characteristics did not differ significantly among the 4 groups. All pain scores were lower in patients in group 1 than in patients in group 2 with significant differences occurring in 3, 4, and 6 hours after drug injection. Patients in group 1 required additional analgesics significantly less often than those in group 2. Group 3 had comparable visual analog scale scores and similar analgesic requirements to group 1. The reduction in pain scores after intra-articularly administered morphine was reversed by naloxone.

Conclusions.—These findings suggest that low-dose morphine given intra-articularly significantly lowers postoperative pain in patients undergoing arthroscopic knee surgery. This effect occurs at the opioid receptors and causes no adverse patient reactions.

▶ In recent years it has become evident that morphine has both a central and a peripheral action, and it is being used widely as a local analgesic, especially in epidural applications. The authors of this study demonstrate that low-dose, intra-articularly administered morphine could be a very useful tool in the management of postoperative pain after arthroscopic knee procedures.—C.B. Sledge, M.D.

Ultrasound, Computed Tomography and Magnetic Resonance Imaging in Patellar Tendinitis
Davies SG, Baudouin CJ, King JB, Perry JD (London Hosp; Hammersmith Hosp, London)
Clin Radiol 43:52–56, 1991   3–7

Background.—High resolution ultrasound can confirm the diagnosis of patellar tendinitis, but there have been few reports of the usefulness of CT and MRI in assessing this condition. All 3 methods were evaluated prospectively in a series of patients with patellar tendinitis.

Methods.—A group of 16 patients (mean age, 29.8 years) referred for imaging of patellar tendinitis were examined. The average duration of symptoms was 1.9 years. All patients underwent sagittal ultrasound, contiguous 4.5-mm CT sections from the apex of the patella to the tibial tuberosity, and 8-mm sagittal MRI scans using 4 sequences. The same MRI sequences were used to study 3 controls with no history of knee disorder.

Results.—Tendon enlargement, usually at the upper insertion, and reduced echogenicity were noted on ultrasound in all 16 patients. Computed tomography typically showed a central tendinous expansion progressing from the insertion for a variable length down the tendon and reduced attenuation of the central portion. Focal tendon enlargement was shown by MRI in all patients, with high signal lesions in 88% of patients. In some cases, focal signal change was noted only on short T1 inversion recovery and partial saturation images. Imaging studies correlated well with surgical findings.

Conclusions.—Ultrasound, CT, and MRI can all demonstrate patellar tendinitis; however, ultrasound should be the initial investigation because the method is quick and easy. Computed tomography and MRI may be used subsequently if necessary to confirm the diagnosis.

▶ Patellar tendinitis, or "jumper's knee," is a very common clinical diagnosis that has been difficult to confirm by objective means. This paper demonstrates that ultrasound can be a very useful diagnostic technique and could obviate the need for much more expensive MRI studies.—C.B. Sledge, M.D.

Dislocation of the Knee
Frassica FJ, Sim FH, Staehell JW, Pairolero PC (Mayo Clinic and Found; Mayo Med School, Rochester, Minn)
Clin Orthop 263:200–205, 1991   3–8

Background.—Knee dislocation is an uncommon but serious injury that can produce disruption of the popliteal vessels as well as the collateral and cruciate ligaments and the posterior joint capsule. Traction injury of the common peroneal nerve also is a possibility. The vascular status of the limb is of prime importance at the time of injury.

Patients.—Twenty patients in an 8-year period had complete knee dislocations, 8 of whom had a total of 23 associated injuries. Three of the 20 were referred with distal limb ischemia after popliteal reconstruction had been done at other centers. Injuries occurred during athletic activity and motor vehicle accidents as well as during farm work. Mean age was 33 years.

Findings.—Of the 17 patients seen initially, 10 had vascular injuries and 9 required surgical repair of the popliteal artery. Most often the vessel had avulsed distally. Two patients had thrombosis in the midpopliteal artery secondary to stretching of the vessel. Intraoperative arteriograms after popliteal artery reconstruction demonstrated both distal thrombosis requiring removal in 5 patients and anastomotic narrowing requiring revision in 2 patients. Vascular reconstruction succeeded in 8 of 9 patients. Eleven of 12 patients had excellent or good results after early open repair of the ligaments of the knee.

Conclusions.—All patients suspected of having traumatic knee dislocation should have vascular assessment of the lower extremities, including Doppler study of the ankle pulses. A younger patient lacking pulses should have immediate femoral arteriography. If the popliteal artery is not normal, it should be explored surgically.

▶ Because knee dislocations are uncommon, clear clinical guidelines for their management have been difficult to develop. Questions about whether one should do arteriography and, if so, when, whether one should explore the popliteal vessel and, if so, when, and how one can avoid unnecessary imaging and exploration are all addressed in this paper. The rarity of the condition is demonstrated by the fact that only 20 patients presented at the Mayo Clinic during an 8-year period and that only 17 of those patients were seen there initially. The authors propose a logical sequence of diagnostic procedures to determine the presence or absence of injury to the vascular structures. In addition, they provide strong evidence in favor of the early repair of all disrupted ligaments. This approach produced good clinical results in 12 patients so treated, as compared to poor results in the 3 who did not have ligamentous repair.— C.B. Sledge, M.D.

Popliteal Arterial Injuries Associated With Fractures or Dislocations About the Knee as a Result of Blunt Trauma

Bryan T, Merritt P, Hack B (Los Angeles County – Univ of Southern California Med Ctr; Glendale Adventist Med Ctr, Calif)
Orthop Rev 20:525–530, 1991   3–9

Background.—Popliteal artery injuries are historically associated with high amputation rates, and a recent review showed a 38% amputation rate with blunt traumatic injuries to the artery. Eleven years of experience with treatment of blunt trauma and associated orthopedic injuries was evaluated.

Methods.—Seventy-three patients including 57 males and 16 females (average age, 26 years) were treated. Seventy percent of the injuries were associated with motor vehicles. Sixty-six percent of fractures were open, 27% of which became infected. There were a variety of associated orthopedic injuries, including knee dislocation, tibial metaphyseal fracture, fracture dislocation with intra-articular proximal tibial fracture, and fracture of both the femur and the tibia. The popliteal artery was repaired, most commonly by end-to-end anastomosis, but in 25 cases by reversed saphenous vein graft, an average of 14.6 hours after injury.

Results.—Fifteen percent of the patients required an amputation. The method of failure was gangrene in 4 patients and recurrent thrombosis in 3. All but 1 amputation occurred in a patient with an open, type III fracture. There was no correlation between amputation and fracture type, delay in diagnosis, or delay in surgery; however, amputation was related to degree of soft tissue trauma. The amputation rate was 22% in 1975–1979 and only 8% in 1980–1985.

Conclusions.—Patients with high-energy blunt trauma to the legs should be suspected of having an injury of the popliteal artery. They must have prompt exploration or arteriography. Patients with massive soft tissue trauma should have prompt external fixation, arterial repair, aggressive débridement, and early soft tissue coverage.

▶ This series combines both direct injury to the popliteal artery and injuries related to fractures and dislocations about the knee. The results demonstrate the seriousness of this group of injuries, with 15% of the patients requiring an amputation as a result of the combination of arterial insufficiency and infection related to the open injuries.— C.B. Sledge, M.D.

Reflex Sympathetic Dystrophy of the Patellofemoral Joint

Finsterbush A, Frankl U, Mann G, Lowe J (Hadassah Univ Hosp, Jerusalem, Israel)
Orthop Rev 20:877–885, 1991   3–10

Introduction.—The number of reported cases of reflex sympathetic dystrophy (RSD) involving the knee is increasing as clinicians become more aware of the disorder. Eighteen patients receiving a diagnosis of RSD of the patellofemoral joint were reviewed.

Patients.—The average patient age was 34 years when the triggering injury occurred and 39 years at the time of final evaluation. Symptoms were present for 5½ years on average. Six patients had diagnoses retrospectively after several operations had failed. In 4 patients there was a previous pathologic condition in the involved knee joint. Eleven patients had direct injury to the knee. Twelve had compensation or liability cases pending.

Clinical Features.—Pain was out of proportion to trauma and was prolonged. It tended to be severe and constant at first and to be initiated by activity later. The patients with no previous diagnosis tended to have an unstable knee or uncontrolled knee motion. Regional osteoporosis was a nearly universal finding (Fig 3–2). Scintigraphy usually showed increased Tc uptake about the knee. Arthroscopy usually revealed synovitis and minor changes in the articular surface of the patella.

Treatment and Outcome.—Patients received continuous epidural nerve block with lidocaine or regional sympathetic block with reserpine, which temporarily relieved pain. Aggressive physical therapy then was instituted. Patients who had RSD diagnosed at a relatively early stage had

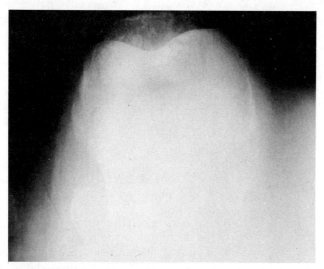

Fig 3–2.—A typical skyline view of the patellofemoral joint during the active phase of RSD. Extreme osteoporotic changes are seen in the patella. (Courtesy of Finsterbush A, Frankl U, Mann G, et al: *Orthop Rev* 20:877–885, 1991.)

the best outcome. The chance of improvement declined when surgery had been carried out, and those with diagnosis at a late stage remained disabled.

Conclusions.—Confidence in the physician is a critically important facet of the management of RSD. Initially, a block is used to reduce pain, and regular physical therapy then is instituted.

▶ Reflex sympathetic dystrophy after knee injury is a commonly overlooked diagnosis: physicians do not think about it, and there is not any reliable early objective diagnostic test. When it is recognized, treatment can be effective, and patients can be spared both unnecessary surgery and the risk of having their symptoms ignored or attributed to psychological factors.—C.B. Sledge, M.D.

Analysis of Subjective Knee Complaints Using Visual Analog Scales
Flandry F, Hunt JP, Terry GC, Hughston JC (Hughston Orthopaedic Clinic; Hughston Sports Medicine Found, Columbus, Ga)
Am J Sports Med 19:112–118, 1991   3–11

Background.—Treatment results can be difficult to measure and analyze, particularly when outcome is related to subjective factors such as pain and functional ability. A system using a possible 100 point numerical score often is used to evaluate knee problems, but this method may have a low degree of sensitivity and interpretation bias. A visual analog scale (VAS) was developed to bring a greater sensitivity and greater statistical power to the analysis of subjective knee complaints.

Methods.—The VAS was tested on 117 consecutive patients who had undergone knee surgery ranging from arthroscopy to total arthroplasty. The validity of the VAS was compared with that of 3 other established subjective evaluation methods: the Lysholm scale, the Noyes knee scale, and the Larson scale. After completing the VAS and 1 of the other scales, each patient was asked to rate the forms and state which form allowed them to best depict their symptoms.

Results.—User understanding was similar for the VAS, Lysholm, and Larson knee scales, but patients were less able to respond satisfactorily to questions posed by the Noyes scale. Eighty percent of the patients who also took the Noyes test found that the VAS was easier to complete. Of those who took the Lysholm knee scale, 43% found the VAS easier to complete and 43% said there was no difference between the scales. The Larson scale was described as being more confusing than the VAS by 58% of the patients.

Conclusions.—The VAS, with its open structure of responses, does not force patients to interpret the definition of the terms mild, moderate, or severe, or to assign themselves to such categories. Because the responses can be converted to objective measures, bias is minimized and statistical power increased. Patient affinity was greater for the VAS than for other scales.

▶ It is becoming obvious that the justification for many orthopedic reconstructive procedures will be improvement in the quality of life through relief of pain. This paper demonstrates that VASs for pain can be used with good statistical validity.—C.B. Sledge, M.D.

Cruciate Ligaments

Knee Function After Surgical or Nonsurgical Treatment of Acute Rupture of the Anterior Cruciate Ligament: A Randomized Study With a Long-Term Follow-Up Period

Andersson C, Odensten M, Gillquist J (Univ Hosp, Linköping, Sweden)
Clin Orthop 264:255–263, 1991   3–12

Background.—There is controversy as to the need to restore the stability of the knee in patients who have anterior cruciate ligament (ACL) rupture. A randomized trial of surgical and nonsurgical treatment for acute ACL rupture was conducted, including a long follow-up period to assess the importance of restoring stability.

Methods.—A total of 167 consecutive patients with acute and complete rupture of the ACL were enrolled, including 119 males and 48 females (mean age, 26 years). Patients were randomized into 3 treatment groups: 50 patients had repair and augmentation of the ACL with an iliotibial strip, 25 had ACL repair without augmentation, and 92 had no surgical treatment of their ACL injury. In all groups, associated meniscal and ligamentous injuries were treated in the same way; 59% of patients had meniscal injuries. Reexamination was done a mean 55 months after injury in 156 patients. A performance test was used to evaluate knee function, and patients were questioned in detail about their subjective complaints. Strength and laxity testing were done.

Results.—Nineteen patients, most in the nonsurgically treated group, required ACL reconstruction during follow-up for severe symptomatic instabilities. Sixty-two percent of patients in the nonsurgical group complained of instability vs. 15% of patients in the repair and augmentation group. Less abnormal laxity was seen in the repair and augmentation group than in either of the other 2 groups. In addition, 63% of patients in the augmentation group were able to return to competitive sports compared to 32% of those in the repair only group and 27% of those in the nonsurgical group. All groups had similar relative hamstrings and quadriceps strength. The repair and augmentation group did better on hop testing, reflecting their superior stability. Running was similar in all groups, but it was correlated with activity level.

Conclusions.—In patients with complete ACL rupture, augmented repair provides better knee function than nonsurgical treatment. Nonsurgically treated patients commonly have instability, but few have problems in activities of daily living. For patients with high functional demands, primary repair and augmentation are indicated. Those with lower demands need not have repair; but, if laxity is pronounced, they will be at risk for subsequent symptoms that will result in deteriorating knee function. Nonaugmented ACL repair is not recommended because the results are no better than nonsurgical treatment.

▶ There is still no clear-cut agreement on when the disrupted ACL should be repaired. In part this is a result of the fact that injury to the ACL often is accompanied by injury to other structures; it is therefore difficult to do comparative studies in which the patient populations have identical associated injuries. A major problem, however, has been the lack of prospective, randomized, controlled trials of surgical vs. nonsurgical treatment. This paper is, therefore, extremely important in that it reports 167 consecutive patients with acute and complete ruptures of the ACL. Patients were randomized into repair with augmentation, repair without augmentation, and nonsurgical management. The distribution of associated injuries in the 3 treatment groups was similar. The patients treated nonsurgically had instability but, if their demands were low, did fairly well. Although it should be noted that 16 of the nonsurgically treated patients had to have late ACL reconstructions because of significant symptomatic instability, patients with repair without augmentation did only slightly better than patients with no surgery. This study confirms that patients who wish to return to high levels of knee function do better with augmented repair of the ACL than with other current treatments.—C.B. Sledge, M.D.

The Conservative Treatment of the Anterior Cruciate Deficient Knee
Bonamo JJ, Fay C, Firestone T (New York Univ)
Am J Sports Med 18:618–623, 1990   3–13

Background.—Physicians still disagree on the best treatment for injury to the anterior cruciate ligament (ACL). The results of conservative care of the ACL deficient knee using arthroscopic surgery for associated meniscal or articular cartilage abnormalities, a comprehensive rehabilitation program, a functional brace for sport, and advice on activity modification were evaluated.

Patients.—Seventy-nine recreational athletes (mean age, 26 years) were treated for complete ACL tears. Follow-up averaged 52 months.

Results.—Six patients (8%) ultimately had ligament reconstruction. These were considered failure of nonreconstructive treatment. In the remaining 73, the results were excellent in 11%, good in 32%, fair in 22%, and poor in 35%. Ninety-seven percent of the patients were satisfied with their results for the activities of daily living, but only 49% were satisfied with their knee for sports. Forty percent had modified their participation in sports significantly. Patient age, sex, interval between injury and treatment, associated meniscal tears, and articular cartilage damage apparently did not affect outcomes. Of the patients with significant pivot shifts, 40% had poor results. Poor results were also associated with multiple repeat injuries, repeat arthroscopy, isokinetic deficits, and increased length of follow-up.

Conclusions.—Conservative management of the ACL deficient knee as described is acceptable only for noncompetitive, recreational athletes willing to significantly modify their future participation in sports. It may also be warranted for those unwilling to risk the possible morbidity of ligament reconstruction.

▶ This paper reports on a carefully documented group of patients with ACL injuries who were managed conservatively by having associated injuries treated arthroscopically and then by participating in a comprehensive rehabilitation program. They can therefore be considered as a benchmark group of patients undergoing conservative management. It is significant that 97% were satisfied with the result of conservative treatment with regard to their activities of daily living but that only about half were satisfied with their knee when it came to participation in sports. The conclusion that conservative management is acceptable only in "the noncompetitive, recreational athlete who is willing to significantly modify future sports activity" appears well justified by this and other studies.—C.B. Sledge, M.D.

Anterior Cruciate Ligament Reconstruction Using Quadriceps Patellar Tendon Graft: Part 1. Long-Term Followup
Howe JG, Johnson RJ, Kaplan MJ, Fleming B, Jarvinen M (Univ of Vermont; Tampere Univ, Finland)
Am J Sports Med 19:447–457, 1991   3–14

Background.—Reconstruction of the anterior cruciate ligament (ACL) of the knee is the primary restraint of anterior displacement and restores knee joint stability. Improvements and refinements in graft material and placement and rehabilitation have lessened morbidity and rehabilitation time. Although the Marshall quadriceps patellar tendon technique is no longer widely used, it was used as an example in reviewing the ACL literature for biases in a review that also describes the long-term follow-up of a single operative procedure.

Methods.—Eighty-three patients who had undergone an ACL reconstruction with the patellar tendon graft were evaluated by physical examination, questionnaire, Genucom analysis, operative note review, and radiographs in a 10-year follow-up. The patients were all treated by the same surgeon.

Results.—Seventy-six percent of the patients had a satisfactory result, and 92% were content with their results, having no more than mild functional deficit. Ninety-three percent of the patients had no significant pain, and 95% did not experience the sensation of "giving way" after reconstruction. On examination 87% of the patients had a negative Lachman test, and 90% had no pivot shift. There was no increase in failure over time of 1–10 years but patients operated on during the first 5 years had more radiographic degenerative changes (table). Two examiners were able to reliably diagnose gross laxity compared to stable ligamentous structures, but they were unable to correlate more specific clinical gradations of laxity accurately.

Conclusions.—The only significant risk factors for a poor recovery

Functional Evaluation

Result	After reconstruction		Before reconstruction	
	No.	(%)	No.	(%)
Satisfied with knee function	76	(92)	0	(0)
Significant pain	6	(7)	35	(42)
Frank subluxation (giving way)	4	(5)	77	(93)
Adequate function (able to perform strenuous activities)	76	(92)	44	(53)
Sports performance level relative to preinjury	64	(77)	27	(32)
Stair climbing >20 without symptoms	67	(81)	36	(43)
Walking >1 mile without symptoms	68	(82)	37	(45)

(Courtesy of Howe JG, Johnson RJ, Kaplan MJ, et al: *Am J Sports Med* 19:447–457, 1991.)

from ACL reconstruction with a quadriceps patellar tendon graft were the lack of a rehabilitation program longer than 4 months or repaired tears of the medial or lateral collateral ligaments.

▶ Early results of ligament reconstruction often deteriorate with time as ligaments and secondary restraints undergo progressive elongation with increasing instability and symptoms. A 10-year follow-up such as that reported in this paper is therefore an important indication of the longevity of an operative procedure for ligamentous injuries to the knee. The findings show excellent stability of the results, with no evidence of deterioration over time. Function appears excellent. Seventy-seven percent of patients were able to return to their preinjury level of sports performance.—C.B. Sledge, M.D.

Reconstruction of the Anterior Cruciate Ligament With An Intra-Articular Patellar Tendon Graft and an Extra-Articular Tenodesis: Results After Six Years
Rackemann S, Robinson A, Dandy DJ (Addenbrooke's Hosp, Cambridge, England)
J Bone Joint Surg 73-B:368–373, 1991   3–15

Background.—For knees with anterior cruciate deficiency, extra-articular reconstruction does not produce long-term functional stability, but intra-articular reconstruction is more invasive and requires longer rehabilitation. A combined procedure has given good short-term and improved long-term results.

Methods.—Seventy-four of 103 patients who underwent combined reconstruction were available for review and examination. The original anterior cruciate ligament (ACL) deficiency resulted from sports activities in 70 patients. The patients all had disabling instability that had failed to respond to conservative measures or correction of internal derangements. The operation consisted of free grafting of the medial third of the patellar tendon to replace the ACL and an extra-articular MacIntosh lateral reconstruction. In the first 28 patients the knees were immobilized in casts; the rest were treated by early mobilization. Follow-up averaged 70 months.

*Results.—*Overall results were satisfactory in 93% of the knees reviewed at 1 year and 92% of those reviewed at 6 years. Sports participation was not restricted in 78% of patients. Final outcome was not associated with cast immobilization, delay between injury and operation, patient age, or severity of preoperative symptoms. Seventeen knees had a block to extension, 12 requiring arthroscopic débridement to improve range of motion.

*Conclusions.—*For symptomatic knees with ACL deficiency that have not responded to conservative treatment, combined intra-articular and extra-articular reconstruction appears to be a safe and reliable procedure. Results are superior to other reported methods of reconstruction, and most patients can return to full sports activity, even at highly competitive levels.

▶ With extra-articular reconstruction for ACL deficiency, long-term follow-up reveals successive deterioration of results as the repair stretches out. This paper reports the results of a combined intra-articular and extra-articular reconstruction with an average follow-up of almost 6 years. The outcome was excellent, but the Lysholm score after this combined operation was only slightly better than that reported for intra-articular repair only; whether or not the additional surgery involved in the extra-articular repair is justified or not remains debatable.—C.B. Sledge, M.D.

Proprioception and Function After Anterior Cruciate Reconstruction
Barrett DS (Royal Natl Orthopaedic Hosp, Stanmore, England)
J Bone Joint Surg 73-B:833–837, 1991   3–16

---

*Background.—*A rupture of the anterior cruciate ligament (ACL) may result in anterolateral instability of the knee with a feeling of instability and a sensation of "giving way." Reconstruction of the ACL is usually necessary to restore stability. In some patients, a poor joint position sense or lack of proprioception continues to cause feelings of instability, although the knee does not sublux on clinical testing. Patients' opinions about their own knee stability were compared with scores of proprioception and standard knee scores in 45 patients in an effort to identify factors that are the most important for the success of anterior cruciate reconstruction.

*Methods.—*Participants were divided into 3 groups: those with normal intact knees, those with anterior cruciate deficient knees, and those with anterior cruciate reconstructed knees. Participants were assessed by the modified knee scoring system of Tegner and Lysholm, clinical ligament testing, the patient's subjective assessment, functional score, and proprioceptive assessment.

Results.—The anterior deficient knees showed significantly poorer joint position sense than the normal knees or the knees with anterior cruciate replacement. The Lysholm scores and clinical assessment of ligaments correlated poorly with patient satisfaction and functional outcomes. Patient satisfaction correlated well with functional outcome. The accuracy of proprioception in the knees after reconstruction correlated well with both patient satisfaction and functional outcome. Proprioception was not related to the "tightness" of the knee.

Conclusions.—Proprioception was the major factor in both the functional outcome and the patient's satisfaction after anterior cruciate reconstruction. Standard knee scoring and clinical assessment of ligaments were poor indicators of objective functional outcome and patient perception of function.

▶ It has long been recognized that there is a difference between subjective and objective results of ACL reconstruction, and a possible explanation is offered by the authors of this study. They report that return of proprioception was the major factor in both functional and subjective outcome after ACL reconstruction. They further suggest that adding an assessment of proprioception would be an important step in improving the quantification of results after ACL surgery.—C.B. Sledge, M.D.

Early Results of the Leeds–Keio Anterior Cruciate Ligament Replacement
Macnicol MF, Penny ID, Sheppard L (Princess Margaret Rose Orthopaedic Hosp, Edinburgh, Scotland)
J Bone Joint Surg 73-B:377–380, 1991   3–17

Introduction.—Early evidence suggests that the Leeds–Keio open-weave polyester ligament is a promising replacement for the anterior cruciate ligament (ACL), with neoligament developing within the prosthetic meshwork in 3–24 months. Twenty patients who had ACL replacement by the Leeds–Keio ligament were reviewed clinically and arthroscopically at least 2 years later.

Patients.—The patients all had disabling knee symptoms resulting from chronic rupture of the ACL. All were men (mean age, 30 years). There was a mean delay of 3.5 years between ACL rupture and replacement. Ligaments were replaced according to the manufacturer's instructions. The knees were splinted for 4–6 weeks postoperatively because of concerns about bone plug fixation. Patients were reassessed 2–4 years postoperatively by examination, and 16 also underwent arthroscopy.

Results.—All of the patients believed that their overall knee function was improved and reported that they no longer had episodes of "giving way" during daily activity. However, objective results were good or excellent in only two thirds of patients. Half of the patients still had a positive pivot shift sign under anesthesia. No functional neoligament was noted on arthroscopic and histologic assessment. All patients had micro-scopic and macroscopic synovitis, mainly around the ligament.

Conclusions.—The Leeds–Keio ACL replacement appears to give gen-erally good subjective results but disappointing objective results. A syno-vitic reaction to polyester particles is a concern. Prosthetic replacement might be augmented by an autograft to avoid gradual deterioration of re-sults.

▶ A substitute ACL would be extremely useful, both as a direct substitute and as a reinforcement after intra-articular repair of rupture of the ACL. Thus far, however, a satisfactory material has not been developed. The authors of this study report that the Leeds–Keio polyester ligament does not produce good objective results, with formation of a new ligament in the scaffold provided by the substitute, and that there may be a problem with synovial reaction to frag-ments from the artificial ligament.—C.B. Sledge, M.D.

Magnetic Resonance Imaging of Meniscal and Cruciate Injuries of the Knee
Boeree NR, Watkinson AF, Ackroyd CE, Johnson C, Southmead Gen Hosp; Bristol Royal Infirmary, Bristol, England)
J Bone Joint Surg 73-B:452–457, 1991   3–18

Objective.—If there were some reliable method of imaging meniscal and cruciate ligament damage, arthroscopy could be avoided for many patients. The reliability of MRI for this purpose was evaluated.

Methods.—One hundred thirty three knees were examined with both MRI and arthroscopy for possible meniscal or cruciate injury during a 2-year period. Proton density images were used for their quick scan times. Patients included 108 males and 25 females (average age, 34 years). Fifty-six percent had a well-described traumatic injury. Magnetic resonance scans were evaluated without knowledge of the patient's his-tory or the original radiologic report.

Results.—Arthroscopy was done for the MRI finding of torn meniscus in 73% of patients; arthroscopy was done despite normal MRI findings in 18%. Although there were false negative and false positive MRI find-ings in the menisci and anterior cruciate ligament (ACL), MRI was quite sensitive, specific, and accurate (table). In the menisci, MRI was able to demonstrate cysts, discoid deformity, and disruption. Findings in the ACL included absence and rupture.

Conclusions.—Magnetic resonance imaging of the knee correlates well with arthroscopic findings and appears to be at least as good as arthrog-raphy in evaluating the menisci and cruciate ligaments. This may allow arthroscopy to be targeted toward the patients most likely to benefit.

▶ The authors of this paper have sought to determine the extent to which MRI could substitute for arthroscopy in evaluating menisci and cruciate ligament in-juries. They found an excellent correlation between the 2 diagnostic modalities

Sensitivity, Specificity, and Accuracy of MRI Judged Against the
Arthroscopic Diagnosis

	Sensitivity		Specificity		Accuracy	
	N/N	*Per cent*	N/N	*Per cent*	N/N	*Per cent*
Medial meniscus	58/60	*96.7*	63/69	*91.3*	121/129	*93.8*
Lateral meniscus	25/26	*96.1*	99/101	*98.0*	124/127	*97.6*
ACL	32/33	*97.0*	89/100	*89.0*	121/133	*91.0*

(Courtesy of Boeree NR, Watkinson AF, Ackroyd CE, et al: *J Bone Joint Surg* 73-B:452–457, 1991.)

and suggest that MRI may be a cost-effective substitute for arthroscopy as a diagnostic procedure, allowing arthroscopy to be reserved for those who would benefit from a concurrent operative procedure.—C.B. Sledge, M.D.

Electrical Stimulation of the Thigh Muscles After Reconstruction of the Anterior Cruciate Ligament: Effects of Electrically Elicited Contraction of the Quadriceps Femoris and Hamstring Muscles on Gait and on Strength of the Thigh Muscles

Snyder-Mackler L, Ladin Z, Schepsis AA, Young JC (Sargent College of Allied Health Professions, Boston)
J Bone Joint Surg 73-A:1025–1036, 1991   3–19

Background.—Postoperative therapy after reconstruction of the anterior cruciate ligament (ACL) consists of early active motion of the knee joint and strengthening weak quadriceps femoris muscles. However, exercising the quadriceps femoris may place increased tension on the graft when these muscles are contracted in isolation, thus provoking the instability of the joint that the operation was intended to correct. Previous reports have shown that neuromuscular electrical stimulation after operation on the knee ligaments improves the torque-generating capability of the quadriceps femoris. The effects of neuromuscular electrical stimulation on the strength of the thigh muscles and on gait were assessed.

Methods.—Ten patients (age, 18–28 years) with recently reconstructed ACLs were assigned randomly to either neuromuscular electrical stimulation plus volitional exercise or to volitional exercise alone. Neuromuscular electrical stimulation was administered 3 days a week from the third through sixth postoperative weeks. Each treatment consisted of 15 maximum, electrically elicited co-contractions of the quadriceps femoris and hamstring muscles. Volitional co-contraction of the thigh muscles was performed 15 times twice daily on off days. Those who did not receive neuromuscular stimulation performed this regimen of volitional contraction 7 days a week. All patients kept an exercise log to check compliance with the exercise regimen.

Results.—The addition of neuromuscular electrical stimulation to the volitional exercise regimen significantly attenuated the usual loss of strength of the quadriceps femoris compared with volitional exercise alone. There was no significant difference between the regimens in any performance measure of the hamstring muscles. Patients who received neuromuscular electrical stimulation had significantly stronger quadriceps muscles, more normal gait patterns, and more normal kinematics than did those in the group engaging in volitional exercise only. Their knees were stronger in the eighth postoperative week than the average strengths reported for such patients months to years after operation.

Conclusion.—Neuromuscular electrical stimulation after ACL repair significantly increased muscle strength and improved the functional use of the muscles more than volitional exercise alone.

▶ One of the problems of rehabilitation of the knee after reconstruction of the ACL has been strengthening of the quadriceps muscle. The authors of this study demonstrate that electrical stimulation can be a useful adjunct to other rehabilitation modalities.—C.B. Sledge, M.D.

The Results of Surgical Repair of Acute Tears of the Posterior Cruciate Ligament
Pournaras J, Symeonides PP (Aristotelian Univ of Thessaloniki, Greece)
Clin Orthop 267:103–107, 1991   3–20

Background.—The importance of the posterior cruciate ligament (PCL) in knee stability remains uncertain. Some reports suggest that the PCL is a prime stabilizer of the knee, whereas others question whether it is necessary for good knee function.

Patients.—The results of repair were reviewed in 20 patients with acute rupture of the PCL who were operated on during the past decade. None of the patients were competitive athletes. Fourteen patients had a midsubstance tear; in 6 patients the ligament was avulsed without bone from its femoral attachment. The study included 17 men and 3 women average age, 26 years). Other knee injuries were seen in 9 of the patients.

Management.—All patients had surgery within 2 weeks after injury. The midsubstance tears were repaired with end-to-end silk sutures. For avulsion injuries, 2 tunnels were opened from the medial side of the medial femoral condyle and directed laterally to the intercondylar notch. A silk suture was then passed through the tunnels and tightened to secure the ligament. A posterior approach was used in 12 patients. A pin was placed through the upper tibia and incorporated in an above-knee cast to prevent posterior displacement of the tibia in the plaster.

Results.—During an average follow-up of 5 years, all the patients returned to their usual daily activities; they were also able to participate in recreational sports. Some patients had occasional mild swelling after activity; none had a poor subjective outcome. In no patient was knee motion limited by more than 10–15 degrees.

Conclusions.—Suturing alone does not restore the PCL; however, a failed repair does not lead to significant functional impairment in normal activities, most likely because it produces single plane (not rotatory) instability.

▶ Although far less common than ACL injuries, injuries to the PCL can produce significant disability. The authors of this paper report a variety of surgical techniques used to repair the ruptured PCL with good subjective recoveries.—C.B. Sledge, M.D.

Miscellaneous Conditions

Osteochondritis Dissecans of the Knee: A Long-Term Study
Twyman RS, Desai K, Aichroth PM (Westminster Hosp, London)
J Bone Joint Surg 73-B:461–464, 1991   3–21

Background.—Some follow-up investigations of osteochondritis dissecans have shown that the condition resolves well in children and does not result in long-term disability or osteoarthritis. However, its management is still debated. The long-term results of osteochondritis dissecans of the knee treated in childhood were examined in middle age.

Methods.—Of 57 patients initially treated, 18 patients with 22 affected knees could be found and examined. Average follow-up was 33.6 years (range, 26–54 years). The average patient age at onset of symptoms was 13 years.

Results.—Twelve patients, including 7 whose knees appeared normal on radiographs, complained of mild pain that did not interfere with activities. One patient complained of moderate pain that reduced her activities and disturbed her sleep. Fixed flexion deformities were seen in 2 knees; the rest had full movement. Graded on Hughston's score, 11 knees were excellent or good, 1 was fair, and 9 were poor or failures. In a 1968 assessment, 14 had been judged excellent or good, 3 were fair, and 4 were poor or failures. The fragment had been excised in 13 knees. None of those with radiographs showing osteochondritis dissecans at the classical site on the medial femoral condyle showed any joint space reduction. However, 4 of the remaining 7, all with osteochondritis dissecans at other sites, had no joint space. One had mild bone attrition. The contralateral knee was normal in all but 3 patients.

Conclusions.—If there is a large region of denuded bone in a weight-bearing position, the long-term outlook is poor. Lesions in the classic position generally have a good outlook as long as any loose fragments are excised.

▶ It is rare in patients coming through total knee arthroplasty to identify osteochondritis dissecans as the initial problem, although osteochondritis dissecans is not a rare childhood condition. This paper suggests that lesions that are large and affect the lateral femoral condyle are much more likely to have osteoarthritis develop.—C.B. Sledge, M.D.

Acromioclavicular Joint Injuries in Sport: Recommendations for Treatment

Dias JJ, Gregg PJ (Derbyshire Royal Infirmary, Derby, England; Glenfield General Hospital, Leicester, England)

Sports Med 11:125–132, 1991   3–22

Background.—The acromioclavicular joint is commonly dislocated in sports, particularly in those with a risk of falling onto the point of the shoulder. Management of this injury and the role of surgical reconstruction are controversial. The anatomy, pathology, diagnosis, and management of acromioclavicular joint injuries were examined.

Pathology and Diagnosis.—Injury is assumed to result from forced acromial depression, but patients are generally unable to describe exactly how they were injured. Detachment of the superior attachment of the intra-articular disk and superior acromioclavicular ligament precedes shelling out of the lateral end of the clavicle from the inferior periosteum, tearing of the coracoclavicular ligaments and clavipectoral fascia, and, in severe cases, stripping of the entire clavicular attachment of the deltoid. The patient has pain and swelling after participation in contact sports. There is acute tenderness over the joint. The severity of the injury may be assessed by resisted flexion of the elbow with the arm by the patient's side to contract the deltoid muscle. A standard posteroanterior radiograph with a 15-degree cephalad tilt shows the injury well. Injuries are classified as type 1, sprain; type 2, subluxation; and type 3, dislocation. A special weight-lifting view designed to contract the anterior deltoid may show 3 patterns of dislocation.

Management and Results.—Type 1 and type 2 injuries are managed first with broad arm slinging for 2–3 weeks and then with gentle mobilization. Treatment of dislocations is controversial, and none of the many surgical techniques described can consistently improve on the results of conservative management. Surgical stabilization may be needed for severe dislocations. The decision relies on the surgeon's judgment; the only indication for acute reconstruction may be displacement of the lateral end of the clavicle to the point where it tents the skin. Patients may have considerable pain and crepitus, although movement is usually unlimited. Excision of the lateral end of the clavicle might be done if symptoms are relieved by lidocaine injection. In the long term, significant disability is uncommon; only 1 of the 9 patients with subluxation had a functional disability. Radiographically, the joint appears to become stable spontaneously.

Conclusions.—Conservative management of acromioclavicular joint injuries yields satisfactory results in most patients. Joint position improves spontaneously in about half of the patients. Most such injuries should be managed conservatively until a specific procedure is shown to produce better results.

▶ Injuries of the acromioclavicular joint have been exposed to a wide variety of treatment modalities over the years because of disagreement regarding optimal treatment. As the authors of this paper state, none of the current surgical techniques can consistently improve on the results of conservative management. Their extensive review of the literature demonstrates a higher complication rate for surgical treatment than for conservative management without a concomitant improvement in results.—C.B. Sledge, M.D.

Traumatic Subluxation of the Hip Resulting in Aseptic Necrosis and Chondrolysis in a Professional Football Player
Cooper DE, Warren RF, Barnes R (The Hosp for Special Surgery, New York)
Am J Sports Med 19:322–324, 1991   3–23

Background.—Aseptic necrosis and posttraumatic arthrosis usually are not associated with subluxation of the hip alone. A professional football player was seen with posterior hip subluxation and subsequent aseptic necrosis and posttraumatic arthrosis.

Case Report.—Man, 23 years, a professional running back, was injured. A fracture fragment at the posterior aspect of the hip was demonstrated and confirmed by CT. Rest and activity modification were prescribed; pain persisted at 6 weeks. Magnetic resonance imaging showed a wedge-shaped focal region of aseptic necrosis in the superior aspect of the femoral head. The patient was treated with nonsteroidal anti-inflammatory medication and stayed on crutches for 4 months. Roentgenograms at 4 months revealed marked loss of the joint space. With the potential for collapse of the femoral head and continued joint space narrowing, the patient was advised of possible progressive arthrosis. He subsequently chose to return to full participation in professional football, and, at 8 months postinjury, he was pain-free and had full range of motion.

Conclusions.—Interruption of the blood supply to the femoral head is a common cause of posttraumatic aseptic necrosis. In a case of subluxation of the hip like this one, when hip congruity is only instantaneously disrupted, aseptic necrosis may be less extensive.

▶ A recent, highly publicized case of avascular necrosis of the hip after subluxation and spontaneous relocation of the dislocated hip has focused attention on this rare condition. The presence of vascular changes in the femoral head after a very brief episode of dislocation refutes the often quoted relationship between duration of dislocation and incidence of avascular changes. It may be that, in susceptible individuals, rupture of the ligamentum teres could result in focal avascularity.—C.B. Sledge, M.D.

Suprascapular Nerve Lesions at the Spinoglenoid Notch: Report of Three Cases and Review of the Literature
Liveson JA, Bronson MJ, Pollack MA (Albert Einstein College of Medicine, New York)
J Neurol Neurosurg Psychiatry 54:241–243, 1991   3–24

Background.—Entrapment of the suprascapular nerve can occur at either the suprascapular notch (SSN) or the spinoglenoid notch (SGN). Failure to distinguish between the 2 lesions (Fig 3–3) can result in surgery to the wrong region. Three young men were treated for SGN lesions and the literature was reviewed.

Patients.—All 3 patients were male athletes in their twenties. In 1 an isolated incident resulted in weakness in the dominant shoulder; the weakness gradually subsided. His right scapula appeared to be losing bulk during this time. He had no numbness or radicular symptoms, but atrophy was evident in the region of the right infraspinatus, with tenderness below the scapular spine. Manual muscle examination revealed no weakness and, as in all 3 patients, sensation was intact. In all 3 patients cranial nerves appeared to be normal, with no Horner's sign. A second patient noted a right shoulder ache without numbness, symptoms of root involvement, or weakness detectable by examination. The third patient had unilateral scapular atrophy on the dominant side, without numbness or cervical symptoms. External rotation of the humerus on the affected side was weak, and atrophy in the infraspinatus region was evident. Electrodiagnostic studies showed isolated denervation in the infraspinatus in all 3 patients. These consisted of fibrillation potentials, positive sharp waves, and single unit recruitment of normal motor unit potentials. Extensive electromyography showed no other abnormalities The motor unit potentials did not suggest myopathy, nor was a diffuse condition of pe-

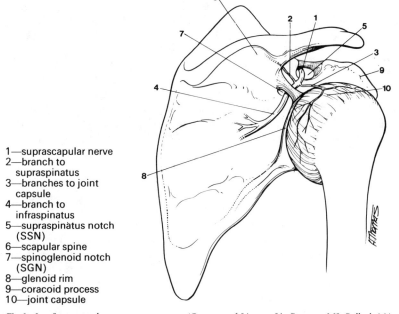

1—suprascapular nerve
2—branch to
   supraspinatus
3—branches to joint
   capsule
4—branch to
   infraspinatus
5—supraspinatus notch
   (SSN)
6—scapular spine
7—spinoglenoid notch
   (SGN)
8—glenoid rim
9—coracoid process
10—joint capsule

Fig 3–3.—Suprascapular nerve entrapments (Courtesy of Liveson JA, Bronson MJ, Pollack MA: *J Neurol Neurosurg Psychiatry* 54:241–243, 1991.)

ripheral nerves detected. In 2 patients the abnormalities were primarily axonal.

Results.—Conservative treatment resulted in normal or near normal strength and functioning in all patients. The SGN lesions usually were preceded by chronic over usage of the shoulder.

Conclusions.—The supraspinatus muscle should be examined to distinguish between lesions at the SSN and the SGN. Involvement of the supraspinatus marks the lesion at the SSN, whereas sparing of this muscle places it at the SGN. Clinically, pain was the initial complaint in SSN lesions, but there is little pain with SGN lesions.

▶ Suprascapular nerve lesions are quite uncommon, but this article suggests that differentiating the site of the lesion can be important as a guide to treatment.—C.B. Sledge, M.D.

Evaluation of the Painful Prosthetic Joint: Relative Value of Bone Scan, Sedimentation Rate, and Joint Aspiration
Levitsky KA, Hozack WJ, Balderston RA, Rothman RH, Gluckman SJ, Maslack MM, Booth RE Jr (Tufts Univ; Thomas Jefferson Univ; Cooper Hosp, Camden, NJ; Univ of Pennsylvania)
J Arthroplasty 6:237–244, 1991   3–25

Background.—The cause of pain in a prosthetic joint may involve infection or aseptic loosening. A diagnosis before revision surgery, which could differentiate between these possibilities, would be especially useful. Patients undergoing total hip or total knee revision surgery were examined prospectively to determine the most useful test for distinguishing between aseptic loosening and deep joint sepsis.

Methods.—Seventy-one patients were evaluated preoperatively with history and physical examination, plain radiographs, 3-phase bone imaging, erythrocyte sedimentation rate, and joint aspiration for culture. Intraoperative cultures and the operative appearance were used to form a diagnosis of definite infection based on findings of unequivocal microbiology and gross sepsis, possible infection based on findings of positive microbiology and gross sepsis, or no infection based on findings of neither positive microbiology nor gross sepsis.

Results.—The single most useful test in establishing a preoperative diagnosis of infection as opposed to aseptic loosening was preoperative joint aspiration (sensitivity, 67%; specificity, 96%). Three-phase bone imaging alone had low sensitivity (33%) and a specificity of 86%; there was little improvement when it was used in conjunction with plain radiographs. A preoperative erythrocyte sedimentation rate greater than 30 had low sensitivity and specificity, but the rate was significantly higher in the joints with significant infection (table).

Conclusions.—Preoperative aspiration is the single most useful test in the workup of a painful total joint arthroplasty. The 3-phase bone imaging was unlikely to provide additional information regarding infection as-

Summary of Results

	3PBI	3PBI and Plain Radiograph	ESR > 30	Joint Aspiration
Sensitivity (%)	33	38	60	67
Specificity (%)	86	41	65	96
Positive predictive value (%)	30	43	25	75
Negative predictive value (%)	88	89	90	94

Abbreviations: 3PBI, three-phase bone imaging; ESR, erythrocyte sedimentation rate.
(Courtesy of Levitsky KA, Hozack WJ, Balderston RA, et al: *J Arthroplasty* 6:237–244, 1991.)

sociated with joint loosening. Erythrocyte sedimentation rate was significantly elevated in infected joints, but the wide range of values restricted its usefulness in predicting infection.

▶ A painful joint replacement can be difficult to diagnose. This study confirms earlier reports suggesting that a positive aspiration of the joint is the most specific and sensitive single test. Although it misses one third of those patients who later are proven to have an infection, a positive preoperative culture is quite definitive. The sedimentation rate and bone scan are much less useful.—C.B. Sledge, M.D.

Metatarsal Head Excision for Rheumatoid Arthritis: 4-Year Follow-Up Of 68 Feet With and Without Hallux Fusion

Hughes J, Grace D, Clark P, Klenerman L (Northwick Park Hosp and Clinical Research Ctr, Harrow, England; Royal Natl Orthopedic Hosp, London; St Bartholomew's Hosp, London)
Acta Orthop Scand 62:63–66, 1991   3–26

Background.—Excision of the metatarsophalangeal joints usually gives good results in rheumatoid feet, but problems may arise from loss of forefoot stability. Consequently, some surgeons perform arthrodesis of the first metatarsophalangeal joint when the lesser metatarsal heads are excised, but this may cause problems because the lateral 4 rays remain shorter that the first ray. Forefoot arthroplasty was compared retrospectively with excision of all metatarsal heads, both with and without fusion of the hallux.

Methods.—Participants were 38 rheumatoid arthritis patients who underwent surgery for painful, deformed feet. A group of 34 feet in 20 patients had excision of all metatarsal heads, and a group of 34 feet in 18 patients had modified forefoot arthroplasty. In the excision group about two thirds of the first metatarsal head was resected, with trimming of the medial exostosis. Fusion of the first metatarsophalangeal joint was done in 24 feet. The lesser metatarsal heads were excised to form a smooth curve, and the plantar condyles were trimmed. Average follow-up was 5 years in the excision group and 4 years in the arthroplasty group.

Results.—One third of the arthroplasty group had failure of fusion of the hallux; these patients had the worst results. Patients who had excision were more likely to have metatarsalgia and plantar callosities develop, but they also had better shoe fitting and correction of deformity. The fusion group had more variable results, and their rates of complication and reoperation were higher.

Conclusions.—In the rheumatoid foot, excision of all 5 metatarsal heads appears to be preferable to fusion arthroplasty. The former procedure is more predictable, technically simple, provides better correction of deformity, and has lower rates of complication and reoperation.

▶ We sometimes forget the old, time-proven operation, such as metatarsal head resection for patients with rheumatoid arthritis, but this careful study documents the usefulness of the procedure and the fact that it is not necessary to complicate the operation by attempting fusion of the first metatarsophalangeal joint.—C.B. Sledge, M.D.

Evaluation of Knee Joint Cartilages and Menisci in Patients With Chronic Inflammatory Joint Diseases: A Prospective Arthroscopic Study Before, Six and Twelve Months After Open Synovectomy
Paus AC, Pahle JA (Oslo Sanitetsforening Rheumatism Hosp, Oslo)
Scand J Rheumatol 20:252–261, 1991   3–27

Background.—Arthroscopy provides detailed information about cartilage, the pannus growth covering the cartilage, and the menisci, with negligible morbidity. Describing and classifying the pathology of chronic inflammatory joint disease will facilitate follow-up studies regarding various treatments. A prospective investigation was done to assess the usefulness of arthroscopy, to classify observed pathology, to assess the changes after synovectomy, and to document areas of the knee that require close attention.

Methods.—In a group of patients with active synovitis of the knee, 70 arthroscopies were done. Clinical evaluation of the patients was based on the University of Colorado Knee score, Steinbrocker, Ritchies score, number of swollen joints, and duration of morning stiffness. Open synovectomy was performed after completion of the first arthroscopy. The knee was divided into 24 areas, and each area was given 3 separate score values according to pathology of the cartilage, pannus growth, and marginal erosions. Each meniscus was given a separate score.

Results.—During 1 year after synovectomy, the number of areas with pathology increased significantly, particularly in the weight-bearing areas of the femur and the tibia, but the areas with pathology at synovectomy did not deteriorate any further. This indicates increased risk of degenerative changes to the cartilages in the first year after synovectomy. With the use of the easy scoring systems, it was possible to compare findings in different patients and in the same patient at different examinations.

Conclusions.—The cartilage destruction after synovectomy is more likely to be a result of osteoarthritis than arthritic changes. After synovectomy, the number of areas with pathology increased significantly, especially in the weight-bearing areas, and the areas with pathology at synovectomy did not deteriorate any further.

▶ Some patients with rheumatoid arthritis will have a large bulk of proliferative synovitis but little radiographic evidence of cartilage destruction, whereas others will show the reverse picture. It is difficult, therefore, to assess the effectiveness of treatment by clinical examination of the joint or estimates of the amount of synovial proliferation. The authors of this report used arthroscopy to evaluate the amount of synovial proliferation and cartilage destruction as well as the state of the menisci. They were able to demonstrate that, after synovectomy, the progression of cartilage destruction was diminished. Indeed, they concluded that further cartilage destruction after synovectomy was more likely related to the mechanical forces acting on already damaged cartilage than to continuation of the inflammatory process. This suggests that biochemical changes in the weight-bearing cartilage occurring during the inflammatory process produce a mechanically deficient cartilage that is unable to withstand the forces of normal activity and that deteriorates in a pattern similar to that seen in osteoarthritis.—C.B. Sledge, M.D.

Cartilage Research

The Potential for Regeneration of Articular Cartilage in Defects Created by Chondral Shaving and Subchondral Abrasion: An Experimental Investigation in Rabbits

Kim HKW, Moran ME, Salter RB (Hospital for Sick Children, Toronto; University of Toronto)
J Bone Joint Surg 73-A:1301–1315, 1991   3–28

Background.—Chondral shaving and subchondral abrasion are commonly performed for chondromalacia, but the healing response of articular cartilage to these procedures has not been scientifically investigated. To address this issue, a rabbit model of chondral shaving and subchondral abrasion was created. The nature of the repair tissue formed after these procedures and whether continuous passive motion after operation would improve the repair tissue were investigated.

Methods.—In 40 adolescent rabbits 1 patella underwent chondral shaving. Forty additional rabbits underwent subchondral abrasion of 1 patella. Both procedures were executed with a round, air-driven burr 1 mm in diameter. The chondral shaving did not extend to the subchondral bone, but the subchondral abrasion penetrated just beyond the chondroosseous junction without entering subchondral cancellous bone. Half the animals in each groups were treated first with continuous passive motion for 2 weeks and then with intermittent active motion; the other half were assigned to intermittent active motion. When the rabbits were killed at 4 or 12 weeks after operation, gross and histologic assessment of the patellae were performed.

Results.—Regardless of the postoperative treatment, no defect produced by chondral shaving was filled with repair tissue at either 4 or 12 weeks. Histologic assessment revealed a moderate degree of degeneration

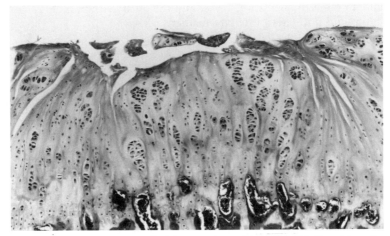

Fig 3–4.—Typical example of superficial fragmentation and formation of shallow clefts at 4 weeks after chondral shaving. Cloning is also present. Hematoxylin-eosin; ×125. (Courtesy of Kim HKW, Moran ME, Salter RB: *J Bone Joint Surg* 73-A:1301–1315, 1991.)

in the underlying cartilage manifested by irregularities in the surface, the formation of clefts, cloning, and hypercellularity (Fig 3–4). In contrast, repair tissue completely filled the defects in 17 of 19 animals at 4 weeks and in 18 of 20 animals at 12 weeks after subchondral abrasion. All animals treated with continuous passive motion after subchondral abrasion had complete filling of the defect after 4 or 12 weeks. Histologic assessment at both times revealed little endochondral ossification or new formation of subchondral bone, but did show mature, hyaline-like cartilage (Fig 3–5).

Conclusions.—According to this rabbit model, chondral shaving cannot be expected to stimulate regeneration of articular cartilage and may

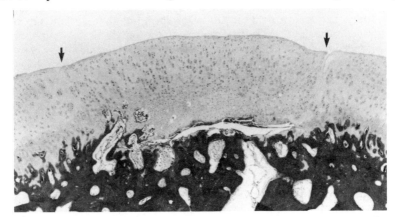

Fig 3–5.—Regenerated cartilage at 4 weeks after subchondral abrasion. There has been good regeneration of articular cartilage. Two edges of defect are indicated by arrows. There is little evidence of new subchondral bone formation or endochondral ossification underneath cartilage. Hematoxylin-eosin; ×50. (Courtesy of Kim HKW, Moran ME, Salter RB: *J Bone Joint Surg* 73-A:1301–1315, 1991.)

result in degeneration of the remaining cartilage. Tissue repair after subchondral abrasion can be excellent and may be enhanced by postoperative treatment with continuous passive motion.

▶ Dr. Salter continues his extensive investigations of the healing potential of articular cartilage after a variety of experimental injuries. As in many previous studies, partial thickness injuries to articular cartilage were not found to heal thickness injuries healed by fibrocartilaginous metaplasia, which, in some instances, produced an acceptable repair tissue.—C.B. Sledge, M.D.

Articular Cartilage Changes Following Meniscal Lesions: Repair and Meniscectomy Studied in the Rabbit Knee
Hede A, Svalastoga E, Reimann I (University of Copenhagen; Royal Veterinary and Agricultural University, Copenhagen)
Acta Orthop Scand 62:319–322, 1991   3–29

Background.—Lesions in the peripheral vascular part of the meniscus are now routinely repaired, as this reduces the risk of long-term articular cartilage degeneration in the knee. It is not known whether the repair of old lesions in the avascular part of the meniscus will prevent cartilage degeneration. The reaction of articular cartilage in rabbits to a meniscal lesion after nontreatment, meniscectomy, and meniscal repair were examined.

Methods.—A well-defined, longitudinal lesion was made during anteromedial arthrotomy of the right knee in 30 adult New Zealand white rabbits. Three months after arthrotomy, 12 rabbits underwent surgical repair of the lesion, 6 had a meniscectomy, and 12 were left untreated. Three untreated rabbits were killed at that time. Another 18 rabbits were killed 6 months after arthrotomy, and the remaining 9 rabbits were killed at 9 months. All 30 right knees were removed for microscopic and macroscopic examination. Fifteen randomly selected left knees were examined as controls.

Results.—None of the 12 untreated meniscal lesions had healed at 3, 6, or 9 months. All 12 surgically repaired meniscal lesions had healed. Five of the 6 knees treated with total meniscectomy had a fibrous meniscal regenerate measuring 2–5 mm. All of the right knees, but none of the 15 control knees, had changes in the medial tibial cartilage. The cartilage changes seen 3 months after meniscectomy were more pronounced than those in surgically repaired knees or in untreated knees. Surgical repair of the meniscal lesion did not reverse the cartilage changes.

Conclusions.—Surgical repair of old lesions in the avascular area of the meniscus does not seem to prevent cartilage degeneration. There was no significant difference between repaired knees examined at 6 months and those examined at 9 months after the lesion.

▶ This paper has 3 interesting conclusions. The first is that chronic tears through the avascular portion of the rabbit meniscus will heal when repaired.

The second is that the changes induced in the articular cartilage by the torn meniscus are not reversed when the meniscus is repaired. The third is that the progression of cartilage degeneration was the same regardless of whether the meniscus was repaired late or excised.—C.B. Sledge, M.D.

The Fate of Meniscus Cartilage After Transplantation of Cryopreserved Nontissue–Antigen-Matched Allograft: A Case Report
De Boer HH, Koudstaal J (De Wever-Hospital Heerlen, The Netherlands)
Clin Orthop 266:145–151, 1991   3–30

Background.—The treatment of patients with an established lateral compartment osteoarthrosis after a total lateral meniscectomy is problematic. A Patient with a disabling lateral compartment osteoarthrosis who could not be helped with a corrective osteotomy and who was too young for an arthroplasty was treated with a meniscal transplantation.

Case Report.—Man, 48, sought medical attention for a painful right knee. Twenty years earlier his lateral meniscus has been removed completely; 10 years earlier the medial meniscus had been partially removed. The patient had lost his job as a housepainter, walked with a crutch, and had pain at rest. His knee was swollen, with a range of motion of 5–130 degrees. Radiographs revealed a lateral compartment arthrosis. A cryopreserved nontissue-antigen-matched meniscus was transplanted. At 6 months, diagnostic arthroscopy was performed. Clinical, histologic, and histochemical examinations demonstrated that meniscal chondrocytes had survived cryopreservation and transplantation. At 1 year postoperatively, the outline of the donor meniscus appeared normal on arthrography.

Conclusions.—In this patient, meniscal chondrocytes survived cryopreservation and transplantation. However, the fate of meniscus cartilage after transplantation of non tissue-antigen-matched allograft in humans remains uncertain.

▶ Two major problems must be solved before widespread use can be made of allograft transplantation of meniscal cartilage: long-term survivorship of the transplanted chondrocytes should be demonstrated, and the problems of mechanical fit must be solved. This paper demonstrates short-term survival of chondrocytes after cryopreservation and a satisfactory clinical result in 1 patient.—C.B. Sledge, M.D.

Neovascularisation of the Meniscus With Angiogenin: An Experimental Study in Rabbits
King TV, Vallee BL (Harvard Med School)
J Bone Joint Surg 73-B:587–590, 1991   3–31

Background.—The blood supply to the menisci of the knee is sparse. The menisci heal poorly after injury. For the first time, biochemically induced neovascularization of the meniscus using angiogenin, a 123 amino acid protein recently isolated and purified, was reported.

Methods.—Angiogenin was derived from human plasma, isolated, and purified to homogeneity. It was implanted into the menisci of 75 experimentally injured New Zealand white rabbits; 22 additional rabbits served as controls.

Results.—Neovascularization occurred in 52% of the menisci treated with angiogenin. In all of these cases, the response was localized to the area of sample implantation. The difference between the angiogenin-treated rabbits and the controls was significant. Neovascularization was seen in 3 of 8 treated rabbits killed before 4 weeks, in 30 of 53 killed between 4 and 10 weeks, and in 6 of 14 killed after 10 weeks. Histologically, neovascularization was characterized by vascular connective tissue invading the meniscus from both the dorsal and ventral surfaces with a thin covering layer of synovial cells. The vessels—arterioles, venules, and capillaries—penetrated the body of the meniscus. Fibroblasts had invaded the area of surgical injury. There were few acute inflammatory cells.

Conclusions.—Angiogenin induces neovascularization in the avascular meniscal body. The localized response results in vigorous vascular fibrous tissue ingrowth. Biochemically induced neovascularization may be useful in enhancing meniscal injury healing.

▶ Meniscal repair is most successful in the peripheral, vascularized rim of the meniscus and much less successful in the avascular midsubstance. The investigators in this study have demonstrated that neovascularization could be induced about half of the time through the use of angiogenin, a protein able to induce new blood vessel formation. Clinical studies using this approach and comparing the results with those using fibrin clots, drill-holes, and other methods of enhancing revascularization are eagerly awaited.—C.B. Sledge, M.D.

Infection

Ultraviolet Radiation Compared to an Ultra-Clean Air Enclosure: Comparison of Air Bacteria Counts in Operating Rooms

Berg M, Bergman BR, Hoborn J (East Hospital, Gothenburg, Sweden)
J Bone Joint Surg 73-B:811–815, 1991   3–32

Background.—Clean air in the operating room is especially important during certain types of surgery, such as joint replacement. Ultra-clean air is usually achieved using laminar-flow ventilation enclosures; however, the needed equipment is expensive and often is not cost-effective. An alternative method is the use of ultraviolet radiation during surgery.

Methods.—The air bacteria counts during hip replacement were compared in an operating room with a Charnley–Howorth air enclosure and in a room equipped with ultraviolet C (254 nm) tubes. The use of occlusive clothing by all operating room personnel also was evaluated. Bacterial air samples were taken during 113 total hip arthroplasties, both at the edge of the wound and at a site 130 cm from the operating table.

Results.—Ultraviolet light proved to be more efficient than use of an ultra-clean air enclosure. The use of occlusive clothing also yielded lower bacteria counts. The bacterial counts did not correlate with either the duration of surgery or the number of individuals in the room.

Conclusion.—The combination of ultraviolet light and occlusive clothing can provide ultra-clean air for joint replacement surgery.

▶ Charnley demonstrated the importance of the operating room environment in joint replacement surgery more than 25 years ago. How best to achieve an appropriate operating room environment has been the subject of much debate. Is it necessary to have an expensive laminar flow system? Are horizontal systems more dangerous than helpful? Are there less expensive alternatives? The frequency of infection after total joint arthroplasty is so low that a clinical study reporting diminished rates of infection would require massive numbers of patients in each arm of the study. Sampling the number of bacteria in the operating room air provides useful information that should allow a comparison between various techniques of achieving an ultra-clean operating room environment. This study demonstrates that the use of ultraviolet light and occlusive clothing is successful in reducing bacterial counts to levels similar to those reached in a laminar flow enclosure and at much less expense.—C.B. Sledge, M.D.

The Importance of Positive Bacterial Cultures of Specimens Obtained During Clean Orthopaedic Operations
Dietz FR, Koontz FP, Found EM, Marsh JL (Univ of Iowa)
J Bone Joint Surg 73-A:1200–1207, 1991   3–33

Background.—Although microorganism isolation depends on culturing the organism when an infection occurs, a positive culture may not be important clinically. The results of a prospective analysis of intraoperative wound specimens were assessed to determine the rate of clinically unimportant intraoperative positive cultures in orthopedic patients.

Methods.—Specimens for culture were collected from 40 consecutive, clean operations on patients who had not received antibiotic treatment. Twenty of these 40 patients then received antibiotics intraoperatively after the specimens were taken. The 40 patients had a mean age of 25 years. All procedures, with 23 done on an extremity, were conducted in conventional, nonlaminar air-flow operating rooms. Two physicians used iodine alone and 1 used iodine and alcohol to prepare the operative field; 2 used paper drapes and 1 used cloth drapes. Follow-up after discharge exceeded 6 months.

Results.—Twenty-three of the 40 patients (58%) had a positive culture from swabbing or tissue biopsy specimens, or both. The proportion of positive cultures fell within 15% of the true amount of positive cultures with a 95% confidence level for the techniques used. Eight of 40 cultures from swabbing specimens and 20 from tissue biopsy specimens were positive. Of these 28 positive cultures, 31 positive blood-agar plates and broth cultures were observed (3 specimens grew different bacteria). The tissue biopsy specimens cultured aerobically in broth demonstrated the highest amount of positivity. Of the 33 identified bacterial organisms, 19 were coagulase-negative *Staphylococcus,* 8 were *Propionibacterium acnes,* and 2 were *Peptostreptococcus.*

Implications.—Clinically unimportant bacteria can grow on culture from specimens obtained from clean orthopedic surgeries. These data suggest that cultures of coagulase-negative *Staphylococcus* may not have clinical importance for the types of wounds observed in this investigation.

▶ Positive wound cultures from clean operative procedures are difficult to interpret. This study suggests that they may bear no relation to postoperative infections and neither predict the fact of a postoperative infection nor the likely organism if one occurs.—C.B. Sledge, M.D.

Changing Pattern of Bone and Joint Infections Due to *Staphylococcus aureus:* Study of Cases of Bacteremia in Denmark, 1959–1988
Espersen F, Frimodt-Møller N, Rosdahl VT, Skinhøj P, Bentzon MW (State Serum Inst; Rigshospitalet; Bispebjerg Hospital, Copenhagen)
Rev Infect Dis 13:347–358, 1991   3–34

Introduction.—The 15,170 cases of *Staphylococcus aureus* bacteremia that occurred in Denmark between 1959 and 1988 included 525 cases of acute hematogenous osteomyelitis and 185 cases of septic arthritis that developed after bacteremia, and 134 cases of contiguous osteomyelitis in which the bacteremia occurred secondarily.

Patterns of Infection.—Although the number of cases of bacteremia increased during the review period, the frequency of bone and joint infections decreased (Table 1). Before 1968 acute hematogenous osteomyelitis

TABLE 1.—Patients with *S. aureus* Bacteremia and Bone or Joint Infections in Denmark, 1959–1988.

No. (%)* of cases

Study period	Bacteremia	Bone or joint infection	Hematogenous osteomyelitis	Contiguous osteomyelitis	Arthritis
1959–1963	776	55 (7.1)	50 (6.4)	0	5 (0.6)
1964–1968	1,699	85 (5.0)	69 (4.1)	5 (0.3)	11 (0.6)
1969–1973	2,648	88 (3.3)	70 (2.6)	7 (0.3)	11 (0.4)
1974–1978	2,664	146 (5.5)	100 (3.8)	25 (0.9)	21 (0.8)
1979–1983	3,348	165 (4.9)	99 (3.0)	34 (1.0)	32 (1.0)
1984–1988	4,035	305 (7.6)	137 (3.4)†	63 (1.6)‡	105 (2.6)‡
Total	15,170	844 (5.6)	525 (3.5)	134 (0.9)	185 (1.2)

*The percentage of cases of bacteremia.
†Decreased frequency in the number of cases (*P* < .05), as compared with the period 1959–1968.
‡Increased frequency in the number of cases (*P* < .01), as compared with the period 1959–1968.
(Courtesy of Esperson F, Frimodt-Møller N, Rosdahl VT, et al: *Rev Infect Dis* 13:347–358, 1991.)

TABLE 2.—The Localization of *S. aureus* Septic Arthritis
in Patients in Denmark, 1959–1988.

Joint of localization	No. (%) of patients
Hip	80 (43)
Knee	45 (24)
Sacroiliac	22 (12)
Shoulder	20 (11)
Other	18 (10)
Total	185

(Courtesy of Esperson F, Frimodt-Møller N, Rosdahl VT, et al: *Rev Infect Dis* 13:347–358, 1991.)

and septic arthritis were chiefly community-acquired infections. Approximately one third of all cases of hematogenous osteomyelitis seen between 1979 and 1983 were hospital-acquired; however, this figure decreased to 19% in the subsequent years. Hospital-acquired arthritis has become prevalent since 1968.

Demographic and Clinical.—Hematogenous osteomyelitis is still prominent in the pediatric age group (age, 1–20 years), especially in young bacteremic infants. Diabetes does not appear to predispose individuals to hematogenous osteomyelitis. More than two thirds of the cases of contiguous osteomyelitis were caused by postoperative infection. Although the femur was the bone most often involved by hematogenous infection earlier in the period, the spine is the most common site today. Septic arthritis most often involved the hip joint (Table 2).

Outcome.—The mortality rate was 5% in cases of hematogenous osteomyelitis; 15% for contiguous osteomyelitis; and 9% for arthritis. The mortality for all *S. aureus* bacteremias was 36%. Today chronic osteomyelitis develops less often in patients with hematogenous infection than it did in the past. Chronic infection occurs more often in females and less often in diabetics.

Implications.—The mortality from *S. aureus* bacteremic infections of bones and joints is low compared with that resulting from other forms of *S. aureus* bacteremia. The increasing prevalence of arthritis might reflect changes in the properties of the bacteria.

▶ This study documents a changing pattern of bone and joint infection after *S. aureus* bacteremia in Danish children. Arthritis became a more common manifestation in later years, and chronic infections became less common.—C.B. Sledge, M.D.

A Bioabsorbable Delivery System for Antibiotic Treatment of Osteomyelitis: The Use of Lactic Acid Oligomer as a Carrier
Wei G, Kotoura Y, Oka M, Yamamuro T, Wada R, Hyon S-H, Ikada Y (Kyoto University, Japan)
J Bone Joint Surg 73-B:246–252, 1991

Background.—Local antibiotic treatment is a key part of treatment of chronic osteomyelitis, along with surgery. A composite of D, L-lactic acid oligomer and dideoxykanamycin B was created in an attempt to provide a means of slowly releasing antibiotic from a biodegradable system.

Methods.—The composite was implanted in the distal part of rabbit femurs, and antibiotic concentrations were measured in the cortex, cancellous bone, and marrow. Test material was inserted into a hole about 4 mm in diameter in the intercondylar region of the bone.

Results.—Antibiotic concentrations in all tissues around the implant exceeded the minimum inhibitory concentration for the organisms that commonly cause osteomyelitis. These levels persisted for 6 weeks. Within 9 weeks of implantation, most implant material had been absorbed, and the marrow appeared nearly normal. There were no systemic side effects. Blood urea nitrogen and serum creatinine levels remained normal.

Conclusions.—Similar experiments will have to be done on diseased bone, but these findings suggest that this type of drug delivery system is clinically applicable. Modifications in the type and loading dose of antibiotic may make it useful in treating other disorders.

▶ The ability to deliver high and local levels of an appropriate antibiotic would be of enormous assistance in the treatment of chronic osteomyelitis. This paper reports on the effect of a biodegradable lactic acid oligomer. Good antibiotic levels were achieved, and there appeared to be no deleterious side effects.—C.B. Sledge, M.D.

Osteoarthritis

Rapid Destructive Osteoarthritis: Clinical, Radiographic, and Pathologic Features

Rosenberg ZS, Shankman S, Steiner GC, Kastenbaum DK, Norman A, Lazansky MG (Hosp for Joint Diseases–Orthopaedic Inst, New York; New York Med College, Valhalla)
Radiology 182:213–216, 1992

3–36

Introduction.—Twenty-four patients with an unusual hip arthropathy have been treated the past 15 years at 1 institution. Radiographs showed marked joint destruction, and pathologic examination yielded the unexpected diagnosis of osteoarthritis. All patients had rapid disease progression.

Patients.—Twenty of the patients were women (mean age, 76 years) and 5 were men (mean age, 70 years). Three patients had bilateral involvement. Mean duration of symptoms was 1.4 years; duration was less than 1 year in 16 patients. Preoperative radiographs suggested a variety of other disorders, including septic arthritis, rheumatoid and seronegative arthritis, primary osteonecrosis with secondary osteoarthritis, or neuropathic osteoarthropathy. Nineteen hips had extreme flattening of the femoral head (Fig 3–6). Superolateral joint space narrowing

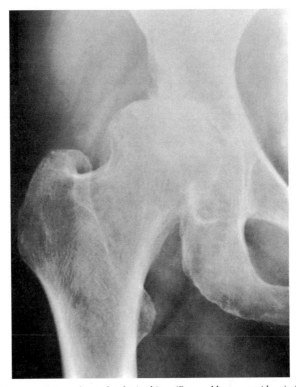

Fig 3–6.—Anteroposterior radiographs obtained in a 67-year-old woman with pain in the right hip. View obtained 3 months after pain began reveals typical osteoarthritis. (Courtesy of Rosenberg ZS, Shankman S, Steiner GC, et al: *Radiology* 182:213–216, 1992.)

was seen, sometimes with subluxation. Impaction sites of the femoral head and acetabulum often showed bone sclerosis. All patients had hip arthroplasty, at which time the diagnosis of osteoarthritis was confirmed. Nine patients had radiographs taken at various intervals before surgery documenting destruction of the hip within a mean of 18 months.

Conclusions.—The clinical, radiographic, and pathologic characteristics described may constitute an uncommon, rapidly destructive subset of osteoarthritis mainly affecting elderly women. It may be confused radiographically with a variety of other entities, but the clinical and pathologic features are different.

▶ The occasional occurrence of a rapidly progressive form of osteoarthritis of the hip has been recognized for many years. Advocates of osteotomies for osteoarthritis of the hip have been aware that the procedure is not likely to be successful in this subset of patients. It is also possible to mistake this rapidly progressive process for an infectious or inflammatory hip disease. In this paper, the authors review the clinical radiographic and pathologic features of this condition.—C.B. Sledge, M.D.

Comparison of an Antiinflammatory Dose of Ibuprofen, an Analgesic Dose of Ibuprofen, and Acetaminophen in the Treatment of Patients With Osteoarthritis of the Knee
Bradley JD, Brandt KD, Katz BP, Kalasinski LA, Ryan SI (Indiana Univ, Indianapolis)
N Engl J Med 325:87–91, 1991   3–37

Background.—Nonsteroidal anti-inflammatory drugs (NSAIDs) often are helpful in relieving joint pain and improving mobility in osteoarthritis, but analgesic agents without anti-inflammatory activity appear to be no less effective. A randomized, double-blind trial was done to compare the efficacy of the NSAID ibuprofen, in either an anti-inflammatory or analgesic dose, with that of the pure analgesic, acetaminophen.

Methods.—Included were 184 patients with chronic knee pain caused by osteoarthritis. They received treatment with either 2,400 or 1,200 mg/day of ibuprofen or 4,000 mg/day of acetaminophen. Outcome measures included the pain and disability scales of the Stanford Health Assessment Questionnaire, visual analog scales for pain at rest and during walking, time needed to walk 50 feet, and the physician's global assessment. Patients were evaluated after a washout period at baseline and again after 4 weeks of treatment.

Results.—The treatment course was completed by 144 patients. Most dropouts resulted from noncompliance or adverse events, with no significant differences noted among the 3 treatment groups. All major outcome variables were improved with each of the 3 treatments; magnitude of improvement was not significantly different among the different treatment groups for most variables. On the pain scale of the Health Assessment Questionnaire, mean improvement on a range of 0–3 was .30 with the analgesic dose of ibuprofen, .33 with acetaminophen, and .35 with the anti-inflammatory dose of ibuprofen. All 3 treatments were well tolerated, and side effects were minor.

Conclusions.—In patients with symptoms of knee pain from chronic osteoarthritis, acetaminophen and high and low doses of ibuprofen appear to have similar efficacy for short-term treatment. Although long-term outcome may be different, this result casts doubt on the practice of giving anti-inflammatory doses of ibuprofen.

▶ Perhaps the most widely prescribed medication in the country today is NSAIDs. This randomized, controlled, double-blind study compares the efficacy of such a drug to that of acetaminophen. Surprisingly, the results in terms of relief of knee pain were similar, although the costs are obviously vastly different.—C.B. Sledge, M.D.

Arthroscopic Débridement of the Knee for Osteoarthrosis
McLaren AC, Blokker CP, Fowler PJ, Roth JN, Rock MG (Univ of Western Ontario, London; Mayo Clinic and Found, Rochester, Minn)
Can J Surg 34:595–598, 1991   3–38

| | Subjective Results | | | | | |
| | Improved | | Same | | Worse | |
	No.	%	No.	%	No.	%
Pain	133	78	33	20	4	2
Disability*	37	22	116	68	17	10
Ambulation limitation	84	49	76	45	10	6
Overall patient assessment	110	65	48	28	12	7

*Disability assessed by patients on a follow-up questionnaire included no restriction, limited recreation and sports, unable to work, and restricted daily activities.
(Courtesy of McLaren AC, Blokker CP, Fowler PJ, et al: *Can J Surg* 34:595–598, 1991.)

Background.—In patients with osteoarthrosis or degenerative joint disease of the knee, joint débridement often is done as a temporizing measure. Arthroscopic débridement is widely used to reduce morbidity, but there have been few reports of its outcome.

Methods.—A group of 119 men and 51 women (mean age, 54 years) were treated with arthroscopic débridement for degenerative joint disease during a 4-year period. Previous treatments, including activity modification, anti-inflammatory drugs, and physiotherapy, were ineffective. The most common indication was aching or pain. Each patient underwent arthroscopic débridement, including lavage, meniscectomy, chondrectomy, and removal of free bodies and limited osteophytes. Outcomes were reviewed at an average of 25 months.

Results.—Improvement of symptoms was reported by 65% of the patients. Pain control was excellent in 38% of patients and function was improved in 22% (table). Twelve percent of patients required an additional surgical procedure. No factor investigated had a significant effect on outcome, including extent of degenerative changes and débridement and patient profile.

Conclusions.—In patients with osteoarthrosis of the knee, arthroscopic débridement is a useful, if temporary, measure. About one third of patients had marked improvement, although it cannot be predicted who will benefit. Patients report a high level of satisfaction with the procedure.

▶ In this retrospective review, 170 patients who underwent arthroscopic débridement for osteoarthritis of the knee were reviewed about 2 years after their treatment. The improvement noticed cannot be distinguished from a placebo effect because there was no control population. The fact that the extent of degenerative changes found in the knee did not correlate with outcome strongly suggests that the observed benefit was either a placebo effect or the temporary effect of removal of debris, inflammatory mediators, and other cellular products from the joint.—C.B. Sledge, M.D.

Prognosis for Patients With Medial Gonarthrosis: A 16-Year Follow-Up Study of 189 Knees
Odenbring S, Lindstrand A, Egund N, Larsson J, Heddson B (University Hospital, Lund, Sweden)
Clin Orthop 266:152–155, 1991
3–39

Background.—Untreated gonarthrosis generally becomes worse. Tibial osteotomy and knee arthroplasty generally are accepted as effective measures for patients with medial gonarthrosis. A group of 157 patients with medial gonarthrosis who had not previously undergone major knee surgery were monitered.

Patients.—Primary medial compartment arthrosis affected 189 knees in 157 patients seen in 1972. Follow-up was maintained through 1988. The patients had a mean age of 65 years.

Findings.—Surgery was done on 118 knees during the follow-up period; 85 had tibial osteotomy, and 33 had arthroplasty. Seventy-one other knees did not undergo surgery. Among 23 surviving patients with 31 affected knees that were not operated on, a majority had an unsatisfactory knee and were capable of only a low level of activity at follow-up. Twenty of the 31 knees were rated as having a poor outcome. Arthrosis worsened roentgenographically in 20 of 24 joints. Patients aged 60 years or younger at the outset had better function at the time of follow-up.

Conclusions.—These observations affirm the generally poor outlook for medial compartment gonarthrosis. A majority of patients eventually will have major knee surgery if it is available. In those who do not, maintaining a low level of activity can limit discomfort.

▶ Clinicians have long suspected that narrowing of the medial compartment of the knee in symptomatic patients was slowly progressive if followed for a long enough period of time. The natural history is important in advising patients with such a condition regarding surgery. If the condition would stabilize, many patients would be happy to tolerate mild-to-moderate discomfort and functional disability. If the lesion will be progressive, however, many patients would elect to have an osteotomy, unicompartmental replacement, or total knee arthroplasty before symptoms become completely disabling or their health does not permit surgical intervention. This study offers strong support for the belief that medial compartment osteoarthritis is a progressive disorder and demonstrates that the majority of patients with such a condition will undergo slow, steady deterioration in function and will eventually require major knee surgery.—C.B. Sledge, M.D.

Techniques of Total Knee Arthroplasty

Subvastus (Southern) Approach for Primary Total Knee Arthroplasty
Hofmann AA, Plaster RL, Murdock LE (Univ of Utah)
Clin Orthop 269:70–77, 1991
3–40

Background.—The subvastus medial arthrotomy, or Southern approach, gives good exposure for total knee arthroplasty (TKA) while preserving the extensor mechanism and maintaining blood supply to the patella. Although it was first described in 1929, it is not mentioned in current orthopedic textbooks. The relevant anatomy, surgical approach, and indications for this approach were examined.

Technique.—A general or spinal anesthetic with complete motor block is recommended. A tourniquet is applied, and the knee is flexed to 90 degrees. A straight anterior midline skin incision is made beginning about 4 finger breadths above the patella. The approach is deep to the superficial fascial layer and under the belly of the vastus medialis obliquus that contains the articular branch of the descending geniculate. The first fascial layer is incised slightly medially to avoid injury to the prepatellar plexus. Blunt dissection is done to raise the vastus medialis off the intermuscular septum to avoid injury to the descending genicular artery and saphenous nerve. The extensor mechanism is lifted anteriorly and laterally, and a curvilinear medial arthrotomy is made from the suprapatellar pouch to the tibial tubercle. With the patella everted and dislocated laterally, the knee is flexed and the muscle belly is bluntly dissected more proximally; this avoids overstretching of the vastus and excessive tension on the patellar tendon insertion. After the knee is prepared, patellar tracking is observed by reducing the patella and putting the knee through flexion and extension. The wound is closed with absorbable suture; the muscle belly need not be reattached to the intermuscular septum. Continuous passive motion is begun in the recovery room.

Conclusions.—The subvastus approach to the knee maintains vascular supply to the patella and preserves the integrity of the extensor mechanism. These considerations make it preferable to the medial parapatellar incision for TKA in the previously unoperated knee; revision arthroplasty is a relative contraindication.

▶ Although the standard straight anterior incision followed by a median parapatellar capsular incision is used by most knee surgeons, there are times when alternative approaches can be helpful. The subvastus approach has strong adherents, and the authors of this paper use it as their standard approach. It does offer less flexibility and cannot be used for revisions. I would anticipate that a particularly deformed knee undergoing even primary arthroplasty might pose some problems.—C.B. Sledge, M.D.

Bilateral Total Knee Arthroplasty: One Cruciate Retaining and One Cruciate Substituting

Becker MW, Insall JN, Faris PM (Hosp for Special Surgery, New York)
Clin Orthop 271:122–124, 1991   3–41

Introduction.—The use of the posterior cruciate ligament (PCL) remains controversial in total knee arthroplasty (TKA). The literature supports the use of cruciate-sacrificing and cruciate-substituting knee replacements. A prospective study was made of patients undergoing paired bilateral TKAs with 1 knee receiving cruciate-retaining replacements and 1 knee receiving cruciate-sacrificing replacements.

Methods.—Thirty patients, 23 women and 7 men, underwent paired bilateral cruciate-retaining and cruciate-substituting TKAs between 1983 and 1987. The patients had an average age of 66 years; 25 had osteoarthrosis, and 5 had rheumatoid arthritis. Surgical results were assessed using a clinical knee score.

Results.—Average preoperative knee scores were poor. Postoperatively, 28 patients had excellent knee scores and 2 had good scores in the cruciate-retaining knees, whereas 27 excellent and 3 good scores were noted for the cruciate-substituting knees. Average postsurgical flexion improved in both treatment groups, and all knees had acceptable alignment. Twenty-five of the 30 patients underwent stair-climbing assessment, 15 used either the railing or nothing at all for balance. Five patients ascended and descended the stairs favoring the cruciate-substituting knee, whereas 4 favored the cruciate-retaining knee. One individual ascended favoring the cruciate-retaining knee but descended favoring the cruciate-substituting knee. Patient opinion overall showed that 10 preferred the cruciate-retaining knee and 8 the cruciate-substituting knee; 12 had no preference.

Conclusions.—These findings, combined with long-term follow-up data concerning the total condylar prosthesis and the Insall–Burstein posterior stabilized prosthesis, suggest that sacrificing the PCL should continue in TKA. This procedure and the use of these 2 prostheses can avoid the problems of PCL tensioning.

▶ The controversy regarding cruciate preservation or substitution continues and will do so for the forseeable future in so far as the results at 10 years from both approaches appear similar. This study used patients as their own control by carrying out a cruciate-substituting arthroplasty in 1 knee and a cruciate-retaining arthroplasty in the contralateral knee. The results were virtually identical as judged by patient satisfaction.—C.B. Sledge, M.D.

Coronal Alignment After Total Knee Replacement

Jeffery RS, Morris RW, Denham RA (Queen Alexandra Hosp, Portsmouth, England)
J Bone Joint Surg 73B:709–714, 1991   3–42

Introduction.—Maquet's line represents the line from the center of the femoral head to the center of the talus body, passing through the middle third of the knee. If this alignment is not achieved during total knee replacement, compression forces on the concave aspect and tensile forces on the convex aspect of the joint can cause loosening. A review was made of the results of 115 Denham knee replacement alignments using intramedullary guide rods and Maquet's line to evaluate coronal alignment in all radiographs obtained during 8 years of follow-up.

Methods.—A total of 139 Denham total knee replacements were performed from 1976 to 1981 using a standard technique. After excluding 24 knees, 115 prostheses in 102 patients underwent assessment. Patients were evaluated clinically and radiographically before and after surgery and on alternate year's until death or removal of the prosthesis. The operative protocol for the Denham knee replacement employed intramedullary guide rods during coronal alignment. The instruments used to prepare the tibial plateau also included an intramedullary guide rod, which was removed after the cement set.

Results.—Before surgery, Maquet's line passed through the middle third of the knee in 13% of the 115 radiographs, whereas this occurred in 68% of early postoperative radiographs and in 65% of the follow-up radiographs taken after 8 years. Failure to achieve Maquet's line alignment was observed in knees with presurgical varus deformity. Eleven of the 115 knees had loosening or early signs of loosening, but no overall association was observed between preoperative malalignment and loosening. When Maquet's line passed through the middle third of the prosthesis in postsurgical radiographs, the incidence of loosening was 3%. When Maquet's line occurred medial or lateral to this point, the incidence of loosening after 8 years was 24%, a highly significant difference.

Conclusions.—Accurate coronal alignment using Maquet's line remains important in the prevention of prosthesis loosening after total knee replacement. Radiographs of the knees of patients with bony deformity or who have had surgery previously are recommended.

▶ There continues to be debate about the proper coronal alignment of the lower extremity after total knee arthroplasty. The authors of this paper use Maquet's line, passing from the center of the femoral head to the center of the talus, as their bench-mark, with the goal of having the line pass through the middle of the knee joint. When that goal was achieved, they had an incidence of component loosening of only 3%, but when they failed to achieve this desired alignment, the incidence of loosening increased dramatically. They do not address the question of whether overall alignment is the only variable or whether individual component alignment in the presence of normal overall alignment is a negative factor.—C.B. Sledge, M.D.

Bone Deficiency in Total Knee Arthroplasty: Use of Metal Wedge Augmentation
Rand JA (Mayo Clinic and Found, Rochester, Minn)
Clin Orthop 271:63–71, 1991   3–43

Background.—There are several options for the management of bone deficiency in total knee arthroplasty (TKA). Bone defects are classified according to symmetry, location, and extent and may be either symmetric or asymmetric. Modular metal wedges attached to the total knee prosthesis can be "customized" intraoperatively to match the defect. The potential complication is the durability of the wedge fixation to the tibial tray.

Metal wedge augmentation used in 25 patients was examined retrospectively.

Patients.—In 25 patients, 28 TKAs with a metal wedge augmentation were evaluated 2–3.5 years after surgery. The patients ranged in age from 55 years to 87 years (mean age, 71 years). The bone defects involved minimal to moderate bone loss. The preoperative bone defect size was 12 mm on the medial size and 8 mm on the lateral side.

Results.—Results were rated excellent in 79% of patients and good in 21%. Mean knee extension increased and mean knee flexion decreased. There were no perioperative complications or reoperations. Although radiolucent lines beneath the metal wedge were seen in 13 knees, none of the radiolucencies were progressive. No failures of the wedge-implant interface were observed.

Conclusions.—Metal wedge augmentation for bone deficiency in TKA offers better load transfer from the implant to bone than cement alone. Another advantage is that metal wedges do not require incorporation by the host as bone grafts do. In older patients, modular metal wedges are recommended for management of peripheral bone deficiency of 3–10 mm remaining after the initial tibial cut has been performed. In younger patients, successful bone grafts offer the potential for restoration of bone stock.

▶ There are a number of ways to restore lost bone when carrying out TKA, including cement, bone graft, or wedges of metal used with the prosthesis. This paper suggests that metal wedges are preferable to cement alone and, indeed, preferable to bone graft in that incorporation of a bone graft may be delayed and restoration of strength of the supporting bone may, therefore, be slow.— C.B. Sledge, M.D.

Influence of Prosthetic Joint Line Position on Knee Kinematics and Patellar Position

Yoshii I, Whiteside LA, White SE, Milliano MT (DePaul Health Ctr, St Louis)
J Arthroplasty 6:169–177, 1991   3–44

Introduction.—Restoring the joint line level is a critical factor in obtaining ideal knee kinematics after total knee arthroplasty (TKA). Prosthetic joint line position was examined using sagittal roentgenograms obtained from 6 fresh frozen cadaver knees.

Methods.—Standard surgical techniques were used to perform TKA. Medium-sized prostheses were used. A special knee testing device was designed that allowed for a controlled angle of flexion while maintaining a constant quadriceps force. Roentgenograms were obtained at 15-degree intervals from 30 degrees to 120 degrees before and after arthroplasty. Pins placed in the medial femoral condyle and patella were used as reference points.

Results.—The bone resection thickness from the femoral, tibial, and patellar surfaces equaled the prosthetic thickness. Correct ligament balance and knee flexibility were achieved without the need for special measurements or tensioning devices. Patellar tracking appeared to be identical before and after knee arthroplasty.

Conclusion.—If all articular surfaces are precisely resected and replaced with implants of equal thickness, then normal patellofemoral kinematics and tibiofemoral positions appear to be assured. However, this investigation dealt with component positioning in the sagittal plane only.

▶ For the knee to function properly through its normal range of motion, the relationship between all of the articular surfaces must be normal. Commonly, after knee arthroplasty the relationship between the articular surface of the femur and the tibia (the joint line) or the relationship between the patella and the joint line, or both, are altered. Methods of achieving joint-line restoration are discussed in this paper.—C.B. Sledge, M.D.

Blood Loss After Total Knee Replacement: Effects of Tourniquet Release and Continuous Passive Motion

Lotke PA, Faralli VJ, Orenstein EM, Ecker ML (Univ of Pennsylvania, Philadelphia)

J Bone Joint Surg 73-A:1037–1040, 1991   3–45

Introduction.—Total knee arthroplasty (TKA) is associated with major postoperative blood loss, for which blood transfusion is often needed. Because of an increasing concern about the safety of blood products, the magnitude of the blood loss associated with total knee replacement was assessed prospectively.

Patients.—The population consisted of 86 women and 35 men aged 41 to 85 years, who were scheduled to undergo unilateral primary total knee replacement with cement. Of the 121 patients, 111 had osteoarthrosis and 10 had rheumatoid arthritis. The patients were divided randomly into 4 groups. In 31 patients (group 1) the tourniquet remained inflated throughout the operation and was released after application of a compressive dressing and a splint that was used for 3 days. Continuous passive motion was started after 3 days. In 36 patients (group 2) the tourniquet was kept inflated throughout operation, but no splint was applied and continuous passive motion was started immediately in the recovery room. In 25 patients (group 3) the tourniquet was released before the prosthesis was inserted. Hemostasis was achieved by electrocoagulation. The tourniquet was reinflated, the bone was irrigated, and the prosthesis was cemented in place. A compressive dressing was applied after wound closure and a splint was used for 3 days. Continuous passive motion was started after 3 days. In 29 patients (group 4) the same procedure as for group 3 was used, except that, instead of a splint, an elastic wrap was applied and continuous passive motion was started immediately in the recovery room. Hemoglobin values and hematocrit were monitored in all patients. Blood loss in suction drainage was recorded, and the total blood loss was calculated.

Results.—The calculated blood loss in the first 3 groups averaged 1,553 mL. There was no statistically significant difference between these 3 groups. The average blood loss in group 4 was 1,793 mL, significantly greater than that in the other 3 groups. Loss in suction drainage correlated with total estimated blood loss and averaged 511 mL. More than half of the patients in the first 3 groups and 75% of the patients in group 4 needed blood transfusions. All 4 groups had similar complication rates.

Conclusion.—The amount of blood loss after TKA is considerable.

▶ Of the several variables related to blood loss during and after TKA (duration of tourniquet use, postoperative immobilization, and time of institution of continuous passive motion), only the combination of letting down the tourniquet before wound closure coupled with the immediate postoperative institution of continuous passive motion produced a statistical increase in blood loss. Patients lost an average of 3 units of blood, of which only 1 unit was in the suction drainage. From the point of view of blood loss, if one wishes to institute continuous passive motion immediately after surgery, it is better not to deflate the tourniquet until after the wound is closed. Whether there would be differences in wound healing with the several approaches evaluated in this study is not addressed.—C.B. Sledge, M.D.

Postoperative Collection and Reinfusion of Autologous Blood in Total Knee Arthroplasty

Majkowski RS, Newman JH, Currie IC (Winford Orthopaedic Hospital, Bristol, England)

Ann R Coll Surg Engl 73:381–384, 1991   3–46

Background.—Morbidity resulting from the use of homologous blood and a decrease in its supply has led to a renewed interest in the use of autologous blood during elective surgery. Postoperative autologous blood salvage and reinfusion were evaluated in 40 patients who underwent primary unilateral total knee arthroplasty (TKA).

Methods.—The Solcotrans orthopedic reinfusion system was used. The system was primed with ACDA anticoagulant, and the reservoir could hold as much as 500 mL. If the blood salvaged exceeded 300 mL, then it was reinfused via a 40-μm filter.

Results.—A mean of 57% of the blood drained in the study group was collected in the reservoirs, and 89% of it (520 mL) was reinfused. All but 2 of the 20 study patients received autologous blood. Only 7 study patients required homologous blood, as did 19 of 20 control patients. The mean number of units of bank blood delivered per patient was .9 units in the study group and 2.5 units in the control group, for an overall saving of 64%. The hemoglobin levels did not differ significantly either before or after surgery. Two patients in each group had deep vein thrombosis. No patient who was given autologous blood had evidence of coagulopathy or impaired renal function.

Conclusions.—Patient requests for autologous transfusion will probably increase as the public becomes more aware of the risks of homologous blood transfusion. Postoperative salvage has proved to be safe in patients undergoing TKA; it has also reduced the need for homologous blood.

▶ As in the previous study, the authors of this paper found an average of about 1 unit of blood recovered in the suction drainage after TKA. By reinfusing that unit, the authors reduced the number of patients requiring blood transfusion from 95% to 35%. An interesting fact is that an average of 1 unit was recovered in the suction drainage. Would that justify the use of a reinfusion unit?— C.B. Sledge, M.D.

Postoperative Use of Continuous Passive Motion, Transcutaneous Electrical Nerve Stimulation, and Continuous Cooling Pad Following Total Knee Arthroplasty
Walker RH, Morris BA, Angulo DL, Schneider J, Colwell CW Jr (Scripps Clinic and Research Found, La Jolla, Calif)
J Arthroplasty 6:151–156, 1991   3–47

Objective.—The effects of 3 rehabilitation methods were compared in patients requiring in-hospital care after unilateral total knee arthroplasty (TKA). The methods included continuous passive motion, transcutaneous electrical nerve stimulation (TENS), and use of a continuous cooling pad in conjunction with continuous passive motion.

Patients.—Twenty-two patients were randomized either to a group receiving continuous passive motion or to a control group after receiving cemented total condylar semiconstrained prostheses. A group of 48 patients was randomized to receive TENS delivering sensory threshold stimulation, TENS delivering subthreshold stimulation, or no TENS. These patients were all treated by continuous passive motion. A total of 30 patients received continuous passive motion with or without a continuous cooling pad.

Results.—The use of continuous passive motion alone significantly reduced the use of pain medication by hospitalized patients. Whether threshold or subthreshold TENS was used with continuous passive motion made no significant difference in the consumption of pain medication. Those patients who used a continuous cooling pad in addition to continuous passive motion required less oral pain medication during hospitalization than did those patients using continuous passive motion only.

Conclusion.—The use of continuous passive motion appears to limit the need for postoperative analgesia in patients undergoing TKA. Use of a continuous cooling pad further enhances this effect.

▶ With various financial pressures forcing the length of hospitalization ever downward, the evaluation of various rehabilitation protocols in an attempt to establish the most efficient means of restoring function after TKA is timely. This paper addresses pain control after knee arthroplasty in patients using either continuous passive motion, TENS, or continuous cooling. Only continuous passive motion was effective in reducing the need for pain medication and, therefore, presumably, in facilitating rehabilitation and earlier discharge.—C.B. Sledge, M.D.

Venous Ultrasonography in the Detection of Proximal Vein Thrombosis After Total Knee Arthroplasty
Woolson ST, Pottorff G (Stanford Univ)
Clin Orthop 273:131–135, 1991   3–48

Background.—An accurate and noninvasive means of detecting proximal venous thrombosis would be useful because of both the substantial risk after total knee arthroplasty (TKA) and the clinical import of venous thrombosis at this site.

Methods.—A group of 61 patients with TKA (in 88 extremities) was examined prospectively to compare the accuracy of real-time B-mode ultrasonography with that of ascending venography. The ultrasound study was done bilaterally, whereas venography was done in the operated extremity only. The studies were done at an average of 8 days postoperatively and within 24 hours of each other. The preventive measures included intermittent pneumatic compression and the use of elastic stockings.

Results.—Both tests gave positive results in 10 extremities with, the findings correlating for thrombus location and size. Five ultrasound studies were false negatives and 1 was a false positive, thereby yielding a sensitivity of 67%, a specificity of 99%, and an overall accuracy of 93%. The overall accuracy was 96% after the vascular laboratory had become experienced in venous imaging.

Conclusions.—Ultrasonography should be used as a routine postoperative screening test in place of venography to rule out the presence of proximal vein thrombosis in patients having TKA. Prophylaxis against deep venous thrombosis is essential for such patients.

▶ Which patients need anticoagulation after TKA? There is no clear consensus on that issue, but virtually everyone would agree that if proximal vein thrombi are demonstrated, anticoagulation is appropriate. Ultrasonography with modern equipment provides an excellent noninvasive means of detecting proximal vein thrombi with an overall accuracy of 96%. This accuracy allows one to select those patients at risk of embolization and treat them rather than having to treat the entire population of patients undergoing knee arthroplasty.—C.B. Sledge, M.D.

Unicompartmental Knee Replacement

Preoperative Diagnostic Protocol to Predict Candidates for Unicompartmental Arthroplasty
Chesnut WJ (Univ of New Mexico, Albuquerque)
Clin Orthop 273:146–150, 1991   3–49

Background.—The unicompartmental knee arthroplasty (UKA) reportedly has several advantages over total knee arthroplasty (TKA), and it is more easily revised. The unicompartmental osteoarthrosis protocol was used prospectively to assess patients who were scheduled for 208 knee arthroplasties.

The Protocol.—A candidate for UKA has a typical history of either pain in 1 compartment or, less often, increasing instability with or without pain. Examination shows mild laxity in the medial or lateral compartment on testing at 30 degrees of flexion. Varus or valgus malalignment can be corrected passively to the midline, and there is no fixed coronal contracture. Hip motion is normal. A 45-degree weight-bearing posteroanterior roentgenograph can detect unicompartmental cartilage loss before it is evident on standing radiographs taken in extension. Moderate degenerative changes of the patellofemoral joint may be present if there are few patellar symptoms.

Surgical Indications.—Patients may be candidates for UKA if they have erosions primarily in 1 compartment and only moderate patellofemoral joint damage. A small erosion may be seen on the opposite femoral condyle. Significant laxity of the cruciate and collateral ligaments requires TKA.

Results.—The unicompartmental arthroplasty protocol predicted localized, unicompartmental osteoarthritic changes in 202 instances, and it proved correct in 207 of 208 arthroplasties. Those patients who had undergone high tibial osteotomies were excluded.

▶ It is difficult to predict preoperatively which patients will be ideal candidates for UKA. The author of this paper proposes an extensive protocol that, in his hands, correctly predicted 207 of 208 candidates. Whether this degree of accuracy will be found by others depends on the criteria for doing a unicompartmental replacement. My own criteria include a normal contralateral compartment including the articular cartilage and a meniscus, no more than grade I chondromalacic changes in the patella, and no erosions in the intercondylar notch of the femur (indicative of subluxation). I do not believe that the proposed protocol would be successful in detecting those subtle changes in all instances. The protocol would be useful, perhaps, in predicting patients *most likely* to be candidates for unicompartmental replacement. With 10-year survivorship studies showing better results from tricompartmental arthroplasty than from unicompartmental arthroplasty, one should seek ideal candidates for unicompartment replacement and carry out tricompartmental arthroplasty in others.—C.B. Sledge, M.D.

The Long-Term Efficacy of Unicompartmental Arthroplasty of the Knee
Stockelman RE, Pohl KP (Miami Valley Hosp, Dayton, Ohio)
Clin Orthop 271:88–95, 1991   3–50

Background.—Unicompartmental knee arthroplasty (UKA) was first reported in 1973 when the Marmor modular knee was introduced. Initial encouraging reports were followed by reports of high failure rates attributable to factors ranging from patient selection to prosthetic design to disease progression. More recent investigations of UKA report high success rates. This investigation reduces as many variables as possible and evaluates the results of UKA performed in a community hospital.

Methods.—Forty-eight patients who had UKA for osteoarthritis confined primarily to the medial compartment were examined retrospectively. All arthroplasties were performed by the same surgeon using cement for fixation of both components. Compartmental II femoral prostheses were coupled with either a Robert Brigham or Compartmental II tibial prosthesis that was greater than 6 mm in thickness. This prosthesis represents an intermediate design; none of the femoral components showed any signs of failure, as the earlier models.

Results.—A total of 44 knees in 33 patients were available for complete follow-up examination, and 3 patients who underwent operation on 3 knees answered a questionnaire only. Follow-up ranged from 5–12 years. Results were satisfactory in 89% of knees fair in 2%. Revisions were required in 8%. In 2 knees there was roentgenographic evidence of disease progression. Most knees were within 4 degrees of neutral, but valgus alignment did not appear necessary for a satisfactory result.

Conclusions.—Results were good or excellent in most patients undergoing UKA. Patient selection is extremely important in preventing UKA prosthesis failure. Young, active, or obese patients should not be considered for this procedure. Unicompartmental knee arthroplasty appears to be successful in treating degenerative arthritis confined to the medial compartment.

▶ Forty-seven unicompartmental arthroplasties were followed for an average of 7 years and had a revision rate of 8—slightly greater than 1% per year. The authors conclude that unicompartmental replacement is indicated in elderly patients who are not overweight, who have medial compartment changes, and who need the shorter rehabilitation and greater range of motion afforded by unicompartmental replacement.—C.B. Sledge, M.D.

Unicompartmental Knee Arthroplasty: Eight- to 12-Year Follow-Up Evaluation With Survivorship Analysis
Scott RD, Cobb AG, McQueary FG, Thornhill TS (Brigham and Women's Hosp, Boston)
Clin Orthop 271:96–100, 1991   3–51

Background.—In 1981, 100 consecutive unicompartmental knee arthroplasties (UKAs) in 86 patients with osteoarthritis were examined. At that time, 2–6 years postoperatively, 92% of the knees were rated good or excellent with average flexion of 114 degrees. The same group of patients was examined again 8–12 years postoperatively, and the quality of results and survivorship for the prosthetic components were evaluated.

Patients.—Since the original follow-up study, 18 patients died and 4 patients were lost to follow-up. In the later follow-up study, 64 knees in

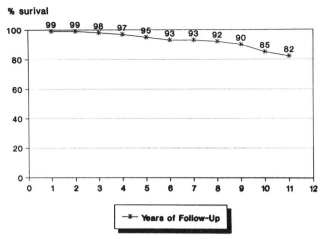

Fig 3–7.—Survival curve for unicompartmental knee arthroplasties. (Courtesy of Scott RD, Cobb AG, McQueary FG, et al: *Clin Orthop* 271:96–100, 1991.)

51 patients were assessed clinically and roentgenographically. Thirteen patients had revision of 13 knees.

Results.—The accumulated survival rate or probability that the prosthesis would remain in place was 90% at 9 years, 85% at 10 years, and 82% at 11 years (Fig 3–7). The improved range of motion after surgery (average, 115 degrees) was maintained in the surviving patients. Of the 51 patients, 87% had no significant pain. Anatomical alignment measured roentgenographically averaged 3 degrees of valgus for knees with preoperative varus alignment and 8 degrees of valgus for knees with preoperative valgus alignment. The patients (average age at second follow-up, 80 years) had decreased mobility, but only 8% of patients implicated the operation. Radiolucent lines were visible at the tibial bone-cement interface in 60% of the patients, but the lines were incomplete in 96%.

Conclusions.—Evaluation of this cohort of elderly patients at 8–12 years after UKA was affected by mortality during the follow-up period and by deteriorating mobility and function resulting from advanced age. However, 87% of the surviving patients had no significant pain. Survivorship analysis shows a possible acceleration in the annual failure rate after 9 years. Of the 13 patients who required revisions, 8 patients would have been excluded from surgery by today's selection criteria.

▶ Sixty-four unicompartmental arthroplasties with follow-up of 8–12 years are reported. Thirteen knees had undergone revision, for a failure rate of almost 20%. Survivorship analysis, however, predicted an 82% survivorship at 11 years, with 87% of the patients without significant pain. The authors suggest that the annual rate of failure of unicompartmental arthroplasty accelerates with time.—C.B. Sledge, M.D.

Unicompartmental Prosthesis for Gonarthrosis: A Nine-Year Series of 575 Knees From a Swedish Hospital

Christensen NO (Central Hosp, Kristianstad, Sweden)
Clin Orthop 273:165–169, 1991
3–52

Methods.—A total of 575 unicompartmental prostheses were implanted for gonarthrosis in 415 patients between 1980 and 1989. The series was consecutive and retrospective. More than half of the prostheses were implanted in patients with arthrosis in both knees; in 115 of the patients, the 2 knees were treated on the same day. Most patients were between 70 and 79 years of age.

Results.—Seven knees (1.2%) were revised and given a different prosthesis. Two other patients required a total knee arthroplasty. Secondary procedures were done in 2.4% of the patients. Good results depended on the state of the ligaments after correction. Secondary wear of the contralateral compartment was not a problem.

Conclusion.—Unicompartmental knee arthroplasty now appears to be indicated in many patients with gonarthrosis, including some with pyrophosphate synovitis or severe arthrosis. Pain relief was good, and the patients were generally satisfied with the results. The procedure involves fixation of a minimum of foreign material with minimal cement, sparing the intact surfaces and ligaments.

▶ A 9-year series of a large number of unicompartmental arthroplasties performed in 575 knees with a 1.2% revision rate is reported. Importantly, the authors report that degenerative changes in the contralateral compartment were not a problem at the time of follow-up.—C.B. Sledge, M.D.

Unicompartmental Versus Total Knee Arthroplasty in the Same Patient: A Comparative Study

Laurencin CT, Zelicof SB, Scott RD, Ewald FC (Brigham and Women's Hosp, Boston)
Clin Orthop 273:151–156, 1991
3–53

Objective.—A group of 24 patients who underwent primary unicompartmental knee arthroplasty (UKA) in 1 knee and primary total knee arthroplasty (TKA) in the other between 1979 and 1987 were examined. Both operations were done at the same admission. All but 1 of the 23 evaluable patients had osteoarthrosis.

Implants.—The Kinematic posterior cruciate-retaining system was used as the total knee replacement system in a majority of patients. Thirteen knees undergoing TKA had no patellar resurfacing. The Robert Brigham unicondylar system was used in 19 patients, and the Unicondylar was used in the other 4.

Results.—There were no intraoperative or perioperative complications. The range of motion improved from a preoperative mean of 106 degrees to 123 degrees on average on the UKA side. The average follow-up was 81 months. In the TKA knees, the mean range of motion improved from 104 degrees to 109 degrees when patellar resurfacing was not done; it remained at 113 degrees in the other knees. Preference for the knee that had UKA was more evident in the patients with resurfaced patellas; however, the difference was not statistically significant.

Conclusions.—Given proper patient selection, UKA can provide better subjective results than TKA, with increased motion and little or no pain. An unresurfaced patellar TKA appears to produce a knee that is more like knees that have undergone UKA than does the resurfaced TKA.

▶ This comparison of UKA verses TKA when carried out on the contralateral knees of a group of 24 patients suggests that UKA provides better patient satisfaction, probably related to better proprioception and kinematics resulting from the retained anterior cruciate ligament and the greater range of motion achieved after UKA.—C.B. Sledge, M.D.

A Comparison of Tricompartmental and Unicompartmental Arthroplasty for the Treatment of Gonarthrosis

Rougraff BT, Heck DA, Gibson AE (Indiana Univ, Indianapolis; Reid Mem Hosp, Richmond, Ind)

Clin Orthop 273:157–164, 1991   3–54

Introduction.—Tricompartmental total knee arthroplasty is an accepted approach to knee arthritis; however, the role of unicompartmental arthroplasty is more controversial. An experience with 120 unicompartmental knee arthroplasties in 98 patients and 81 tricompartmental arthroplasties in 66 patients was reviewed. The respective average follow-up intervals were 78 and 68 months.

Prostheses.—Two generations of the Zimmer implant were used for unicompartmental surgery. The most common types of implant used for tricompartmental arthroplasty were the Porous Coated Anatomic and Variable Axis prostheses. Non metal-backed polyethylene tibial components were used in the unicompartmental operations.

Results.—The postoperative prosthetic survivorship was 97% at 5 years and 65% at 10 years after tricompartmental arthroplasty. The respective figures for patients undergoing unicompartmental arthroplasty were 99% and 92%. There were no significant group differences in aseptic loosening. The need for transfusion was much less in patients having unicompartmental arthroplasty. Patient satisfaction and subjective pain scores were not significantly different between the 2 groups. A total of 5 knees undergoing unicondylar arthroplasty and 16 knees undergoing tricompartmental arthroplasty required reoperation.

Conclusions.—Unicompartmental arthroplasty can give results comparable to those achieved by tricompartmental knee arthroplasty in elderly patients with less severe arthritis. The range of motion is better, and the initial postoperative morbidity is lower with unicompartmental arthroplasty.

▶ Unlike the previous study (Abstract 3–53), this study compares UKA and TKA, not in the same patient, but in 2 similar groups of patients. Like the previous report, however, they report better patient satisfaction after UKA.—C.B. Sledge, M.D.

Results of Total Knee Arthroplasty

Survivorship Analysis of Total Knee Arthroplasty: Cumulative Rates of Survival of 9200 Total Knee Arthroplasties
Rand JA, Ilstrup DM (Mayo Clinic and Found, Rochester, Minn)
J Bone Joint Surg 73-A:397–409, 1991   3–55

Background.—Many variables influence success rates in total knee arthroplasty (TKA), including implant design, previous operations, diagnosis, revision vs. primary procedure, type of fixation, and patient age. The effects of these factors on the results of TKA were assessed in 9,200 operations.

Methods.—Data were drawn from the Mayo Clinic's Total Joint Registry which contains information on all patients undergoing total joint replacement. Patients are assessed by examination, telephone, or mail at 1, 2, and 5 years postoperatively and every 5 years thereafter. The registry included 8,069 primary and 1,131 revision TKAs performed during 16 years. Sixty-one percent of operations were done in women. Sixty-eight percent of the knees were affected by osteoarthrosis, and 31% had rheumatoid arthritis. Eighteen percent of the primary arthroplasties were preceded by 1 or more other operations. Nine general categories of implants were used. Actuarial analysis was performed to estimate cumulative survival rates. A proportional hazard, general linear model was used to identify independent variables associated with a significantly lower risk of failure.

Results.—Four variables associated with a significantly lower risk of failure were identified: primary arthroplasty, a diagnosis of rheumatoid arthritis, age of 60 years or older, and use of a metal-backed tibial condylar prosthesis. A patient with all of these characteristics had a 97% chance of a functioning implant at 5 and 10 years. Ten-year survival rates were 81% for primary and 72% for revision arthroplasties. For primary procedures, patients aged 60 years and older had an 83% survival rate at 10 years vs. a 77% survival rate for younger patients. Ten-year survival rates were 82% for rheumatoid arthritis, 79% for osteoarthrosis, and 63% for posttraumatic arthritis. Use of the condylar metal-backed prosthesis increased survival regardless of diagnosis.

Conclusions.—Favorable prognostic factors for survival of TKA are primary operation, diagnosis of rheumatoid arthritis, age 60 years or older, and use of a condylar prosthesis with a metal-backed tibial component. The surgeon should still use caution when considering TKA for younger patients.

▶ This 10-year follow-up of a large number of knee arthroplasties confirms that the ideal candidate is a patient who is older than 60 years of age, has rheumatoid arthritis, is undergoing TKA as the primary operation on the knee, and has an implant with a metal-backed tibial component. If all 4 of these favorable factors are present, there is a 97% chance that the implant will be functioning 10 years after implantation. At 5 years the survivorship of uncemented implants was not as good as the survivorship of cemented implants, and the difference was significant.—C.B. Sledge, M.D.

Survivorship Analysis and Confidence Intervals: An Assessment With Reference to the Stanmore Total Knee Replacement
Lettin AWF, Ware HS, Morris RW (St Bartholomew's Hosp, London)
J Bone Joint Surg 73-B:729–731, 1991   3–56

Background.—Survival analysis has been widely used to calculate the annual failure rate of implants and the proportion that survive after long-term follow-up. In 1984, survival analysis was completed on 210 Stanmore total knee replacements performed in 163 patients between 1972 and 1979. The same cohort was evaluated in 1988 and 1989. The 8- and 15-year survival analyses were compared to demonstrate the limitations of survival analysis when the standard error and confidence limits of the calculations are not considered.

Findings.—Sixteen knees were lost to the 8-year follow-up. The estimated annual failure rate and cumulative success rate of 194 knees were calculated with success defined as the prosthesis remaining in situ. The total number of known failures was 26. No further failures were recorded for the first or second years of follow-up, but 1 additional knee failed in each of the third, fifth, sixth, tenth, 11th, and 13th years, and 2 additional knees failed in the eighth year. During the first 5 years of both studies, the cumulative success rate was almost identical, and it differed only slightly at the 8-year follow-up. The standard error of the 7-year cumulative success rate calculated from data available in 1984 was 12.1%. In the last review, the standard error for 7-year survival became 3.1% instead of 12.1%. The new confidence interval is considered a more reliable estimate of long-term success. It is possible to predict an 80% rather than a 60% chance of the prosthesis surviving for 7 years.

Conclusions.—To estimate properly the expected life span of the Stanmore prosthesis, a long-term, disciplined follow-up of many patients receiving the same prosthesis is required. These data are based on surgery completed in 1973. With the same level of operative skill and similar patient populations, about 80% of Stanmore prostheses can be expected to remain in situ for at least 10 years.

▶ This follow-up study reports the results of a hinge replacement of the knee: 80% of the implants were functioning 10 years after surgery! In addition to this somewhat surprising information, the authors also provided an extensive discussion of the pitfalls of survivorship analysis.—C.B. Sledge, M.D.

TABLE 1.—Survival Rates for Failure: Revision

	ON			OA		
Years Postoperatively	*Knees Remaining in Study*	*Survival*	*Standard Error of Survival*	*Knees Remaining in Study*	*Survival*	*Standard Error of Survival*
0	32	100%	0%	63	100%	0%
1	31	100%	0%	57	100%	0%
3	21	100%	0%	41	100%	0%
5	8	100%	0%	31	100%	0%
7	4	83%	15%	17	100%	0%

(Courtesy of Ritter MA, Eizember LE, Keating EM, et al: *Clin Orthop* 267:108–114, 1991.)

The Survival of Total Knee Arthroplasty in Patients With Osteonecrosis of the Medial Condyle

Ritter MA, Eizember LE, Keating EM, Faris PM (Ctr for Hip and Knee Surgery, Mooresville, Ind; Louisiana State Univ, Shreveport)
Clin Orthop 267:108–114, 1991   3–57

Background.—No reports have correlated spontaneous osteonecrosis of the femoral condyle with the prognosis of total knee arthroplasty (TKA). Osteonecrosis is often incorrectly diagnosed as osteoarthrosis, and the 2 are commonly considered together in studies of TKA. Osteonecrosis of the medial compartment was distinguished from osteoarthrosis and its relation to survival after TKA was investigated.

Methods.—During an 11-year period, TKA was performed in a group of 43 knees with idiopathic osteonecrosis of the medial femoral condyle and in a group of 132 knees with osteoarthrosis of the medial compartment. Women predominated in the osteonecrosis group, so only the women in both groups were compared. These deletions and the patients lost to follow-up, resulted in 32 assessable TKAs in 23 women in the osteonecrosis group (mean age, 75 years) and 63 assessable TKAs in 42 women in the osteoarthrosis group (mean age, 73 years). Results were evaluated by means of the Kaplan-Meier survival analysis, with failure categories of revision; revision or radiolucency; revision, radiolucency, or

TABLE 2.—Survival Rates for Failure: Pain

	ON			OA		
Years Postoperatively	*Knees Remaining in Study*	*Survival*	*Standard Error of Survival*	*Knees Remaining in Study*	*Survival*	*Standard Error of Survival*
0	32	100%	0%	63	100%	0%
1	31	94%	4%	57	96%	2%
3	21	94%	4%	37	90%	4%
5	8	82%	12%	27	90%	4%
7	4	82%	12%	12	90%	4%

(Courtesy of Ritter MA, Eizember LE, Keating EM, et al: *Clin Orthop* 267:108–114, 1991.)

pain. Mean follow-up was 3.9 years in the osteonecrosis group and 4.6 years in the osteoarthrosis group.

Results.—The operation was generally beneficial in both groups, and there were few complications. Survival analysis showed no significant differences between the 2 groups (Tables 1 and 2). At 5 years pain was relieved in 82% of the osteonecrosis group and 90% of the osteoarthrosis group.

Conclusions.—Good immediate and long-term results can be expected with TKA performed on knees with spontaneous osteonecrosis of the medial femoral condyle. Although there appears to be no difference in survival rate between patients with osteonecrosis and those with osteoarthrosis, the sample size was small.

▶ The authors raise the question, "does osteonecrosis as the presenting diagnosis affect the outcome of TKA?" In this small group of patients the authors were unable to demonstrate any effect of this diagnosis on implant survivorship.—C.B. Sledge, M.D.

Knee Replacement in Morbidly Obese Women
Pritchett JW, Bortell DT (Univ of Washington)
Surg Gynecol Obstet 173:119–122, 1991   3–58

Background.—Traditionally, morbidly obese patients have not been considered satisfactory candidates for total joint replacement. However, many obese patients complain that their efforts to lose weight are hindered by painful knees, and they believe that knee replacements will enable them to be more active and lose weight. The results of total knee replacement in a series of morbidly obese patients were evaluated.

Methods.—The results of 66 total knee replacements in 50 obese women with osteoarthritis were compared with those of 64 knee replacements in 50 nonobese women. A group of 50 obese women not undergoing knee replacement surgery was also used for comparison. All obese patients were counseled by a dietician for weight loss. Five obese women with 6 knee replacements and 4 nonobese women were lost to follow-up. Mean follow-up was 33 months in the remaining patients.

Results.—There was no significant weight loss in the obese women who had knee surgery or in those who did not have surgery. Of the nonobese patients undergoing surgery, 86% had excellent or good results compared with 57% of the obese patients. Two infections occurred in obese patients compared with none in nonobese patients. Two revision operations were needed in the obese patients, and 1 was required in the nonobese patients.

Conclusions.—Total knee replacement appears to be safe and reasonably effective in morbidly obese persons. However, the results are not comparable with those in nonobese patients, and there is no evidence that knee replacement will facilitate weight loss.

▶ Excessive weight is often mentioned as a contraindication to total knee arthroplasty. Most studies demonstrate a higher failure rate in overweight women. In this study, with follow-up of less than 3 years, 86% of nonobese patients had good results, as compared to only 57% of obese patients. With longer follow-up, it would be expected that even more of the arthroplasty in the overweight population would fail. Incidentally, no one has reported much success in achieving weight loss in patients before they undergo knee arthroplasty or in patients after they have received a knee arthroplasty.—C.B. Sledge, M.D.

Total Knee Replacement for Metastatic Destruction of the Proximal Tibia
Tillman RM, Smith RB (Royal Preston Hospital, Preston, England)
J Bone Joint Surg 73-B:516–517, 1991   3–59

Background.—Unlike the hip, the proximal tibia only rarely has metastatic deposits requiring operation. Prophylactic total knee replacement is a challenging procedure in such patients, and has been reported only 1 time previously. The procedure was used successfully in a terminally ill patient.

Case Report.—Man, 46, had advanced myeloma and was wheelchair-bound by a painful, large lytic metastasis in the right proximal tibia. Only the cortical shell was left intact, along with the collateral ligaments and patellar tendon. Total knee replacement was performed using a kinematic long-stem "stabilizer" prosthesis with a 21-mm tibial component. They used a triple mix of cement for the tibia, holding a plastic spatula to form a mold where the posterior cortex was completely destroyed and removing the spatula when the cement hardened. Satisfactory alignment and stability were achieved, and the patient was discharged to home 8 days postoperatively, free of pain and able to walk. Nine months later, he was readmitted for terminal care with the prosthesis intact.

Conclusions.—The proximal tibia is a rare site of metastatic lesions, for which total knee arthroplasty can be a rewarding procedure. The treatment goal is to improve quality of life, and the procedure is worthwhile if survival of even a few months is expected.

▶ This is an interesting case report, in which a grossly destroyed proximal tibia in a patient with malignancy was replaced by a combination of implant and a larger amount of cement. Because of the expected short duration of life in the patient, this approach has much to recommend it in terms of expediency and cost.—C.B. Sledge, M.D.

Functional Improvement and Costs of Hip and Knee Arthroplasty in Destructive Rheumatoid Arthritis
Jonsson B, Larsson S-E (Univ Hosp, Linköping, Sweden)
Scand J Rheumatol 20:351–357, 1991   3–60

Background.—Endoprosthetic reconstruction of the hip and knee has greatly improved the outlook for patients who have destructive rheumatoid arthritis. However, increasing medical costs make it necessary to analyze resource use, especially with respect to the functional improvement that can be achieved at different stages of rheumatoid disease.

Patients.—The functional results and costs of treatment were examined in 54 patients with destructive rheumatoid arthritis who underwent 31 knee and 23 hip arthroplasties. The 38 women and 16 men had a mean age of 63 years. The mean surgical stay was similar for hip and knee arthroplasty; however, a longer period of inpatient rehabilitation was required after knee arthroplasty.

Results.—Significant improvement was evident both objectively and subjectively 6 months after surgery. Patients of both genders and all ages improved. Less pain, better walking ability, and improved sleep all contributed to a better quality of life. The hospital costs were greater for knee arthroplasty. Home help costs declined by nearly one third. Many patients used fewer analgesics and nonsteroidal anti-inflammatory drugs after surgery. The use of walking aids was greatly reduced, and approximately 80% of the patients walked more than 90 minutes per week.

Conclusions.—Both functional ability and quality of life appear to improve significantly after hip or knee arthroplasty in patients with destructive rheumatoid disease. The cost benefits are substantial. Surgical reconstruction should be undertaken before the patient is seriously incapacitated.

▶ As cries for cost containment in medical care increase, it becomes ever more important to demonstrate the cost-effectiveness of elective reconstructive orthopedic surgery. This is the first demonstration, to my knowlege, of the cost savings made possible by hip and knee arthroplasty. The paper stresses the need to carry out these operations before the patients have been disabled too severely and for such a long period of time that return to independence is unlikely.—C.B. Sledge, M.D.

Patellar Problems

The Metal-Backed Patella: An Invitation for Failure?
Peters JD, Engh GA, Corpe RS (Fitzsimons Army Med Ctr, Aurora, Colo; Anderson Orthopaedic Research Inst, Arlington, Va)
J Arthroplasty 6:221–228, 1991   3–61

Background.—One of the newer designs for components for total knee arthroplasty (TKA) is metal backing applied to ultra-high molecular weight polyethylene. The metal backing has been used in tibial and patellar implants, but, recently, there is a disturbing incidence of metal-backed patellar component failure (Fig 3–8). The potential adverse outcome and the clinical spectrum of events associated with component failures were examined.

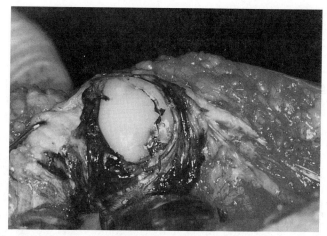

Fig 3–8.—Ultra-high molecular weight polyethylene wear on fragmentation. Intraoperative photograph of a fragmented plastic portion of the patellar component. (Courtesy of Peters JD, Engh GA, Corpe RS: *J Arthroplasty* 6:221–228, 1991.)

Methods.—Thirty-one cases of failed metal-backed patellar components requiring revision surgery were evaluated. Eighteen men and 13 women (average age, 66 years) underwent TKA for osteoarthritis or rheumatoid arthritis. Five types of manufacturer's components were used in these patients.

Results.—Factors contributing to failures of the metal-backed patellar components, as described by Stulberg, et al., included patellar implant design, patellar and femoral component size, surgical technique, clinical characteristics of patients, and femoral component design. Implant failure had either a gradual or sudden onset. In both modes there were delays in patient presentation and diagnosis of the failed component. A triad of symptoms of anterior knee pain, grating crepitance, and the presence of an effusion should be evaluated carefully in any patient with a metal-backed patellar implant.

Conclusions.—Onset of metal-backed patellar failure may be insidious, and the physician must be alert to the symptom complex associated with the onset of implant failure. The consequence of delayed diagnosis may be complete TKA revision. Discontinuing the use of metal-backed patellar components in TKA is recommended. If patellar resurfacing is performed, only an all-polyethylene prosthesis should be used. Both the patient and the physician should be aware of the triad of diffuse anterior knee pain, grating crepitance, and the presence of an effusion, which is characteristic of the failed metal-backed patella syndrome.

▶ Here is another paper suggesting that metal-backed patellar implants should be abandoned because of their propensity to wear through and produce severe destructive metal synovitis.—C.B. Sledge, M.D.

All-Polyethylene Patellar Components Are Not the Answer
Collier JP, McNamara JL, Surprenant VA, Jensen RE, Surprenant HP (Dartmouth College)
Clin Orthop 273:198–203, 1991   3–62

Background.—Metal backings for polyethylene-bearing prosthetic surfaces were developed to replace a worn bearing surface without separating the component from its cement mantle. However, recent reports of frequent polyethylene failure have increased interest in the use of cemented, all-polyethylene implant designs.

Methods.—A total of 104 retrieved patellar components of metal-backed and all-polyethylene designs were examined for wear. Using pressure-sensitive film, patellofemoral contact stress was measured as a function of flexion angle for unused components.

Results.—Significant wear was evident in 65% of the metal-backed designs and in 78% of the all-polyethylene components. Severe wear was present in 39% and 44% of instances, respectively. Severe wear was significantly less frequent in congruent designs than in noncongruent designs. Contact stress analysis showed that a dome-type geometry typically produced stresses that exceeded the yield strength of polyethylene; more congruent designs produced significantly less stress.

Conclusions.—If the goal of patellar design is to produce components that maintain their geometry over time, then the all-polyethylene dome-type patella is not the answer. Increased conformity will reduce both contact stress and the trend toward creep deformation. A highly congruent patella carries a low risk of polyethylene fatigue failure and allows cementless fixation.

▶ This paper, somewhat of a counterpoint to the preceding paper, suggests that all-polyethylene patellar components have their own problems and that the issues are more complex than whether or not there is a metal backing and include factors such as the contact area, stresses on the surface, and stresses on the fixation.—C.B. Sledge, M.D.

Polyethylene Wear

The Dominance of Cyclic Sliding in Producing Wear in Total Knee Replacements
Blunn GW, Walker PS, Joshi A, Hardinge K (University College, Stanmore, England; Wrightington Hosp, Appley Bridge, England)
Clin Orthop 273:253–260, 1991   3–63

Background.—Contact stress in condylar total knee replacements can exceed the yield strength of ultra-high molecular-weight polyethylene; such stress can lead to rapid breakdown of the plastic. Many retrieved knees exhibit marked damage that may extend through to the metal base plates. The range of surface damage is often quite wide—even for a particular prosthetic design.

Methods.—A test machine was developed that was applied to spherical-ended metal "femoral" components acting on a flat polyethylene "tibial" plateau. Loading was cyclical at 2.2 kilonewtons for 10 million cycles using a distilled water lubricant.

Results.—Cyclic loading produced a shiny depression. Oscillating and sliding motions, which were superimposed on cyclic loading, produced marked surface and subsurface cracking that resulted in high wear. Rolling motion produced a shiny wear track with minimal cracking. There was little surface damage in the cyclic load specimens.

Conclusions.—Low-confirmity prosthetic components that are inserted with high ligamentous laxity are vulnerable to anteroposterior sliding that leads to high wear. Moderate-to high-confirmity components are less susceptible to wear because they limit sliding and reduce contact stress.

▶ Polyethylene is exposed to different types of stress depending on whether it is subjected to rolling or sliding contact. This retrieval study, coupled with bench tests, suggests that sliding contact between polyethylene and metal produces more wear than does rolling. These findings have clear implications in the design of implants.—C.B. Sledge, M.D.

The Arthroscopic Evaluation and Characteristics of Severe Polyethylene Wear in Total Knee Arthroplasty

Mintz L, Tsao AK, McCrae CR, Stulberg SD, Wright T (Univ of Iowa; Northwestern Univ; Univ of Pennsylvania, Wyomissing, Pa; Hosp for Special Surgery, New York)
Clin Orthop 273:215–222, 1991

3–64

Background.—Polyethylene wear is an increasing concern in patients who undergo total knee arthroplasty (TKA). High contact stresses that are secondary to a lack of surface conformity, especially in malaligned implants or in those implants given to large, active patients, can lead to accelerated polyethylene wear, synovitis, pain, and ultimately, a loosened implant.

Patients.—Among a group of 487 porous-coated anatomical total arthroplasties performed by the same surgeon during an 8-year period, effusion, pain, or limited motion developed in 43 patients after a period of pain-free function. The symptoms developed an average of 4½ years after surgery. A total of 33 patients underwent arthroscopy; of these, 32 eventually required revision surgery.

Results.—Aspirated synovial fluid contained high-density polyethylene crystals that were best seen by polarized microscopy. Extensive wear and delamination were evident at arthroscopic examination. Although wear was most extensive on the medial tibial plateau, patellar polyethylene wear was also noted. Substantial abrasion of the femoral component was seen in areas where the tibial and patellar base plates had been exposed. Diffuse granulomatous synovial tissue exhibited a foreign-body giant-cell reaction to the polyethylene particles. Symptoms were temporarily lessened after arthroscopy in all patients. Subsequent revision surgery provided an opportunity to confirm the arthroscopic findings. Wear was most pronounced in younger, larger, and more active patients; in the presence of nonconforming femorotibial articular surfaces; and when the polyethylene was thin. In addition, nonrigid mechanical attachment of polyethylene to the metal base plate promoted wear.

Conclusions.—Younger and more active patients must be watched closely for evidence of polyethylene wear after TKA. Arthroscopy can help diagnose and determine the extent of polyethylene wear.

▶ Thirty-three patients with symptomatic TKAs were subjected to arthroscopic evaluation to see if there was a correlation between wear as assessed by arthroscopic exam and that found at subsequent surgery. The authors determined that arthroscopy is a reliable way of determining the presence and extent of polyethylene wear and may be a useful technique in evaluating patients with symptomatic knee arthroplasties in whom other examinations, including radiography, are noninformative.—C.B. Sledge, M.D.

Complications of Total Knee Arthroplasty

The Infected Knee Arthroplasty: A 6-Year Follow-Up of 357 Cases
Bengtson S, Knutson K (Lund Univ, Sweden)
Acta Orthop Scand 62:301–311, 1991   3–65

Introduction.—A retrospective, multicenter investigation, of the treatment of infected knee arthroplasties was conducted. The included patients were those treated in the community and reported to the Swedish Knee Arthroplasty Project.

Methods.—From October 1975 through 1985, 12,118 primary knee arthroplasties were reported, of which 1,214 underwent 1,518 revisions during the same period because of aseptic loosening or instability. Deep infection had been reported after primary arthroplasty in 309 knees and after a noninfected revision arthroplasty in 48 knees. Systemic antibiotics alone were primarily used in 225 knees. The infection healed in 44 of these, 20 of which had a functioning prosthesis at final follow-up. Soft tissue surgery was performed in 154 knees, with healing in 37 knees, 15 of which had a functioning prosthesis. Resection arthroplasty was carried out in 22 knees, with healing in 11 knees. Revision arthroplasty was performed in 107 knees, with healing in 81 knees, 36 of which had a functioning prosthesis. Arthrodesis was attempted in 135 knees, with eventual healing of the deep infection in 120 knees and fusion in 105. An above-the-knee amputation was performed in 22 patients.

Outcome.—At final follow-up, deep infection was considered clinically healed in 315 knees (88%), 271 after surgery and 44 after systemic antibiotics alone. However, only 71 knees (20%) had recovered with a functioning prosthesis, and 8 patients had died of infection.

Conclusions.—In primary knee arthroplasty, attention should be focused on prophylactic measures directed toward potential soft tissue problems by avoiding conflicting skin incisions, by handling periarticular soft tissues gently, by avoiding the use of constrained prostheses and oversized compartmental prostheses, by letting wound healing take priority over motion in knees with compromised soft tissue, and by using prophylactic antibiotic treatment for skin ulcers until these have healed.

▶ Infection remains the most dreaded complication of knee arthroplasty. The authors of this paper stress the importance of preventive measures because corrective measures are not entirely satisfactory.— C.B. Sledge, M.D.

Treatment of Acutely Infected Arthroplasty With Local Antibiotics
Davenport K, Traina S, Perry C (Marquette Gen Hosp, Mich; Orthopedic Associates, Denver; Washington Univ)
J Arthroplasty 6:179–183, 1991   3–66

Background.—Infection involving a total joint arthroplasty can result in an unacceptably high level of patient morbidity. The treatment of acutely infected arthroplasty with local antibiotics was examined.

Methods.—Twenty-two patients with acutely infected total joint arthroplasties—9 in the hip and 13 in the knee—were treated. After the organisms were identified and the patients' general medical condition was assessed, the patients were treated with an implantable antibiotic pump that permitted delivery of a high concentration of antibiotic solution to a localized area. Systemic antibiotic levels were kept to a minimum to eliminate the potential serious side effects of antibiotic treatment.

Results.—Local concentrations exceeded the minimal inhibitory concentration eightfold to tenfold in all patients. Of the 20 patients with follow-up of at least 30 months, 17 were judged free of infection. Three treatment failures occurred. Organisms treated included gram-negative, gram-positive, and some mixed infections.

Conclusions.—The results of local antibiotic treatment of acutely infected arthroplasty are encouraging. Additional patients are continually being enrolled in the investigation.

▶ It is possible to achieve high local levels of antibiotic with the use of an implantable pump. This appears to be a useful method for treating some cases of infected knee arthroplasty. It is important to note that the patients in this study had acute infections, defined as presentation within 3 months of joint implantation. In this group of patients it was possible to retain the prosthesis in a functional manner in 17 of 20 patients treated.— C.B. Sledge, M.D.

Suppressive Antibiotic Therapy in Chronic Prosthetic Joint Infections
Tsukayama DT, Wicklund B, Gustilo RB (Hennepin County Med Ctr, Minneapolis)
Orthopedics 14:841–844, 1991   3–67

Background.—The best treatment for chronically infected prosthetic joints is implant removal and systemic antibiotic treatment; however, implant removal has its own risks and morbidity. Thirteen patients receiving prolonged suppressive antibiotic treatment for chronic prosthetic joint infection were evaluated to determine whether this treatment can allow joint salvage and to assess the rate of treatment-related complications.

Patients.—Eight patients had chronic infections with total knee arthroplasty, and 5 had chronic infections with total hip arthroplasty. Management was with suppressive antibiotic treatment, surgical débridement, and 4–6 weeks of intravenously administered antibiotics. Seven patients had underlying rheumatoid arthritis, and 6 had degenerative joint disease. All infections had lasted at least 3 months, with a mean follow-up of 38 months from the start of suppressive therapy. Pathogens recovered included coagulase-positive staphylococci in 7 patients, coagulase-negative staphylococci in 6 patients, *Salmonella choleraesuis* in 1 patient, and *Proteus mirabilis* in 1 patient.

Results.—Prostheses were salvaged in only 3 patients, with follow-up times of 24, 34, and 45 months. Two had recurrent episodes of inflammation, but none had wound breakdown or drainage. Of the 10 patients who required removal of the prosthesis, mean time to removal was 16 months for hip and 27 months for knee prostheses. Intravenously administered antibiotics were given for 4–6 weeks after implant removal. Three hip patients were managed with resection arthroplasty and 2 were managed with revision arthroplasty; 3 knee patients had arthrodesis, 1 had delayed revision arthroplasty after removal of the prosthesis and 1 had pseudoarthrosis after removal of the prosthesis. There were 3 instances of recurrent infection and 3 instances of adverse side effects, with 38% of patients requiring a change in antibiotic.

Conclusions.—In patients with chronic joint prosthesis infections, suppressive antibiotic treatment is of limited effectiveness. There is also a significant incidence of adverse effects. Management of these patients should include prosthesis removal; innovative approaches are needed for patients in whom this is not feasible.

▶ In patients with chronic infection after total knee arthroplasty it may not always be possible or desirable to remove the implant, manage the infection, and do a delayed reimplantation. In such instances suppressive antibiotic treatment is attractive. This paper suggests, however, that such management is fraught with difficulties and cannot be recommended when any other approach is possible.—C.B. Sledge, M.D.

Radiographic Detection of Metal-Induced Synovitis As a Complication of Arthroplasty of the Knee
Weissman BN, Scott RD, Brick GW, (Brigham and Women's Hosp, Boston)
J Bone Joint Surg 73-A:1002–1007, 1991   3–68

Background.—Metal-induced synovitis is a reported complication of total knee arthroplasties (TKAs) in which hinged knee prostheses are implanted. Metal-induced synovitis after total knee replacement may be caused by wear of a metal-backed patellar or tibial component. The radiographs of 18 patients with diagnosed metal-induced synovitis after TKA were reviewed.

Methods.—Multiple sets of radiographs were available for 11 patients, and 1 set of radiographs was available for the other 7. All radiographs were examined for the presence of a dense line outlining a portion of the capsule or articular surface of the knee joint, called a metal-line sign. Histologic sections of resected synovial tissue were available for 15 patients. Bone and articular cartilage specimens were available for 8 patients.

Findings.—A metal-line sign associated with wear was found in the radiographs of 11 patients. Specimens for histologic examination were available for 9 of these 11 patients. All 9 specimens had dense depositions of metal particles in the synovial tissue. In contrast, 5 of 6 specimens from patients who did not have a metal-line sign on their radiographs contained only slight amounts of metal in the synovial tissue, and the sixth specimen contained only a moderate amount of metal.

Conclusion.—The appearance of a radiographic metal-line sign after TKA is essentially diagnostic, particularly when seen on radiographs obtained a year or more after operation.

▶ When metal articulates with metal in a knee arthroplasty, minute amounts of material are shed into the joint cavity and are eventually picked up by macrophages in the synovial lining. When the metal debris reaches a sufficiently high concentration, it can be visualized on radiographs as a linear density outlining the synovial lining. When detected, it is a useful diagnostic clue when the patient with a TKA has a chronic effusion.—C.B. Sledge, M.D.

Periprosthetic Fractures of the Femur After Total Knee Arthroplasty: A Literature Review and Treatment Algorithm
DiGioia AM III, Rubash HE (Univ of Pittsburgh)
Clin Orthop 271:135–142, 1991

3–69

Background.—Supracondylar fractures of the femur after total knee arthroplasty (TKA) can cause significant problems in the outcome of knee arthroplasty. The literature was reviewed for reports of such fractures, and treatment approaches proposed in the past decade were assessed. Predisposing factors, injury mechanisms, and fracture characteristics for this problem were identified.

Literature review.—In 1981, case reports of distal femoral fractures after TKA began to appear in the medical literature. Most of these patients underwent immediate cast immobilization for nondisplaced breakages and open reduction and internal fixation for other types of fractures. Notching of the anterior femoral cortex often was associated with these fractures. A review of 22 patients with 24 ipsilateral supracondylar femur

TREATMENT ALGORITHM

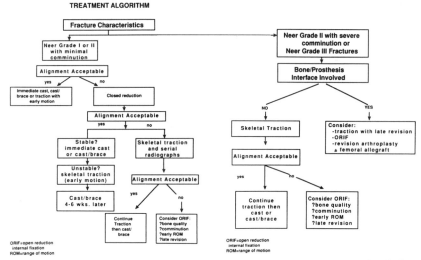

Fig 3–9.—Proposed algorithm for the treatment of periprosthetic femoral fracture based on the fracture characteristics and degree of comminution. (Courtesy of DiGioia AM III, Rubash HE: *Clin Orthop* 271:135–142, 1991.)

fractures occurring above the TKA demonstrated the overall incidence of these breakages to be 1.8%. Treatments for these 22 patients included cast immobilization, open reduction and internal fixation, and custom TKA (e.g., external fixator application, distal femoral allografts, and immediate primary arthrodesis). The latter approach stressed avoidance of anterior femoral notching and bypassing such a notch using an uncemented stem.

Recommendations.—Based on the literature review, a treatment protocol was derived from a modified Neer classification of the distal fracture and overall fracture characteristics (Fig 3–9). Under this treatment plan, a grade I fracture with acceptable position would be immobilized immediately in a cast, with subsequent early cast bracing. If the fracture position is unacceptable, other treatments may be tried, particularly closed reduction under anesthesia. Use of open reduction and internal fixation should be based on bone quality and degree of comminution at the fracture site.

Conclusions.—Treatment for supracondylar fractures of the femur after TKA requires the consideration of many factors to establish a workable protocol for all patients involved.

▶ Fractures about the knee after TKA are uncommon and difficult to manage. The authors of this paper suggest that some patients can be treated by temporary immobilization, that others will require closed reduction followed by immobilization, and that some will require open reductions and internal fixation. A treatment algorithm is proposed to facilitate decision-making in this complex issue.—C.B. Sledge, M.D.

4 Hip Reconstruction and Osteoporosis

Introduction

The literature of 1992 focuses on certain aspects of the imaging of the hip and on the documentation of the results of total hip arthroplasty and dwells to a great degree on the deleterious effects of particulate debris in total joint replacement. We are now entering an era where clinical and radiographic data can be collected in a uniform manner, thus allowing comparison of results from many centers. Digitization of radiographs and their semiautomated analysis will greatly facilitate these types of studies. It is apparent that global scores do not convey adequate information about the results of hip replacement, and, therefore, contemporary reporting of the results of hip replacement must use standard definitions and address specific areas of function and radiographs. Importantly, increasing emphasis is now being placed on the patient's assessment of the results of surgery, so outcome assessment will be a vital part of the analysis of the results of this type of surgery.

A number of papers report on newer treatment protocols for indomethacin and radiation in the prevention of heterotopic bone. New strategies aimed at reducing deep vein thrombosis and pulmonary emboli are also reviewed. Some very provocative laboratory studies point the way to biologic replacement of tissues rather than prosthetic replacement. There is still much work to be done to realize the potential of biologic replacement, but these studies clearly represent the beginning steps along that path.

Robert Poss, M.D.

The Acetabular Rim Syndrome: A Clinical Presentation of Dysplasia of the Hip
Klaue K, Durnin CW, Ganz R (Inselspital, Berne, Switzerland)
J Bone Joint Surg 73-B:423–429, 1991   4–1

Background.—The acetabular rim syndrome can precede osteoarthritis of the hip secondary to acetabular dysplasia. Tears of the limbus, with or without an associated bone fragment, can occur after traumatic hip dislocation or may occur without a history of injury. The nature of this syndrome, as seen in 29 patients, was described.

Clinical Features.—None of the 29 patients were asymptomatic. The patients, mostly young adults, described sharp pain in the groin and a

155

feeling that the hip was locking after either sitting or walking. Often the pain was relieved by shaking the extremity. When questioned, some patients recalled a long past incident in which the hip had been stressed in rotation, producing sudden pain and a "dead" leg feeling. Pain usually could be produced by passively moving the thigh into full flexion, adduction, and internal rotation. Imaging did not always document a labral tear.

Surgical Findings.— A all clinical diagnoses of a torn limbus were confirmed at operation, with the tears being found at the anterosuperior quadrant of the acetabular rim. Intraosseous ganglia were seen from within the joint and extraosseous ganglia, when present, extruded through the limbal defect.

Management.— The goal of surgery was to correct deficient acetabular coverage of the femoral head by means of a periacetabular osteotomy. Twelve patients had the limbal tear repaired, and 12 others had the torn limbus resected. Patients who underwent repair recovered more slowly than the others, and 2 of them required revision to remove a reruptured limbus.

Conclusions.— Refixing the torn limbus to the bony acetabular rim is not of definite value. Resection of the limbus may impair joint lubrication and thereby promote degenerative change. The best treatment remains elusive.

▶ The acetabular rim syndrome is a physical sign associated with dysplasia of the hip. The importance of this paper is that it points out that the appropriate treatment must address restoration of sufficient bony coverage of the femoral head. The torn or displaced labrum and its clinical manifestation are best treated as part of the comprehensive approach to the dysplastic hip.— R. Poss, M.D.

Measurement of Hip Prostheses Using Image Analysis: The MAXIMA Hip Technique
Hardinge K, Porter ML, Jones PR, Hukins DWL, Taylor CJ (Wrightington Hosp, Wigan, England; Univ of Manchester, England)
J Bone Joint Surg 73-B:724–728, 1991   4–2

Background.— Angular and linear measurements from plain radiographs are an important part of orthopedic research, but manual measurements of this type are tedious and subjective. A computerized image analysis system, the Manchester X-ray image analysis (MAXIMA) technique, was developed to measure parameters in patients who have had total hip replacement.

The System.— The system relies on a frame grabber card contained in a personal computer that converts camera output into a digital image. The system software can improve the quality of the image, including the enhancement of areas of special interest, and can quantify predetermined parameters, some of which are generated automatically and some of which are identified in interaction with the software. Several measurements from coronal plane radiographs are programmed into the system. Images are recorded on cartridges, each of which are capable of storing 50 images.

Applications.—The system can easily detect bending of the femoral component by successive measurements of the angle between the midline of its neck and stem. Measurements between the proximal and distal transverse lines of the stem can be made to assess stem subsidence. Cup migration and wear can be measured by automatic and interactive reference points. The user can generate and automatically plot Shenton's line on the image, and the cortical thickness of the femoral shaft can be measured easily and reliably. System reproducibility is within .01 mm, and accuracy is within .5 mm.

Discussion.—The MAXIMA system of radiographic analysis was used to study important sequential features in total hip replacement. Prospective clinical trials of the system are in the planning stages.

▶ In the next few years we will increasingly benefit from the application of computer technology to the documentation of orthopedic procedures. In this paper, the authors introduce a semiautomated method of analyzing digitized radiographs. The eventual use of computerized clinical and radiographic databases will greatly enhance the accuracy and efficiency of assessing the results of total hip replacement in particular and the outcome of the treatment of muscukoskeletal problems in general.—R. Poss, M.D.

The Effect of Stem Stiffness on Femoral Bone Resorption After Canine Porous-Coated Total Hip Arthroplasty
Bobyn JD, Glassman AH, Goto H, Krygier JJ, Miller JE, Brooks CE (Montreal Gen Hosp)
Clin Orthop 261:196–213, 1990   4–3

Background.—Fracture fixation devices and prostheses tend to deprive bones of normal physiologic stresses, inducing osteopenia. This so-called stress shielding increases with both stem size and increasing amount of porous coating. Flexible implants have been developed, but their effect on stress shielding has not been documented. A canine model was developed using porous-coated hip prostheses to evaluate the relationship between stem stiffness and stress-related bone resorption.

Methods.—Two porous-coated canine hip stems of identical configurations and external dimensions were compared. The first was made of a cobalt–chromium alloy, and the second, made of titanium alloy, was hollowed out to a wall thickness of 1 mm. The differences in stiffness between the 2 were 5.4-fold axially and 3.6-fold in bending and torsion. Staged bilateral total hip arthroplasties were performed on 8 dogs, with each receiving 1 prosthesis of each type. After implantation and recovery, the dogs underwent roentgenography for evidence of bone remodeling; after death the femora was studied histologically. Bone ingrowth and remodeling were quantified by computer-aided image analysis.

Results.—Within each dog there was consistently increased resorption on the stiff stem size. Bone resorption was evidenced by cortical thinning and change in cross-sectional size and geometry. This remodeling was apparent within the first 6–9 postoperative months, with no noticeable changes occurring after that time. Femora with flexible stems had an average of 25% to 35% more cortical bone area than those with stiff stems. The degree and extent of bone ingrowth appeared similar for the 2 types of stems. All implants showed bone ingrowth fixation at multiple points along the implant length.

Conclusion.—Stem stiffness has a strong influence on absorptive bone remodeling of the canine femur. Use of a flexible stem results in more uniform load transfer and reduced stress shielding.

Quantifying Bone Loss From the Proximal Femur After Total Hip Arthroplasty
McCarthy CK, Steinberg GG, Agren M, Leahey D, Wyman E, Baran DT (Univ of Massachusetts, Worcester)
J Bone Joint Surg 73-B:774–778, 1991   4–4

Background.—Resorption of bone from the proximal femur contributes significantly to the failure of total hip arthroplasty (THA). The natural history of bone resorption was defined around the femoral stem of a THA.

Methods.—Using dual-energy x-ray densitometry, the bone mineral content (BMC) and bone mineral density (MBD) were measured in 28 patients with unilateral THA, 18 age-matched controls, and 7 patients with osteoarthritis. The measurements were made inside the lesser trochanter (box 1) and 4.8 cm distal to it (box 2); they were then compared in the affected femur and the contralateral femur (Fig 4–1).

Results.—In the patients undergoing THA, the average BMC and BMD in box 1 and box 2 were significantly lower in the prosthetic femur than in the nonoperated femur. There was a significant difference in BMC at box 1 and box 2 between the patients undergoing THA and the normal age-matched controls and osteoarthritic controls. Between 1 and 3 years after THA there was a 40% loss in BMC in box 1 and a 29% loss in BMC in box 2. At 7–14 years after THA there was a 47% loss in box 1 and a 49% loss in box 2, suggesting a progressive cortical bone loss in the proximal femur adjacent to the femoral prosthesis after THA. The majority of the loss appeared to occur within 3 years of THA, with continuing loss at 7–14 years, particularly in box 2.

Conclusion.—The bone loss around a femoral prosthesis appears to be significant and progressive, and it may occur in a proximal-to-distal pattern.

▶ The degree to which prosthetic design and materials influence the response of bone is dramatically demonstrated in the paper by Bobyn et al. (Abstract

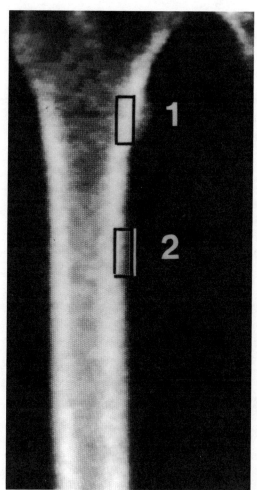

Fig 4–1.—The location of sample boxes 1 and 2, scanned by the Lunar DPX bone densitometer. (Courtesy of McCarthy CK, Steinberg GG, Agren M, et al: *J Bone Joint Surg* 73-B:774–778, 1991.)

4–3). Implant stiffness is determined in large part by the properties of the material and, perhaps more importantly, by the geometry of the implant, because stiffness is directly proportional to the fourth power of the diameter. In this study, stiffer stems produced 25% to 35% more cortical bone resorption than their more flexible counterparts. The results of the study by Bobyn et al. using dogs is corroborated in humans with the use of dual energy x-ray densitometry. McCarthy and associates found that 3 years after cementless THA there was approximately a 40% loss in average bone mineral content at the level of the lesser trochanter and that 7–14 years after surgery there had been no quantitative adaptive response to compensate for that loss. A consequence of canal-filling, metallic femoral prostheses is bone loss. The degree to which this proximal osteopenia may limit the longevity of hip implants remains to be determined.—R. Poss, M.D.

Fixation and Loosening of Hip Prostheses: A Review
Mjöberg B (Uppsala Univ Hosp, Sweden)
Acta Orthop Scand 62:500–508, 1991   4–5

Background.—The good results of cemented hip arthroplasty deteriorate as mechanical loosening occurs. Radiographic signs of loosening may occur late; this has led to the restriction of the term "loosening" to clinical and radiographic failure. Issues related to the fixation and loosening of hip prostheses were reviewed.

Discussion.—Based on the results of roentgen stereophotogrammetry and bone scintigraphy, a broad definition of prosthetic loosening may be proposed: migration. This implies a narrow definition of fixation: nonmigration. In cemented hip arthroplasty, the acetabular component migrates more commonly than the femoral component does. Studies using roentgen stereophotogrammetry suggest that loosening begins at an early stage when it occurs. Even in patients without symptoms, roentgen stereophotogrammetry may reveal migration of 1 or both components in the first year after implantation. Some of these components are likely to fail with time. Instability and progressive resorption of bone may occur if initial fixation is insufficient or fixation is lost by resorption of a layer of heat-injured bone. Shear stress is greater on the femoral than on the acetabular component; fixation of the femoral component may not be achieveable more than occasionally without the use of bone cement. Heat injury does not occur in uncemented prostheses, but debris from external wear of the polyethylene cup can contribute to resorption. Although the prosthetic collar might help prevent subsidence of the uncemented femoral component, it will not prevent axial rotation of the femoral component; once the initial prosthetic fixation is lost, it probably cannot be re-established.

Conclusions.—In hip prostheses, late loosening appears to result from late detection rather than delayed loss of fixation. Important causes of loosening in epidemiologic studies, such as body weight, physical activity, and varus/valgus position, may have only a secondary influence. Other proposed causes, such as responses to wear products, metal sensitivity, stress-shielding, and immunologic responses, are probably results of loosening.

▶ Roentgen stereophotogrammetry is an exquisitely sensitive method of determining migration of components. By using this technique, all loose prosthetic components are seen to have been migrating and no nonmigrating component is found to be loose. The author has found that migration begins early in the postoperative course and is probably the result of failure of a number of aspects of surgical technique and of the quality of bone. So called risk factors (increased weight, increased activity) are then superimposed on the initial suboptimal mechanical fixation and result in late loosening.—R. Poss, M.D.

The Initiation of Failure in Cemented Femoral Components of Hip Arthroplasties

Jasty M, Maloney WJ, Bragdon CR, O'Connor DO, Haire T, Harris WH (Massachusetts Gen Hosp, Boston; Harvard Med School)

J Bone Joint Surg 73-B:551–558, 1991   4–6

Objective.—To define the mechanisms involved in initiating the loosening of cemented femoral components, 16 femora were harvested at the postmortem examination from 12 patients who had undergone a satisfactory cemented total hip arthroplasty from 2 weeks to 17 years before death. Morphological and fractographical studies of the cement and its interfaces were performed.

Findings.—Only 1 specimen had definite radiographic evidence of loosening. In the remaining 15 specimens, the implants were stable to mechanical testing. None of the 16 specimens had morphological evidence of loosening at the cement–bone interface, and all but 1 had minimal fibrous tissue formation. However, some debonding at the cement–prosthesis interface and fractures in the cement mantle were common. The most common early feature was debonding of the cement from the metal, seen at the proximal and distal ends of the prosthesis. Debonding tended to be extensive in those specimens that were retrieved late; it was complete in 2 specimens retrieved at 118 and 156 months. Fractures in the cement mantle were common in prostheses that had been in use for more than 3 years. These fractures were oriented either circumferentially near the cement–metal interface or radially extending from the interface into the cement and sometimes to the bony interface. Both types of fractures were associated with debonding of cement from metal. The most extensive cement fractures appeared to have started at or near sharp corners in the metal or where the cement mantle was thin or incomplete. The fractures also appeared to originate from voids in the cement.

Conclusion.—Long-term failure of the fixation of cemented femoral components appears to be primarily mechanical, starting with debonding at the interface between the cement and the prosthesis, and continuing as slowly developing fractures in the cement mantle.

▶ Postmortem examination of total hip replacement in patients who had well-functioning hips has provided invaluable insights into the mechanisms of bone adaptation and the failure of fixation with time. In this study, the authors find that femoral loosening is initiated at the metal cement bone, where the cement mantle was not of optimum thickness or where there was suboptimal homogeneity of the cement. Contemporary cemented total hip replacement is vastly superior to the first generation of total hip replacements but can be improved even further by optimizing the metal–cement bond, insuring a cement mantle adequate in both thickness and homogeneity.—R. Poss, M.D.

Range of Motion in Contemporary Total Hip Arthroplasty: The Impact of Modular Head–Neck Components

Krushell RJ, Burke DW, Harris WH (Brigham and Women's Hosp; Massachusetts Gen Hosp, Boston)
J Arthroplasty 6:97–101, 1991   4–7

Background.— Most contemporary hip arthroplasty systems incorporate a Morse taper in the femoral neck, thereby allowing the use of modular femoral head components of varying neck lengths. Many of the components with longer neck lengths have a flange or skirt. These changes in implant geometry presumably can influence the prosthetic range of motion.

Methods.— The range of motion of 2 modular total hip arthroplasty systems (Zimmer HGP and Howmedica PCA) and of an older nonmodular system (Howmedica HD-2) was estimated by using an apparatus that incorporates a 3-dimensional protractor to stimulate compressive force across the hip joint.

Findings.— The modular systems had a smaller range of motion than the nonmodular system, most obviously because of the flanges of longer head–neck components. The limiting effect was more evident as head size decreased. The total arc from maximal flexion to maximal extension was as little as 113 degrees (for the PCA).

Conclusions.— Modular head–neck components may carry a substantially smaller range of motion than older hip arthroplasty systems and have an increased risk of prosthetic impingement. If instability is noted during the reduction of trial components, the options include repositioning the component, using a longer necked femoral component with a shorter head–neck component that lacks a flange, and using a larger sized femoral head if the acetabulum is large enough.

Corrosion of Modular Hip Prostheses

Mathiesen EB, Lindgren JU, Blomgren GGA, Reinholt FP (Karolinska Inst, Huddinge, Sweden)
J Bone Joint Surg 73-B:569–575, 1991   4–8

Objective.— Cobalt-chromium alloys have been used successfully as orthopedic implant materials. Previous trials have shown in vivo corrosion of surgical implants. A group of 9 uncemented madreporic hip prostheses that had been revised was examined to analyze the retrieved components and the adjacent tissues.

Setting.— All the hip modular prostheses were made of cast cobalt-chromium alloys. These prostheses had been revised after a mean of 52 months as a result of late infection in 2 patients, femoral stem loosening or fracture in 2, loosening of threaded cups in 3, and protrusion of bipolar cups in 2.

Results.— At surgery 4 hips showed discoloration of bone and soft tissues and had black deposits at the junction between the head and neck of

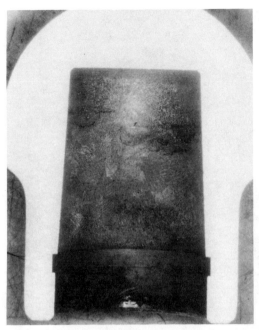

Fig 4–2.—The interior channel of a modular Lord head. The head has been cut in half to show the rough appearance of the surface. (Courtesy of Mathieson EB, Lindgren JU, Blomgren GGA, et al: *J Bone Joint Surg* 73-B:569–575, 1991.)

the prostheses. Similarly, the interior channel and the corresponding taper of the femoral neck showed discoloration and a rough appearance (Fig 4–2). The other 5 prostheses were not affected. In most hips histologic examination showed extensive necrosis and histiocytic proliferation, as well as mononuclear infiltration. Obliterative vascular changes were uncommon, but metal particles were often found in these areas. Scanning electron microscopy of the soft tissue with energy dispersive analysis showed peaks of cobalt, chromium, molybdenum, calcium, and phosphorus. Metallographic examination of the prosthetic heads showed structural imperfections and inhomogeneity in the corroded heads with discoloration but not in the modular heads without discoloration.

Conclusion.—These findings suggest that the crevice between the head and the neck is a potential site of corrosion in modular designs.

Corrosion at the Interface of Cobalt-Alloy Heads on Titanium-Alloy Stems
Collier JP, Surprenant VA, Jensen RE, Mayor MB (Dartmouth College; Dartmouth–Hitchcock Med Ctr, Hanover, NH)
Clin Orthop 271:305–312, 1991   4–9

Background.—Press-fit and biologic fixations are commonly done with the combination of a cobalt-alloy head on a titanium-alloy femoral hip stem. However, corrosion has been observed recently around the neck of a titanium-alloy femoral component and inside the tapered recess of the

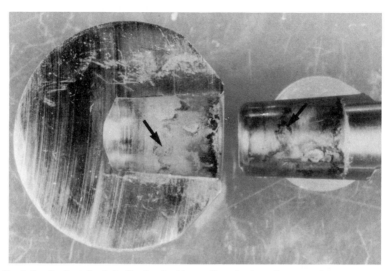

Fig 4–3.—Section of cobalt-alloy head with matching titanium-alloy tapered stem (3×), which shows crevice corrosion of large area of both surfaces *(arrows)*. This device was removed with head tightly fixed 54 months after operation because of pain. (Courtesy of Collier JP, Surprenant VA, Jensen RE, et al: *Clin Orthop* 271:305–312, 1991.)

mated cobalt head. Modular head hip prostheses were reexamined to evaluate the extent and magnitude of corrosion of this interface.

Methods.—Eighty-eight uncemented, porous-coated femoral hip prostheses were examined, including 49 composed of a cobalt-alloy stem and head, 30 composed of a titanium-alloy stem and cobalt-alloy head, and 9 composed of a titanium-alloy stem and head. The neck of the femoral component and the matching tapered recess of the head were carefully examined for corrosion. If any was found, the head was sectioned to detail its location and extent.

Results.—No corrosion was found in any of the matched cobalt-alloy heads on cobalt-alloy stems or titanium-alloy heads on titanium-alloy stems. However, 57% of the cobalt-alloy–titanium-alloy prostheses showed evidence of crevice corrosion. Duration of implantation ranged from .5 to 67 months and was significantly correlated with percentage of corrosion found on the femoral head component. On the tapered interface between the components, corrosion was identified by the loss of material and the elimination of machining marks (Fig 4–3). Loss of material into host tissue was plainly seen, and pitting was visible on electron microscopic examination.

Conclusions.—Corrosion may occur in mixed-alloy femoral hip prostheses. This represents a previously unsuspected source of metal ion release from prostheses. In the long-term, corrosion could also result in loss of head-to-stem fixation.

▶ Modularity in contemporary total hip and total knee systems brings with it the obvious advantages of versatility and a reduced inventory but also carries a number of problems that are a source of complications. The increased diameter of prosthetic femoral necks, particularly those longer necks that require a collar, result in a decreased impingement-free range of motion. The immediate consequence of this increasing impingement can be dislocation, and a long-term consequence can be the generation of particulate polyethylene debris. Other problems associated with modular femoral necks are fretting corrosion and, in some instances, fracture of the prosthetic femoral neck. While all metal–metal interfaces (distal sleeves, modular collars, proximal modular bodies) are sources for the generation of metal particulate debris, the most troublesome area thus far identified is the head–neck interface.— R. Poss, M.D.

Effect of Short-Course Indomethacin on Heterotopic Bone Formation After Uncemented Total Hip Arthroplasty
McMahon JS, Waddell JP, Morton J (St Michael's Hosp; Univ of Toronto)
J Arthroplasty 6:259–264, 1991   4–10

Background.— A recent prospective trial showed that 75 mg of indomethacin administered daily for 6 weeks is effective in reducing the incidence and the severity of heterotopic bone formation after cemented total hip arthroplasty (THA). Whether a shorter course of indomethacin can effectively suppress bone formation, thereby reducing the risk of side effects, and whether indomethacin can be used after uncemented arthroplasty were investigated.

Methods.— A group of 200 consecutive primary THAs was examined using the uncemented madreporic St. Michael's THA system. A group of 108 patients received no indomethacin prophylaxis, and a group of 92 patients received 25 mg of indomethacin 3 times daily for 10 days starting on the first postoperative day. Pain, range of motion, and radiographs of the hip were evaluated up to 24 months postoperatively.

Results.— The incidence and severity of heterotopic bone formation were significantly decreased among patients who received indomethacin prophylaxis as compared with controls. Among those patients who received indomethacin, 80% had no heterotopic ossification, only 1 patient had grade 3 involvement, and none had grade 4 involvement. In contrast, among those patients who received no prophylaxis, only 30% were free of heterotopic ossification, and 24% demonstrated grade 3 or grade 4 ectopic bone formation. Radiographs of the hip showed that indomethacin did not interfere with bone–prosthesis interface in the 2 groups; furthermore, indomethacin did not adversely affect the postoperative pain scores.

Conclusion.— A 25 mg dosage of indomethacin given 3 times daily for 10 days can effectively reduce the incidence and severity of heterotopic ossification without adversely affecting the stability of the St. Michael's madreporic system.

Single-Dose Radiation Therapy for Prevention of Heterotopic Ossification After Total Hip Arthroplasty

Healy WL, Lo TCM, Covall DJ, Pfeifer BA, Wasilewski SA (Lahey Clinic Med Ctr, Burlington, Mass)
J Arthroplasty 5:369–375, 1990   4–11

Background.—Heterotopic ossification (HO) is a recognized complication of total hip arthroplasty (THA) that can compromise the surgical outcome by limiting hip motion. Multidose radiation protocols have proved effective in preventing HO after hip arthroplasty.

Methods.—The efficacy of single-dose radiation therapy in a dose of 700 cGY was examined in 31 patients with 34 hips at high risk for HO. The most frequent risk factors were previous HO (in 27 hips) and ankylosing spondylitis (in 10 hips). Nineteen hips had primary, and 11 had revision arthroplasty; 4 underwent excision of HO. Radiation treatment was administered as soon as possible after surgery, most often on the first postoperative day. All patients were treated with 4- or 10-megaelectron volt radiation.

Results.—No patient had clinically significant HO after radiation treatment. Two hips had recurrent disease, for a 94% radiographic success rate. There was 1 late wound infection, and 2 of 6 patients who had transtrochanteric osteotomy for revision arthroplasty had nonunion of the greater trochanter.

Conclusions.—Single-dose radiation treatment can prevent HO after hip arthroplasty. It is less expensive than multidose treatment and is more easily administered.

▶ Regardless of the method used for heterotopic bone prophylaxis, virtually all authors have maintained that to be successful treatment must be initiated early in the postoperative course. During the past 4 years a number of papers have appeared advocating indomethacin as an effective agent for this prophylaxis. The trial described in Abstract 4–10 suggests that a course of only 10 days, so long as it is begun on the first postoperative day, seems to be as effective as previous protocols that called for a longer course of treatment. In Abstract 4–11, a single dose of radiation of 700 cGy was found to be effective in the prevention of heterotopic bone when administered as soon as possible after surgery, usually on the first postoperative day.—R. Poss, M.D.

Should Nonsteroidal Anti-Inflammatory Drugs Be Stopped Before Elective Surgery?

Connelly CS, Panush RS (Univ of Florida; St. Barnabas Med Ctr, Livingston, NJ)
Arch Intern Med 151:1963–1966, 1991   4–12

Background.—There is considerable concern about the safety of administering nonsteroidal anti-inflammatory drugs (NSAIDs) to patients in the perioperative period. Such drugs might increase the risk of bleeding-

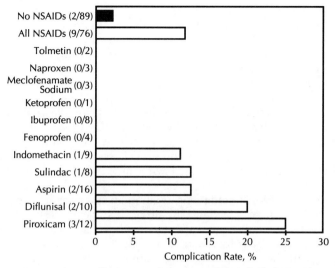

Fig 4–4.—Postoperative complication rates for patients taking individual NSAIDs. Complication rate (numbers in parentheses) is expressed as number of complications-number of patients taking that NSAID. (Courtesy of Connelly CS, Panush RS: *Arch Intern Med* 151:1963–1966, 1991.)

events and increase morbidity. This issue was investigated in patients undergoing total hip arthroplasty (THA).

Patients.—Included were 165 patients who had primary THA during a 4-year period. Fifty-one percent were men. At admission 76 patients were taking NSAIDs and 89 were not. Mean age was 60 years in the group

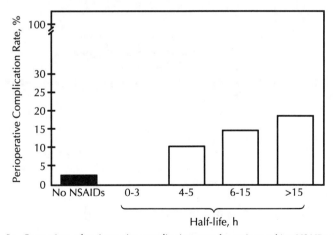

Fig 4–5.—Comparison of perioperative complication rates for patients taking NSAIDs. Drugs are grouped by pharmacologic half-lives (for aspirin, the half-life of the effect on platelet function was used). Differences between groups were statistically significant. Drugs with a half-life of 0 to 3 hours included fenoprofen, ibuprofen, meclofenamate sodium, and tolmetin; those with a half-life of 4 to 5 hours were indomethacin and ketoprofen; those with a half-life of 6 to 15 hours were diflunisal, naproxen, and sulindac; and those with a half-life of more than 15 hours were aspirin and piroxicam. (Courtesy of Connelly CS, Panush RS: *Arch Intern Med* 151:1963–1966, 1991.)

taking NSAIDs and 59 years in the group not taking NSAIDs. There were no significant differences in sex or diagnoses between the 2 groups.

Results.—There were no significant differences in intraoperative fluid administration, intraoperative transfusions postoperative wound drainage, maximum decrease in hematocrit, or length of hospital stay between the 2 groups. The group taking NSAIDs tended to have more intraoperative bleeding, but the difference was not significant. Of 11 postoperative bleeding complications, 9 occurred in patients taking NSAIDs and 2 occurred in the non-NSAID group. Use of NSAIDs was a significant risk factor for perioperative complications such as low blood pressure or postoperative gastrointestinal bleeding. The NSAIDs with half-lives of more than 6 hours were associated with an increased risk of complications (Figs 4–4 and 4–5).

Conclusions.—Nonsteroidal anti-inflammatory drugs appear to pose a risk of perioperative bleeding in surgical patients, especially those NSAIDs with long half-lives. Patients who have elective surgery should cease taking these drugs long enough before surgery to allow their elimination. Patients who need NSAIDs should switch to drugs with short half-lives. It would be inappropriate to conduct a prospective trial in which patients receive NSAIDs preoperatively.

▶ Nonsteroidal anti-inflammatory drugs are associated with increased perioperative bleeding if continued up to the time of surgery. It is recommended that these agents be discontinued in time to allow elimination of the drug before surgery, and, toward that end, NSAIDs with short half-lives should be used preoperatively. In Figure 4–5 the incidence of perioperative complications is shown as a function of the half-lives of commonly used NSAIDs.—R. Poss, M.D.

Intermittent Pneumatic Compression to Prevent Proximal Deep Venous Thrombosis During and After Total Hip Replacement: A Prospective, Randomized Study of Compression Alone, Compression and Aspirin, and Compression and Low-Dose Warfarin
Woolson ST, Watt JM (Stanford Univ)
J Bone Joint Surg 73-A:507–512, 1991   4–13

Background.—Prophylaxis against deep venous thrombosis is important in patients who have had hip arthroplasty. A trial was conducted to determine whether intraoperative and postoperative use of intermittent pneumatic compression reduces the rate of deep venous thrombosis and to compare the frequency of this complication with 3 prophylactic measures.

Methods.—A group of 196 patients older than 39 years of age who underwent 217 total hip arthroplasties were examined. Patients started walking by the third day after operation. The procedure was performed to revise a previous hip replacement or endoprosthesis in 28% of patients. Patients were randomized into 3 groups: intermittent pneumatic compression alone was used in 76 hips, compression and aspirin were used in 72 procedures, and compression and low-dose warfarin were used in 69. Venography was performed before discharge and an average of 7 days postoperatively to determine whether deep venous thrombosis was present.

Results.—Proximal deep vein thrombosis occurred at a rate of 12% in the compression-alone group, at a rate of 10% in the group receiving compression and aspirin and at a rate of 9% in the group receiving compression and warfarin; the differences were not significant. Increased age was a significant risk factor, but revision and history of deep venous thrombosis were not. The overall relative frequency of 10% was significantly lower than the 20% to 50% frequencies reported for the control groups of other trials.

Conclusions.—In patients with total hip replacement, intermittent compression during and after surgery reduces the rate of proximal vein thrombosis. Combination of this prophylaxis with orally administered aspirin or low-dose warfarin does not appear to augment this effect; however, the sample size in this trial was small.

Prevention of Deep-Vein Thrombosis and Pulmonary Embolism After Total Hip Replacement: Comparison of Low–Molecular-Weight Heparin and Unfractionated Heparin
Eriksson BI, Kälebo P, Anthmyr BA, Wadenvik H, Tengborn L, Risberg B (Gothenburg Univ, Sweden)
J Bone Joint Surg 73-A:484–493, 1991   4–14

Background.—Animal studies have shown that low–molecular-weight heparin has less interaction with platelets and less effect on overall ex vivo clotting than regular heparin. The safety and efficacy of low–molecular-weight and standard heparin were compared in a prospective, randomized, double-blind analysis of 136 patients with total hip replacement.

Methods.—The patients were allocated randomly into 2 groups. Low–molecular-weight heparin, 5,000 IU/day, was administered to 67 patients, and unfractionated sodium heparin, 5,000 IU 3 times per day, was administered to 69 patients. Treatment began 12 hours preoperatively in the group receiving low–molecular-weight heparin and 2 hours preoperatively in the group receiving standard heparin and continued for 10 days. Bilateral ascending phlebography was performed in 122 patients and pulmonary scintigraphy was performed in 127 patients 12 days after surgery.

Results.—Deep vein thrombosis occurred in 44 patients, affecting 19 (30%) receiving low–molecular-weight heparin and 25 (42%) receiving standard heparin. All but 4 patients, 2 in each group, were asymptomatic (Fig 4–6). The difference in total rate of thrombosis was insignificant, but 6 patients (10%) receiving low–molecular-weight heparin had thrombosis in the thigh, compared with 18 patients (31%) receiving stan-

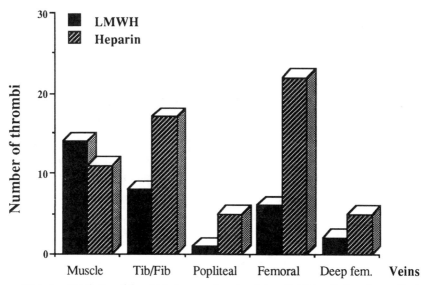

Fig 4–6.—Distribution of thrombi in the muscular veins of the calf, tibial or fibular veins, popliteal vein, femoral vein, and deep femoral vein. The multifocal character of the thrombotic process is illustrated. Six patients who received low-molecular-weight heparin and 15 who received standard heparin had 1 or several thrombi in more than 1 section of the venous system. (Courtesy of Eriksson BI, Kälebo P, Anthmyr BA, et al: *J Bone Joint Surg* 73-A:484–493, 1991.)

dard heparin. Pulmonary embolism occurred in 27 patients, affecting 8 (12%) receiving low–molecular-weight heparin and 19 (31%) receiving standard heparin. Only 3 patients had clinical signs of embolism. Those receiving low–molecular-weight heparin had significantly less total blood loss and less blood transfused.

Conclusions.—Although the overall incidence of deep venous thrombosis is not significantly different with low–molecular-weight vs. standard heparin, low–molecular-weight heparin is superior in preventing femoral thrombosis and pulmonary embolism. Use of low–molecular-weight heparin also reduces blood loss and transfused blood, thus improving safety.

A Comparison of General Anesthesia and Regional Anesthesia as a Risk Factor for Deep Vein Thrombosis Following Hip Surgery: A Critical Review

Prins MH, Hirsh J (McMaster Univ; Hamilton Civic Hosp Research Ctr, Canada)
Thromb Haemost 64:497–500, 1990   4–15

Methods.—To determine whether the incidence of postoperative deep vein thrombosis after hip surgery is lower with regional than with general anesthesia, the literature was critically reviewed. Only articles that included the method of anesthesia used (either spinal or epidural) and mandatory venography in patients who underwent elective or fractured hip surgery were reviewed. The level of evidence provided by a study was graded based on the quality of study design.

Results.—For patients who did not receive antithrombotic prophylaxis against venous thromboembolism 3 studies provided a high level of evidence. The incidence of postoperative deep vein thrombosis ranged from 53% to 77% in patients who had general anesthesia and from 29% to 40% in patients who had regional anesthesia, for a significant relative risk reduction of 46% to 55% with regional anesthesia. Among patients who received prophylaxis, there were no randomized studies that directly compared the incidence of postoperative deep vein thrombosis. However, between-study comparisons failed to show even a trend towards a reduction in the incidence of postoperative deep vein thrombosis with regional anesthesia.

Conclusions.—In patients who do not receive antithrombotic prophylaxis, the incidence of postoperative deep vein thrombosis is significantly lower with regional anesthesia than with general anesthesia after hip surgery. However, the incidence of postoperative deep vein thrombosis is still substantial in the unprotected patient, indicating that regional anesthesia should not be regarded as a substitute for effective primary antithrombotic prophylaxis.

▶ These 3 papers (Abstracts 4–13, 4–14, and 4–15) address various aspects of the prophylaxis of deep vein thrombosis. In the first paper, by Woolson et al. (Abstract 4–13), the efficacy of intermittent pneumatic compression, even without oral anticoagulants, is suggested. In the second paper, by Eriksson et al. (Abstract 4–14), low–molecular-weight heparin is proposed as a superior anticoagulant when compared to unfractionated heparin. Although the total incidence of thrombosis was not significantly different when the 2 agents were compared, thrombosis in the thigh was less frequent in the low–molecular-weight group, and pulmonary embolism was significantly less frequent in the group that received low–molecular-weight heparin. In addition, blood loss was less in the low–molecular-weight heparin group. Finally, patients received subcutaneous low–molecular-weight heparin only once daily in comparison to administration of standard heparin 3 times a day. In the third paper, by Prins and Hirsh (Abstract 4–15), a review of the literature finds that the incidence of postoperative deep vein thrombosis is decreased when regional anesthesia is used. It should be stressed, however, that the incidence of deep vein thrombosis is still high in unprotected patients and that other methods of prophylaxis should be used in addition to regional anesthesia.—R. Poss, M.D.

The Effect of Intravenous Fixed-Dose Heparin During Total Hip Arthroplasty on the Incidence of Deep-Vein Thrombosis: A Randomized, Double-Blind Trial in Patients Operated on With Epidural Anesthesia and Controlled Hypotension

Sharrock NE, Brien WW, Salvati EA, Mineo R, Garvin K, Sculco TP (Hosp for Special Surgery, New York)

J Bone Joint Surg 72-A:1456–1461, 1990   4–16

Introduction.—Because of the high risk of deep vein thrombosis, anti-coagulation treatment is often administered postoperatively to patients who have undergone total hip replacement. The effect of intravenous administration of low doses of heparin preoperatively and throughout the operation was investigated. All patients were having a unilateral primary total hip replacement under epidural hypotensive anesthesia.

Methods.—Of 150 patients randomly assigned to treatment groups, 24 were excluded. Data were available for 66 patients who received saline solution intravenously and for 60 who received heparin. Mean arterial pressures were maintained at 50–60 mm Hg. Heparin was administered in fixed doses 5 minutes before the operative incision and every 30 minutes throughout the operation. All patients received aspirin daily during hospitalization. On postoperative day 7, ascending venograms of the affected extremity were obtained.

Results.—The 2 patient groups did not differ significantly in the amount of blood that was transfused or in average length of hospital stay. Based on the amount of bleeding, surgeons could not tell during the operation which patients had received heparin. However, deep vein thrombosis differed significantly between the 2 groups. Venograms were positive in 16 patients in the control group and in 5 in the heparin group. At 6-month follow-up no further deep vein thrombosis or pulmonary embolus developed.

Conclusions.—Low-dose administration of heparin during total hip replacement operation was successful in reducing the incidence of deep vein thrombosis. This regimen may be less effective in other operations or with a different method of anesthesia.

▶ Intravenous fixed-dose heparin during total hip arthroplasty was shown to decrease the incidence of deep vein thrombosis. The authors postulate that intraoperative administration of heparin may reduce the venous stasis and tissue damage associated with positional obstruction of the femoral vein during total hip replacement.—R. Poss, M.D.

Patients' Recall of Preoperative Instruction for Informed Consent for an Operation

Hutson MM, Blaha JD (West Virginia Univ, Morgantown)
J Bone Joint Surg 73-A:160–162, 1991   4–17

Background.—Previous trials report the lack of recall by patients of preoperative instructions. A trial was conducted to determine whether intensive preoperative teaching by a patient–educator would improve later recall of information given while obtaining informed consent.

Methods.—Thirty-eight consecutive patients (mean age, 62 years) who were admitted for total joint replacement were evaluated. Before the operation all patients received instruction on the diagnosis, alternative treatments, risks and benefits of alternative treatments, and the recommendation of the attending surgeon. A verbal questionnaire was then administered to assess the patients' recall. If answers were not correct, the educator tutored the patient until all questions were answered correctly, and only then was the consent document presented for signature. Patients were interviewed again 6 months after the operation to determine the recall of items taught during the instruction for informed consent.

Results.—At the time they signed the consent document, 100% of patients recalled all the information, including risks and benefits. Six months after operation the number of patients who recalled the risks ranged from 9 (25%) who remembered the risk of infection to only 1 who remembered the risk of damage to an artery or nerve. More patients recalled the potential benefits: 8 (22%) remembered discussing relief of pain and improved function, and another 5 (16%) remembered discussing improved function. Thirty-four patients (94%) recalled what treatment had been recommended, and all patients reported that all their questions were answered before the operation.

Conclusion.—Despite the preoperative instruction and tutoring, patients' recollections after operation about the risks and benefits of the operation are not reliable.

▶ A sobering assessment of patients' selective memory of risks and benefits despite an intensive preoperative education program.—R. Poss, M.D.

Long-Term Results After Implantation of McKee-Farrar Total Hip Prostheses

Jantsch S, Schwägerl W, Zenz P, Semlitsch M, Fertschak W (Centre of Pulmology of the City of Vienna; Ludwig Boltzmann Institute of Orthopaedic and Rheumatoid Surgery, Vienna)
Arch Orthop Trauma Surg 110:230–237, 1991   4–18

Methods.—The McKee-Farrar total hip prosthesis is a metal-to-metal endoprosthesis that is made of a cast cobalt–chromium–molybdenum alloy. The edge of the spherical cup has a lip that prevents the plastic cement from overflowing into the cup during implantation; together with the small studs at the outer surface, it provides an adequate thickness of the cement mantle and has a favorable effect on the stability of the cement–implant combination (Fig 4–7). Between 1973 and 1976, 330 McKee-Farrar total hip prostheses were performed in 248 patients. Of these patients, 81 with 100 total hip prostheses in situ (according to the Mayo Clinic hip score) and 36 who had undergone 36 revision operations had complete records of the radiologic changes at the bone–implant or bone–cement interface, thereby allowing evaluation of the long-term results of these prostheses.

Results.—The mean follow-up period was 14 years in the 81 patients without revision. Revision operations with replacement of the prosthesis were performed at an average of 6 years after the primary operation. The clinical rating was excellent to good in 62% and satisfactory in 16%. Ra-

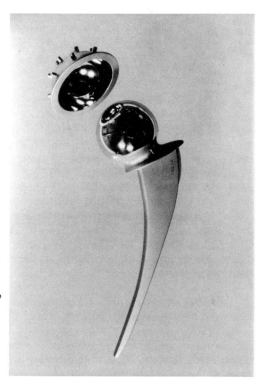

Fig 4–7.—The metal-to-metal cup of a McKee-Farrar total hip system. (Courtesy of Jantsch S, Schwägerl W, Zenz P, et al: *Arch Orthop Trauma Surg* 110:230–237, 1991.)

diologically, 66% of cups were stable. The combined clinical and radiologic ratings were less favorable. All stable implants showed hardly any loosening between the 2 interfaces, and only 3% showed cement fracture. Small cup sizes, valgus implantation, and strong medialization with damage of the floor cup were more frequent in loose, presumed loose, and replaced cups than in stable cups. Loosening began with disconnection of cement and bone, followed by migration of cup, including the complete, intact cement mantle. Metallosis was extremely rare, and abrasion of the cup and the head was only 1 μm per year.

Conclusions.—These long-term results confirm the advantages of the McKee-Farrar total hip prostheses. The design of the metal cup with metal studs at the outer surface provides a favorable effect on the stability of the implant–cement combination.

▶ Because of the widespread concern regarding particulate polyethylene debris, there is renewed interest in metal–metal articulations. This review, a 15-year result with one of the original total hip replacements, the McKee-Farrar, finds that in only 1 of 36 revision operations was there any sign of metal abrasion and generation of particulate metal debris. Wear at the cup and at the head amounted to only 1 μm per year.—R. Poss, M.D.

Hydroxyapatite Coating of Prostheses

Morscher EW (Orthopäichische Universitäitsklinik Basel, Basel, Switzerland)
J Bone Joint Surg 73-B:705–706, 1991 4–19

Background.—The use of hydroxyapatite ceramic as a coating for the femoral components of hip arthroplasties has been investigated recently. The material has been found to enhance osseointegration. In addition, chemical bonding may occur between hydroxyapatite and bone. Therefore, the tensile forces may also be transmitted. However, hydroxyapatite is applied to metal implants by a plasma spray process, and a full coating cannot be achieved in the depths of porous surface cavities. Other basic questions also need to be answered.

Bond Strength.—The long-term strength of the bond between hydroxyapatite and various implant surfaces is still unknown. Hydroxyapatite is very brittle and has a high modulus of elasticity; therefore, there is a risk of separation from more elastic materials when the composite is subjected to bending. Chemical and physical disintegration of hydroxyapatite over time has been reported. Granules may be transported away from the implant surface by the macrophages. If these very hard granules enter a joint space, then extensive abrasion of polyethylene and metal will occur. Although such a disaster has not yet been reported, it is still a matter of concern. Another theoretical possibility is the development of excessive paraarticular ossification.

Long-Term Outcomes.—The long-term clinical outcomes of implants coated with hydroxyapatite will depend on various factors, including coating thickness, chemical purity, bonding strength, and porosity. Thicker coatings are more porous and brittle, but thinner coatings are more likely to be resorbed. Even where hydroxyapatite eventually disappears from the surface, osseointegration would be maintained by the bioinert properties of the underlying titanium. The advantages of early osseointegration must be balanced against the possible problems associated with a weak interface.

Conclusions.—With this biomaterial, bonding at the molecular level is evident. However, the use of this material in clinical practice requires more research. Success with this material would mean a shift in orthopedics from the age of mechanics to an age of molecular biology.

Hydroxyapatite-Coated Femoral Stems: Histological Analysis of Components Retrieved at Autopsy

Bauer TW, Geesink RCT, Zimmerman R, McMahon JT (Cleveland Clinic Found)
J Bone Joint Surg 73-A:1439–1452, 1991 4–20

Background.—Plasma-sprayed hydroxyapatite coatings are biocompatible. Because of their osteoconductive properties, they may contribute to early fixation of total joint prostheses. This interface was analyzed histologically.

Methods.—A group of 5 hydroxyapatite-coated femoral stems was analyzed. The stems and the surrounding bone were retrieved from 3 individuals at autopsy. The femoral components had been in place for a mean of 12 months; they had been inserted for osteonecrosis in 2 cases, osteoarthrosis in 2 cases, and as an uncemented revision for failure of a cemented stem in 1 case. The 3 patients had a good or excellent clinical result after implantation, and all had died of causes unrelated to the joint arthroplasty.

Results.—A hydroxyapatite coating could be identified on each stem. The amount of apposition of bone varied from 32% to 78% of the available surface per section. Bone deposition was most marked on the surface of the prosthesis close to the endosteal surface of the bone, particularly in the anterior and medial aspects of the implant and at the lateral-oblique corners. Some foci of bone remodeling around the implant were noted, including osteoclast-mediated removal of the hydroxyapatite coating along with the adjacent bone. Some ceramic particles were also present within the macrophages in the adjacent bone marrow. Other areas showed new bone formation, with a few areas of bone directly against the metal substrate.

Conclusions.—These histologic findings suggest that the implants were mechanically stable, with bone remodeling at the surface of the bone–implant interface. Additional electron microscopy studies are needed to further characterize the intracellular and extracellular material next to the hydroxyapatite.

Fixation of Hip Prostheses by Hydroxyapatite Ceramic Coatings
Furlong RJ, Osborn JF (London; Univ of Bonn)
J Bone Joint Surg 73-B:741–745, 1991   4–21

Background.—When a cementless prosthesis is driven into the femur, stability is immediately produced by limited areas of interference fit, often against crushed and necrotic trabeculae. The strength of the hold declines with time as necrotic bone is removed. The success of long-term fixation relies on the speed and completeness of new bone formation. The outcomes of prostheses with a coating of hydroxyapatite ceramic were examined.

Methods.—A group of 4 postmortem specimens were evaluated. The specimens were obtained 10 days, 17 days, 7 weeks, and 19 weeks after implantation of the hydroxyapatite-coated femoral components of the hip arthroplasties. Nondecalcified ground sections stained with toluidine blue were used for microscopic examination.

Findings.—Early deposition of woven bone on the hydroxyapatite ceramic was noted; it was identical to that found on surviving cancellous trabeculae. The space between the deposits became bridged from both sides by new trabeculae. There was no evidence of an inflammatory reaction or fibrous tissue formation.

Conclusions.—These findings confirm that, with hydroxyapatite coatings, the repair time is halved by the simultaneous development of new bone on both the implant and the femur. In addition, the induction of osteogenesis apparently produces permanent fixation within a few days or weeks. If the hydroxyapatite ceramic coating remains stable and strong in the long term, then the process of bonding osteogenesis could produce stability analogous to primary fracture healing in healthy cancellous bone, with its potential for permanent union.

Bonding of Hydroxyapatite-Coated Femoral Prostheses: Histopathology of Specimens From Four Cases

Hardy DCR, Frayssinet P, Guilhem A, LaFontaine MA, Delince PE (Univ Hosp Saint-Pierre, Brussels)
J Bone Joint Surg 73-B:732–740, 1991   4–22

Background.—Arthroplasties of the hip must withstand loads as great as 5 times an individual's body weight. Therefore, bonding to bone is a matter of concern. The biologic behavior of hydroxyapatite-coated hip prostheses and the nature of the interfaces were investigated.

Methods and Findings.—Specimens of hydroxyapatite-coated femoral prostheses were obtained from 4 patients who had died within 9 months of implantation for fractured neck of the femur. Histologic assessment showed newly formed immature bone overlying the hydroxyapatite coating. In addition, there was new trabeculae-bridging to the endosteal bone layer. In the diaphysis, where contact between the hydroxyapatite and cortex had been, a dense, firmly anchored bone with a haversian architecture was noted. The newly forced bone had a trabecular structure in other locations, containing bone marrow tissue with normal cellularity. Biologic osseointegration appeared to have occurred.

Conclusions.—This biomaterial appears to possess remarkable biologic properties. Its biocompatibility was confirmed by the absence of any inflammatory process or adverse tissue reaction. The use of hydroxyapatite may be a major advance in the technology of uncemented implants.

▶ The early clinical results of hydroxyapatite coatings to metallic implants are encouraging. An osteoconductive response is generally seen and confers, at least in the short-term, satisfactory clinical and, perhaps, even enhanced radiographic results. However, many questions must be answered before the role of hydroxyapatite in cementless total joint replacement is assured. The concerns are addressed in the paper by Morscher (Abstract 4–19) and provide an important perspective against which to assess the significance of the early findings reported by Hardy et al. (Abstract 4–22), Furlong et al (Abstract 4–21) and Bauer et al. (Abstract 4–20).—R. Poss, M.D.

Polyethylene Wear From Retrieved Acetabular Cups
Weightman B, Swanson SAV, Isaac GH, Wroblewski BM (Imperial College, London; Wrightington Hospital, Wigan, England)
J Bone Joint Surg 73-B:806–810, 1991   4–23

Background.—As the Charnley hip prosthesis is used in younger, more active patients, the number of revision operations is increasing, most often necessitated by component loosening and tissue reaction to the debris of wear. Polyethylene wear is a significant factor that is not adequately understood. Laboratory wear tests were performed on specimens prepared from acetabular cups removed from hip replacement patients after varying periods of implantation.

Methods.—Twelve Charnley acetabular cups had been implanted for 10 months to 17.5 years (mean, 8.5 years). Cylindrical specimens of polyethylene were taken from the worn and unworn regions of the cups to test separately for the effects of degradation and fatigue. The loss in weight of polymer specimens was measured to assess wear.

Results.—There was no relationship between the penetration rate of the cups and the wear resistance of polyethylene. A wide variation was noted in clinical penetration rates that could not be explained by batch-to-batch variation in the wear resistance of the material. In 2 specimens, the wear coefficients were about 1 order of magnitude higher than the others; no satisfactory explanation could be found for this result. There were no signs of time-dependent degradation in the wear resistance of the polyethylene material.

Conclusions.—The differences between worn and unworn regions of these cups results from an increase in wear resistance in the worn region rather than a reduction in wear resistance in the unworn region. These differences probably result from the different surface finishes of the polyethylene.

▶ There was a wide range of polyethylene wear in patients with total hip replacement, and these differences cannot be explained merely on the basis of batch-to-batch variation of polyethylene or the patient's activity or weight. The authors proposed that differences in wear resistance may be the result of different surface finishes of the polyethylene. This hypothesis is intriguing in light of the recent information regarding different surface finishes in total knee prosthesis. It has been noted recently that heat-pressed finishing of tibial polyethylene components renders that surface more likely to undergo early degradation than similar surfaces that were machine-finished.—R. Poss, M.D.

The Biomechanical Problems of Polyethylene as a Bearing Surface
Collier JP, Mayor MB, Surprenant VA, Surprenant HP, Dauphinais LA, Jensen RE (Dartmouth College, Hanover, NH)
Clin Orthop 261:107–113, 1990   4–24

Background.—The use of metal backings for polyethylene modular acetabular components reduced deformation of all-polyethylene components, but metal-backed components can also fail. Polyethylene and metal-wear debris and implant loosening can occur with these components. These biomechanical and biomaterial concerns were reviewed.

Methods.—The 85 retrieved polyethylene acetabular components of various types, including 81 with metal backings, were examined microscopically. Samples of bulk, medical grade, ultra-high molecular-weight polyethylene of 3 different grades were machined into test shapes and studied for tensile measurements and creep properties.

Results.—More than 40% of the retrieved polyethylene acetabular components showed burnishing and abrasion, more than 25% had pitting, and 17% showed severe wear. There was frequent evidence of significant motion between the polyethylene inserts and the metal backings. In most components, spherical voids were seen internally, sometimes containing inclusions and often associated with cracking. There was significant creep and deformation of the polyethylene in 4 components after less than 5 years of wear. Bulk polyethylene samples had variable yield strengths and tensile strengths and extremely variable creep and elongations to break.

Conclusions.—Surface replacement prostheses appear to be at great risk for creep, polyethylene separation, and cracking as a result of reduced polyethylene thickness. The polyethylene performance of acetabular components may vary with the type and grade of polyethylene.

▶ Polyethylene wear of acetabular components is a multifaceted problem that includes both the material properties of the polyethylene and the design of the polyethylene metal-backed composite. In this investigation bulk polyethylene samples had variable mechanical properties. Of great importance, however, was the discovery of polyethylene damage between the polyethylene inserts and their metal backings in many of the components. Additional risk factors to the longevity of the polyethylene acetabular component included the thickness of the polyethylene and the accuracy and stability of fit of the polyethylene liner into its metal-backed shell.—R. Poss, M.D.

Metal Wear and Tissue Response in Failed Titanium Alloy Total Hip Replacements

Witt JD, Swann M (Wexham Park Hospital, Slough, England)
J Bone Joint Surg 73-B:559–563, 1991   4–25

Background.—Metal debris from titanium alloy prostheses may contribute to loosening of the components or cause a soft tissue reaction. The long-term metabolic, bacteriologic, immunogenic and oncogenic effects of the metal components in total joint replacements are also worrisome. The findings from 13 total hip replacements with titanium alloy femoral components (all requiring revision for loosening) were assessed.

Patients.—All patients underwent revision total hip arthroplasty after implantation of a McKee-Farrar titanium alloy femoral prosthesis fixed with polymethyl methacrylate bone cement. All the patients had osteoarthritis; the average patient age was 67 years. At an average of 2 years after implantation, each replacement required revision. The patients had pain on weight bearing and loosening documented radiographically.

Results.—Heavy black staining of the periprosthetic tissues and a proliferative reaction of the synovial tissues were seen at all revision operations. The blackened membranes had infiltrated the cement–bone interface, loosening the femoral component and, in 7 cases, the acetabular component. Patches of the shot-blasted surface coating of the femoral stems had been rubbed off. Histologic study showed that the black, fibrous, affected tissues were fibroblastic. Black fragments were seen within the histiocytes and giant cells, and they were heavily deposited extracellularly. Atomic absorption analysis of the stained tissues of 1 patient showed that metals were present in approximately the same ratio as in the alloy, except for increased aluminum. Energy dispersive x-ray analysis of the unabraded region of the removed femoral stem showed an increased amount of aluminum resulting from embedded particles of aluminum oxide grit.

Conclusions.—The early failure of these implants may have been caused in part by tissue reaction to the metal-wear debris. The shot-blasted finishes of these prostheses were abraded, perhaps by micromotion; this contributed to the failures. The ability of the surfaces of such implants to withstand abrasive wear or to create injurious debris should be considered.

▶ Metallic particulate debris invokes a biologic reaction that results in osteolysis and loosening of total hip prosthesis.—R. Poss, M.D.

An Improved Technique for Cement Extraction in Revision Total Hip Arthroplasty
Chin AK, Moll FH, McColl MB, Hoffman KJ, Wuh HCK (Origin Medsystems, San Mateo, Calif; Southern California Orthopaedic Inst, Van Nuys)
Contemp Orthop 22:255–264, 1991   4–26

Introduction.—Removing polymethyl methacrylate (PMMA) cement in revision total hip arthroplasty may be a tedious procedure and can produce many complications, including femoral fracture. An improved method of cement removal involves the application of newly mixed bone cement to the old mantle, which permits segmental extraction of the mantle.

Technique.—The inner surface of the old cement mantle is abraded with a steel wire brush after removing the femoral component. It then is irrigated with saline and dried thoroughly. An extended plug, if present distal to the femoral step, is drilled under fluoroscopic control. Low-viscosity PMMA cement is then injected into the distal part of the old mantle, and the rest is filled retrograde to the level of the lesser trochanter. A thread-forming rod is centered within the cement canal and, after the new cement has polymerized, the rod is unscrewed from the femur. The proximal cement mantle and cancellous bone are removed to allow extraction of the mantle without obstruction. A series of extraction rods are used to sequentially extract the cement mantle.

Results.—This technique was used to extract successfully cement mantles in 113 of 130 femoral component revisions performed in 129 patients. Complications included 3 femoral fractures and 1 inadvertent cortical window.

Conclusions.—Cement-assisted mantle removal is a simple and effective means of extracting old PMMA cement when revising loosened femoral components. The method is relatively safe and does not preclude conventional instrumentation should it fail.

Revision Arthroplasty Facilitated by Ultrasonic Tool Cement Removal: II. Histologic Analysis of Endosteal Bone After Cement Removal

Caillouette JT, Gorab RS, Klapper RC, Anzel SH (Univ of California, Irvine)
Orthop Rev 20:435–440, 1991

4–27

Objective.—The effects of ultrasonic removal of cement from the canine femur on the underlying endosteal bone were examined. Polymethyl methacrylate (PMMA) cement was used in all instances.

Findings.—No significant damage to cortical bone was evident after the use of ultrasonically driven tools to remove PMMA cement. Microfractures and fissures were not seen after treatment of cortical windows with a high-speed burr. Osteonecrosis was less evident at ultrasonic sites than where a high-speed burr was applied. Osteoclastic activity was reduced at sites of ultrasonic cement removal. Osteoid formation and osteoblastic rimming suggested new bone formation along the endosteal surface and filling of part of the intramedullary defect.

Conclusions.—Ultrasonic cement removal is a safe procedure. These findings are in accord with the results of temperature analysis in human cadaveric femurs subjected to ultrasonic cement removal.

▶ Two methods are described for removal of cement from femoral canals. As with all new techniques, the surgeon should be thoroughly familiar with the advantages as well as the disadvantages and should be technically proficient with its use before its clinical application.—R. Poss, M.D.

Management of the Recalcitrant Total-Hip Arthroplasty Wound

Meland NB, Arnold PG, Weiss HC (Mayo Clinic and Found, Rochester, Minn)
Plast Reconstr Surg 88:681–685, 1991

4–28

Background.—Between 10% and 20% of all patients who undergo girdlestone arthroplasties for infections complicating total hip arthroplasty (THA) will preset with chronic, nonhealed, draining hip wounds. Between 1977 and 1988, 27 patients with 28 infected THAs that did not respond to removal of the prosthesis and cement and closure were seen. The management of this complication was reported.

Patients.—The average patient age was 64 years. The patients had undergone an average of 4.2 (range, 1–21) operative débridements before wound closure. The most common organisms were *Staphylococcus aureus* and group A streptococcus. Virtually all of the infections were polymicrobial.

Management.—All patients underwent multiple operations for implant removal, débridement, complete removal of all the methyl methacrylate, and culture-directed antibiotic treatment. Wound care included high-pressure lavage and curettage. A total of 33 muscles was used for wound closure in the 27 patients, including the rectus femoris in 23 instances, vastus lateralis in 8, tensor fasciae latae in 1, and combined latissimus doris–serratus anterior free-tissue transfers in 2. Multiple combinations of transpositions and free flaps were used.

Results.—At an average follow-up of 6.4 years (range, 1–10 years), all of the patients had a healed, noncomplicated wound. A group of 18 patients walked with the assistance of a cane, walker, or crutches and, with minor pain, 4 ambulated unassisted. All of these patients had reimplantation of their hip arthroplasty at least 12 months after the muscle-flap procedure. Three patients were nonambulatory.

Conclusion.—Muscle, either by transposition or free-tissue transfer, is an ideal choice for obliteration of the recalcitrant THA wound.

Treatment of Chronic Infected Hip Arthroplasty Wounds by Radical Debridement and Obliteration With Pedicled and Free Muscle Flaps

Jones NF, Eadie P, Johnson PC, Mears DC (Univ of Pittsburgh)
Plast Reconstr Surg 88:95–101, 1991   4–29

Background.—Chronic infection after total hip arthroplasty (THA) is often seen with a deep, extensive, nonhealing wound extending from the lateral thigh into the depths of the acetabulum. Successful treatment of chronic osteomyelitis of the tibia has been achieved by serial débridement of the infected bone and the surrounding soft tissues followed by obliteration of the resultant defect with free muscle flaps. The same principles were applied in the treatment of 9 patients with chronic infection of the hip joint after failed THA.

Methods.—The patients, aged 33–82 years, had chronic extensive wounds of the hip joint after THA internal fixation of femoral head or neck fractures, or hematogenous osteomyelitis of the hip joint. The infected implants and internal fixation devices were removal in all patients with conversion to a Girdlestone arthroplasty. The patients had undergone between 4 and 32 previous surgical attempts at wound closure. All of the patients underwent multiple radical débridement to remove the devitalized bone in the proximal femur, the remnants of bone cement, and the chronic scar tissue; débridement was done until both bone and soft tissue cultures were sterile. The resultant defect of the hip was obliterated with either pedicled muscle flaps or free muscle flaps. Subcutaneous or transpelvic transposition of the rectus abdominis muscle flaps was preferred for smaller defects, and the free latissimus dorsi muscle flap provided sufficient volume of tissue to obliterate the more extensive hip defects. Systemic antibiotics were administered for 14 days postoperatively.

Results.—All 9 muscle flaps healed primarily without infection, and all of the wounds were completely healed within 21 days of surgery. During a follow-up of 6 months to 3¼ years, none of the patients had a recurrence of infection. One patient walked unaided after reimplantation of a second custom hip prosthesis into the vascularized bed of a free latissimus dorsi muscle flap. Of the remaining 8 patients with Girdlestone arthroplasties, 1 walked unaided and 7 walked with the assistance of a cane or walker.

Conclusion.—Chronic infection of the hip joint after failed THA can be treated successfully by radical débridement and obliteration of the cavity using either a pedicled rectus abdominis muscle flap or a free latissimus dorsi flap.

▶ Chronic infection will heal only in the presence of a properly vascularized tissue bed. Increasingly, plastic reconstructive procedures such as vascularized muscle or myocutaneous flaps are being used in these most difficult clinical situations.—R. Poss, M.D.

Long-Term (Twelve to Eighteen-Year) Follow-Up of Cemented Total Hip Replacements in Patients Who Were Less Than Fifty Years Old: A Follow-Up Note
Collis DK (Orthopedic and Fracture Clinic of Eugene, Ore)
J Bone Joint Surg 73-A:593–597, 1991   4–30

Objective.—In a report in 1984 on 45 cemented total hip arthroplasties (average follow-up, 7½ years), the revision rate was 9%. Extended follow-up data now are available on 43 of these patients, all of whom were younger than age 50 years at the time of replacement.

Findings.—Thirty-one unrevised hips were available for follow-up an average of 15 years after surgery. No reduction in clinical function had occurred since follow-up assessment in 1983. Only 4 patients occasionally used external support. Hip flexion averaged 110 degrees. No hip exhibited definite loosening of the acetabular cup, and there was no measurable migration of a femoral component. However, 3 hips had definite loosening of the femoral component. Six of 10 replacements done on patients in their thirties required revision.

Conclusions.—Cemented total hip replacement has been successful in most patients, even with the techniques and prostheses available in the early 1970s. When revision has been necessary, the results have been good.

▶ Well-performed cemented total hip replacement in this cooperative group of patients, even though they were younger than 50 years of age at the time of surgery, produced satisfactory long-term results. Using revision as the end point, the rate of survival was 69% at 15 years in this series.—R. Poss, M.D.

Proximal Femoral Allografts in Revision Hip Arthroplasty
Allan DG, Lavoie GJ, McDonald S, Oakeshott R, Gross AE (Mount Sinai Hosp, Toronto)
J Bone Joint Surg 73-B:235–240, 1991   4–31

Background.—Massive femoral bone deficiency is frequently encountered in patients undergoing revision total hip arthroplasty (THA) after multiple previous revision procedures. Various treatment options for this problem have been described, including the use of cadaveric bone allografts. Long-term data on cadaveric allografts in revision arthroplasties with bone loss were reviewed.

Methods.—During a 6-year period 51 women and 18 men aged 29–83 years underwent 78 proximal femoral allografts in 73 hips. In 4 patients, the operations were bilateral and 5 hips received 2 allografts. Follow-up lasted 29–68 months. All operations were performed in laminal flow ventilation, with the surgical team wearing body exhaust suits. The transtrochanteric approach was the most common. Three types of allografts were used, including calcar grafts of less than 3 cm in length to restore moderate bone loss proximally, large fragment proximal allografts, and cortical strut grafts. Prophylactic cephalosporin was administered intravenously for 5 days and by mouth for another 5 days. Because most patients had already undergone several previous revisions, 83% required concomitant acetabular allografting. The mean intraoperative blood loss was 2,249 mL, requiring an average of 4.6 blood units for replacement.

Results.—The overall mean hip score improved considerably, from 39.1 before operation to 68.3 after operation. Calcar grafts in 31 patients were clinically successful in 81%, but resorption of one third to one half of the graft occurred in 10% of the hips, and resorption of more than half of the graft occurred in 40%. In several hips virtually the entire allograft was resorbed. Resorption of more than one third of the graft was seen in 79% of grafts where polymethylmethacrylate cement was not used but in only 10% of grafts cemented to the prosthesis. Thus, cement within the calcar allograft appears to reduce the risk of resorption. Large fragment proximal allografts in 40 hips and cortical strut allografts in 7 hips were successful in 85%. Deep sepsis developed in 5 hips (6.8%).

Conclusions.—Large proximal femoral allografts and cortical strut allografts provide dependable reconstruction of bone stock deficiencies during revision THA. Small calcar grafts are less reliable because resorption is common.

▶ Large proximal femoral allografts and cortical strut allografts are uniformly successful in reconstruction of large bone defects associated with failed total hip replacement. Grafts smaller than 3 cm in length undergo significant resorption and are not recommended.—R. Poss, M.D.

A Comparison of Quality of Life Before and After Arthroplasty in Patients Who Had Arthrosis of the Hip Joint
Wiklund I, Romanus B (Östra Hosp, Gothenburg, Sweden)
J Bone Joint Surg 73-A:765–769, 1991   4–32

Objective.—The quality of life a year after total hip arthroplasty was compared with that before surgery in 56 patients younger than age 80 years with hip joint arthrosis. The 35 women and 21 men had a median age of 65 years.

Methods.—The functional impairment of the hip joint was estimated objectively using the Charnley-Merle d'Aubigné Score. The Nottingham Health Profile served to assess the health-related quality of life before and after arthroplasty.

Results.—The quality of life improved significantly after arthroplasty with respect to pain, energy, sleep, and social isolation. Health-related problems pertaining to housework, hobbies, social life, family life, and sexual function were all significantly reduced after surgery. Postoperative adjustment did not relate significantly to age, duration of symptoms, or severity of disease. Single patients were more socially isolated and had more emotional problems than those who were married.

Conclusion.—Total hip arthroplasty can achieve good practical results regardless of the age of the patient or the history of symptoms.

▶ The evaluation of total hip replacement will increasingly be measured with outcome instruments that seek to measure the patient's assessment. In this important study, a highly significant improvement in the patient's quality of life is demonstrated on a patient assessment instrument, while the more traditional "objective" assessment is shown to be relatively insensitive.—R. Poss, M.D.

Total Hip Replacement With Cemented, Uncemented, and Hybrid Prostheses: A Comparison of Clinical and Radiographic Results at Two to Four Years
Wixson RL, Stulberg SD, Mehlhoff M (Northwestern Univ, Chicago)
J Bone Joint Surg 73-A:257–270, 1991.   4–33

Objective.—To determine the effectiveness of fixation of total hip replacements by bony ingrowth without the use of cement, 144 consecutive primary total hip replacement in 131 patients were followed prospectively for 2–4 years.

Methods.—A cemented or a hybrid prosthesis consisting of a cemented femoral component and an uncemented acetabular component was used in men older than age 70 years, in women (older than age 60 years, and in younger patients in whom adequate fixation required cement. All other patients received uncemented porous-surfaced implants. In all, a group of 52 hips received cemented, a group of 65 received uncemented, and a group of 27 received hybrid implants.

Results.—The 3 groups had comparable overall clinical results. Mean Harris hip ratings were 90 or higher in all groups and pain scores were 42–43 points. Two prosthetic stems designed for bony ingrowth had aseptic loosening. About one fourth of the patients receiving a femoral component to allow bone ingrowth had mild thigh pain at 1 year. Component migration was more frequent when the acetabulum received a cemented component instead of a cup that permitted bony ingrowth. There was 1 late infection.

Conclusions.—When cemented implants are used out of necessity, the results are comparable to those achieved in younger patients receiving uncemented implants. It is not clear how cemented and uncemented prostheses compare in younger patients or whether older patients benefit from uncemented implants.

▶ Cemented, uncemented, and hybrid fixation of the same total hip system were compared. When one uses global scores to assess the results, few differences among the 3 methods of fixation are noted. This study points out the insensitivity of global scores in reporting the results of joint replacement procedures. Only when individual, functional, or radiographic criteria are evaluated and compared can meaningful differences be noted. For example, in examining for thigh pain, there are significant differences in the uncemented vs. the cemented femoral components. The results of total joint replacement are obscured when global scores are used.—R. Poss, M.D.

Somatosensory Evoked Potential Monitoring in the Surgical Management of Acute Acetabular Fractures

Helfet DL, Hissa EA, Sergay S, Mast JW (Florida Orthopaedic Inst, Tampa; Willoughby, Ohio; Tampa, Fla; Warren, Mich)
J Orthop Trauma 5:161–166, 1991   4–34

Background.—A high rate of iatrogenic sciatic–peroneal nerve injury is a major risk of acetabular surgery. The role of somatosensory evoked potential (SSEP) monitoring was examined in patients having surgery for acute acetabular fracture.

Methods.—Twelve patients, 3 of whom had preoperative neuropraxia, comprised a retrospective series. Subsequently, 38 patients were managed prospectively. Most had complex fracture patterns. Electrodes were applied to the posterior tibial nerve on both sides, and needle electrodes were placed subdermally in the lumbar region and scalp.

Results.—Thirteen patients (26%) had a loss of sciatic–peroneal neurologic function preoperatively, most often involving a decrease in motor power. Fourteen patients (28%) had changes in SSEP during surgery. In the prospective series, 6 of 10 patients with preoperative neurologic loss had intraoperative changes in SSEP. All of these patients had an injury involving the posterior acetabulum and required a posterior surgical approach. Two patients with persistent SSEP alterations had minor peroneal palsy postoperatively that was transient. In 2 patients technical problems precluded accurate intraoperative monitoring.

Conclusions.—Somatosensory evoked potential monitoring is an effective means of lowering the risk of sciatic–peroneal nerve injury in patients operated on for acute acetabular fracture. None of the patients examined had a permanent neurologic defect.

Somatosensory-Evoked Potential Monitored During Total Hip Arthroplasty

Black DL, Reckling FW, Porter SS (Univ of Kansas, Kansas City)
Clin Orthop 262:170–177, 1991

4–35

Objective.—Because of the serious import of sciatic palsy complicating hip surgery, the value of monitoring somatosensory evoked potentials (SSEPs) was examined.

Methods.—A group of 100 consecutive patients were admitted for elective total hip arthroplasty. A posterolateral surgical approach was used in 83 patients. The SSEPs were elicited by percutaneous stimulation of the peroneal nerve at the fibular neck on both sides, and they were recorded with an electrode on the scalp.

Results.—Eighteen patients had latency changes suggesting neural compromise. All but 2 of them had surgery by a posterolateral approach. Half of the patients had been operated on previously. Eight of these patients had a totally flat tracing at some point. In all patients but 2, the baseline tracing returned after repositioning the extremity or the retractors. Intraoperative changes related most closely to femoral reaming and implant placement. Monitoring caused no complications.

Conclusions.—Monitoring of SSEPs is an effective means of assessing sciatic nerve function during hip arthroplasty. Sciatic palsy correlates with a loss of activity that persists to the time of closure. Monitoring is expensive and requires specially trained personnel, and, therefore, is not warranted on a routine basis.

Nerve Palsy Associated With Total Hip Replacement: Risk Factors and Prognosis

Schmalzried TP, Amstutz HC, Dorey FJ (Univ of California, Los Angeles)
J Bone Joint Surg 73-A:1074–1080, 1991

4–36

Background.—There is a reported .6% to 3.7% incidence of nerve palsy after total hip replacement, most commonly affecting the sciatic nerve or its peroneal division. There are many possible causes of these injuries, but the true cause is usually not discovered.

Patients.—Data on 52 affected patients treated during a 17-year period were reviewed. The 52 patients, with 53 neuropathies in the ipsilateral lower extremity, were identified from a series of 3,126 consecutive total hip replacements. Follow-up was 12–198 months.

Results.—The overall incidence of neuropathy was 1.7%, and the incidence after primary arthroplasty was 1.3%. There was a 5.2% incidence in patients who had primary arthroplasty for congenital dislocation or dysplasia of the hip, and a 3.2% incidence in patients with all diagnoses who had revision surgery. Only part of the increased prevalence with these procedures could be ascribed to limb lengthening. The sciatic nerve was involved in 48 neuropathies, and the cause of the injury was unknown in 30. At follow-up 7 patients were neurologically normal, 33 had a mild deficit, and 13 had a major deficit. Neurologic recovery always occurred by 21 months. Of 36 patients assessed at least 24 months postoperatively 7 were normal, 23 had a mild deficit, and 6 had a major deficit. All patients had decreased ability to walk, with the most serious disabilities in patients who had a primary hip replacement at age 48 years or younger. Recovery was good in all patients who had some motor function immediately after the injury or recovered some while in the hospital. Recovery was not good in any of the 5 patients who had severe dysesthesias.

Conclusions.—Risk factors for nerve palsy after total hip replacement include congenital dislocation or hip dysplasia, revision surgery for any cause, and primary operation in patients aged 48 years or younger. The only factor related to prognosis is the severity of the nerve injury. Nerve palsy is the most troubling complication of hip replacement surgery, and the patient's dissatisfaction will preclude a good result.

▶ Somatosensory evoked potential monitoring may play a useful role in monitoring nerve function in complex surgery about the hip.—R. Poss, M.D.

Antibiotic Resistance of Biomaterial-Adherent Coagulase-Negative and Coagulase-Positive Staphylococci
Naylor PT, Myrvik QN, Gristina A (Wake Forest Univ, Winston-Salem, NC; Natl Hosp for Orthopaedics and Rehabilitation, Arlington, Va)
Clin Orthop 261:126–133, 1990   4–37

Background.—Microbial adhesion to biomaterial substrata is responsible for many resistant biomaterial-localized infections. Although the mechanisms by which bacterial surface populations acquire antibiotic and biocide resistance is unclear, it is clear that surface populations have different physiology and behavior than suspension populations. The antibiotic sensitivity and killing kinetics of pathogens retrieved from the surface of biomaterials in human infections were compared with those of suspended bacterial populations.

Methods.—Three strains each of coagulase-positive and coagulase-negative staphylococci were evaluated. Each was grown in suspension culture in the presence of surgical-grade stainless steel, ultra-high molecular weight polyethylene, or polymethylmethacrylate; adherent and nonadherent bacteria were exposed to standard reference preparations of cefazolin, vancomycin hydrochloride, Daptomycin, Gentamycin, and Nafcillin.

Results.—For coagulase-negative organisms in suspension, the minimum bacterial concentrations for the relevant antibiotics were equal to or lower than those for biomaterial-adherent organisms. The difference was organism- and biomaterial-specific. Bacteria bound to hydrocarbon polymers had higher resistance than those bound to stainless steel. For all strains studied, bacterial killing for adherent organisms was time- and biomaterial-dependent. Slime-producing strains did not have higher antibiotic resistance than nonslime-producing bacteria.

Conclusions.—Antibiotic resistance of staphylococci involved in biomaterial-localized infections appears to be related to surface adhesion and the specific surface material. The presence or absence of slime does not appear to be related to antibiotic resistance.

▶ Bacterial resistance in the presence of implants is a function of microbial adhesion to the biomaterial. Bacteria in suspension are far more susceptible to antibiotics than are bacteria that are adherent to a substrate.—R. Poss, M.D.

Natural History of Nontraumatic Avascular Necrosis of the Femoral Head
Ohzono K, Saito M, Takaoka K, Ono K, Saito S, Nishina T, Kadowaki T (Osaka University; Sumitomo Hospital; Osaka Kosei-Nenkin Hospital, Japan)
J Bone Joint Surg 73-B:68–72, 1991   4–38

Background.—Nontraumatic avascular necrosis of the femoral head (ANFH) may progress rapidly to collapse or remain fairly static. Because the natural history of ANFH has not been well described, it is difficult to predict the fate of the hip, select appropriate treatment, or evaluate the various treatment outcomes.

Methods.—To define the natural history of ANFH based on its radiographic characteristics, the radiographs of 87 patients (age, 18–70 years) with ANFH in 115 hips were examined. The ANFH was steroid-induced in 69 hips, caused by excessive alcohol intake in 21 hips, and idiopathic in 25 hips. The period between symptom onset and the initial diagnosis of ANFH ranged from 1 month to 8 years. Average follow-up was 5 years 3 months. Progress to collapse of the femoral head was related retrospectively to the cause of ANFH, disease stage, extent at initial diagnosis, and to the site and extent of the necrotic lesion in the femoral head. Affected femoral heads were first classified into 4 stages based on the presence of radiographic abnormalities and then classified into 6 types based on site and extent of the necrotic lesion in the femoral head, degree of flatness of the weight-bearing surface on anteroposterior radiographs, and the presence or absence of cystic lesions.

Results.—During follow-up none of the 5 hips without necrosis occupying the weight-bearing surface of the femoral head collapsed. In contrast, all 5 hips in which the necrotic lesion occupied the entire weight-bearing surface of the femoral head collapsed. Flatness of the femoral head resulting from subchondral fracture was an early manifestation of collapse.

Conclusion.—The use of radiographic criteria for the typing of ANFH has a high sensitivity for the prognosis of the hip. This classification is useful when planning treatment and projecting treatment outcome.

▶ A radiographic classification has been devised that relates a poor prognosis with the osteonecrotic fragment or cyst in the weight-bearing sector.— R. Poss, M.D.

Synthetic Polymers Seeded With Chondrocytes Provide a Template for New Cartilage Formation

Vacanti CA, Langer R, Schloo B, Vacanti JP (Massachusetts Gen Hosp, Boston; Children's Hosp, Boston; Massachusetts Inst of Technology, Cambridge; Deborah Heart and Lung Inst, Brown Mills, NJ)
Plast Reconstr Surg 88:753–759, 1991   4–39

Background.—There have been several reports of new cartilage formation using naturally occurring polymers. A method using synthetic biodegradable polymers onto which chondrocytes are seeded and which are then implanted into an animal was examined. By this method, exact engineering of matrix configuration was achieved, thus allowing formation of large 3-dimensional masses of precisely shaped and sized cartilage.

Methods.—A chondrocyte suspension in a concentration of 5×10^7 cells/cc from the articular cartilage of newborn calves was prepared. Synthetic bioabsorbable suture material, or polymer fiber, was made in braided threads so as to create interfiber distances of between 0 and 200 μm while keeping the unit intact (Fig 4–8). Twenty-eight fibers were seeded with 100 μL of chondrocyte solution, and 22 were not exposed to chondrocytes. After culture for 3 or 10 days, 21 experimental and 16 control fibers were implanted subcutaneously to the base of the neck in nude mice. Some animals were injected with chondrocyte unattached to polymers. Specimens were excised at specified points in time for immunohistochemical evaluation.

Results.—In 19 of 21 animals, cartilage plates as large as 100 mg were created. Average weights were 60–70 mg and peaked at day 49, by which time there was little evidence of an inflammatory response or polymer remnants. Type 3 collagen was seen through day 49. The chondrocyte-injected animals showed no signs of cartilage formation.

Conclusions.—A polymer fiber template method of new cartilage for-

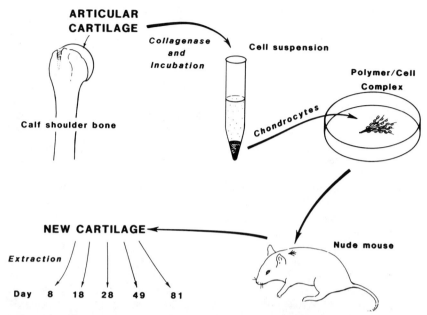

Fig 4–8.—The implantation of the cell-polymer constructs into nude mice after chondrocyte isolation from articulating surface of calf shoulder and adherence to polymer fibers in vitro. Chondrocytes were harvested from the articular surfaces of newborn calf shoulders as described by Klagsbrun M: *Methods Enzymol* 58:560, 1979. One hundred microliters of the chondrocyte suspension, concentrated to 5×10^7 cells/mL, was seeded onto braided threads of polyglactin 910 of approximately 17 mm in length and kept in vitro for either 3 or 10 days. Fibers containing chondrocytes were then surgically implanted subcutaneously on the dorsum of 37 male nude mice, 4–5 weeks of age, in the midline at the base of the neck. After being implanted for specified periods of time, the implants were excised and fixed in 10% buffered formalin phosphate. To classify the type of collagen present in the specimens, immunohistochemistry was performed using antibodies to bovine collagen types 1–4. (Courtesy of Vacanti CA, Langer R, Schloo B, et al: *Plast Reconstr Surg* 88:753–759, 1991.)

mation in vivo was devised. The use of synthetic polymers, prepared to provide a large surface area for cell attachment and to promote cell function and survival by diffusion of nutrients, has yielded stable and mature cartilage in mice. The new cartilage maintains the approximate dimensions and configuration of the original template.

▶ It has now been demonstrated in the laboratory that, by providing a sufficient artificial scaffold, chondrocytes can populate this structure and maintain, at least for a period of time, a chondrocyte phenotype.—R. Poss, M.D.

Familial Aggregation of Paget's Disease of Bone
Siris ES, Ottman R, Flaster E, Kelsey JL (Columbia Univ, New York; Columbia Presbyterian Med Ctr, New York)
J Bone Miner Res 6:495–500, 1991   4–40

Background.—A familial aggregation for Paget's disease of bone has been reported previously. An epidemiologic study investigated the extent to which Paget's disease of bone aggregates in families, the cumulative incidence of the disease in first-degree relatives of patients throughout life, and the influence of the age at diagnosis and the presence of bone deformity in the patient on the risk of Paget's disease in relatives.

Methods.—Individuals with Paget's disease were recruited through an announcement in the newsletter of the Paget's Disease Foundation in the United States. Questionnaires were completed by 788 individuals and 387 spouse controls. The final study population also included 2,930 relatives of individuals with Paget's disease and 1,360 relatives of controls.

Findings.—A positive family history of Paget's disease in first-degree relative (parents or siblings) was reported by 12.3% of the patients and 2.1% of the controls. The rate of Paget's disease was about 7 times as high in the relatives of the individuals with Paget's disease as in the relatives of the controls; this increased risk did not differ according to the gender of the patient or control or to the gender of the relatives. The cumulative incidence of Paget's disease to 90 years of age in relatives of the individuals with Paget's disease was 8.9%, which was much higher than the 1.8% risk in the relatives of the controls (Fig 4–9), regardless of the gender of the patient or relative and the relationship (parent vs. sibling) to the patient. In relatives of patients, the risk of Paget's disease was associated with diagnosis before 55 years of age, with presence of bone deformity, and with presence of an affected parent. The risk of Paget's disease was greatest (20.7%) among relatives of patients with both bone de-

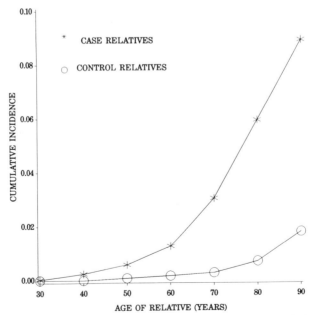

Fig 4–9.—The cumulative incidence of Paget's disease in relatives of patients and relatives of controls, by age of the relatives. (Courtesy of Siris ES, Ottman R, Flaster E, et al: *J Bone Miner Res* 6:495–500, 1991.)

formity and early age at diagnosis, it was least (3.6%) among the relatives of patients without bone deformity who had late age at diagnosis. The risk in siblings of individuals with Paget's disease was 22.1% when 1 parent was affected, compared with 6.7% when both parents were affected.

Conclusion.—First-degree relatives of patients with Paget's disease of bone have an increased risk of the disorder, contracting particularly if the affected relatives have early age at diagnosis or bone deformity.

▶ This study of familial aggregation of Paget's disease suggests that a genetic predisposition may play a role in the manifestation of this disorder.—R. Poss, M.D.

The Proliferative and Synthetic Response of Isolated Calvarial Bone Cells of Rats to Cyclic Biaxial Mechanical Strain

Brighton CT, Strafford B, Gross SB, Leatherwood DF II, Williams JL, Pollack SR (Univ of Pennsylvania, Philadelphia)
J Bone Joint Surg 73-A:320–331, 1991   4–41

Background.—Most tests of bone response to mechanical stress do not account for the amount of strain or deformation on the substrate or membrane on which the bone was growing. In addition, there have been no reports of the strain amplitudes that are present on the cellular level within or on bone. A series of experiments were performed to examine the proliferative and synthetic response of bone cells to cyclic biaxial mechanical strain.

Methods.—Using specially constructed culture chambers and polyurethane membranes, isolated bone cells were grown from the calvaria of 1–2-day-old Sprague-Dawley rats. Cyclic biaxial mechanical strains of .02%, .04%, and .1% were applied at a frequency of 1 Hz; these strains corresponded to 200, 400, and 1,000 microstrain, respectively. The strains were applied for periods of 15 minutes to 72 hours.

Results.—Measured as an index of proliferation, DNA content was increased at a strain of .04% applied for a duration of 15 minutes, 24 hours, and 48 hours (Fig 4–10). No such increase was noted at the other strain amplitudes nor at strain applications of over 48 hours. At a strain amplitude of .04% and durations of 15 minutes and 24, 48, and 72 hours, there were significant decreases in indicators of macromolecular synthesis, including collagen, noncollagenous protein, and proteoglycan synthesis and alkaline phosphatase activity. None of the other strain amplitudes affected macromolecular synthesis. There was a significant increase in prostaglandin E_2 content but no change in net cyclic adenosine monophosphate content at a strain of .04% at 5, 15, and 30 minutes; the increased proliferation and decreased macromolecular synthesis observed were mediated at least in part by prostaglandin E_2.

Conclusions.—Bone cells respond to a mechanical strain of .04% with cell proliferation and, to a lesser degree, with decreased macromolecular

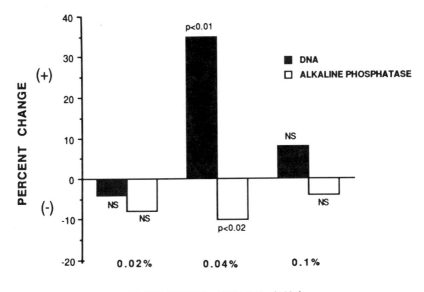

MECHANICAL STRAIN (1Hz)

Fig 4–10.—Graph depicting the percentage change in DNA content and activity of alkaline phosphatase of bone cells that were subjected to biaxial mechanical strains of .02% (200 microstrain), .04% (400 microstrain), and .1% (1,000 microstrain) for 24 hours at a frequency of 1 hertz. Note that DNA content is significantly increased at a strain of .4%, and that activity of alkaline phosphatase is significantly decreased at that level of strain. Changes in the percentage of collagen either were not significant or were inconsistent. (Courtesy of Brighton CT, Strafford B, Gross SB, et al: *J Bone Joint Surg* (73-A:320–331, 1991.)

synthesis. These changes can occur with very brief durations of strain and occur with increased prostaglandin E_2 synthesis. The clinical aspects of bone remodeling can be understood through a knowledge of the response of isolated cells to such strain and of the mechanisms involved in physiologic response.

▶ A long asked question of critical importance is "what is the osteoblast transducer that converts mechanical signals into a biologic response?" This paper is one of a number of studies being conducted at various laboratories that used isolated osteoblasts in a controlled mechanical environment and studies their response to altered strains. This field of investigation will blossom in the next few years.— R. Poss, M.D.

Tissue Transformation Into Bone In Vivo: A Potential Practical Application
Khouri RK, Koudsi B, Reddi H (Washington Univ, St. Louis; Natl Inst of Dental Research, Bethesda, Md)
JAMA 266:1953–1955, 1991   4–42

Background.—Few of the recent breakthroughs in cell biology have found their way into the surgical armamentarium. Mesenchymal tissue such as muscle can be induced to transform into bone by osteogenin, a recently purified osteoinductive factor. An investigation in rats tested the possibility of transforming muscle flaps into vascularized bone grafts of various shapes for use as skeletal replacement parts.

Methods.—In 23 Lewis rats, thigh adductor muscle island flaps pedicled on the femoral vessels were dissected from the ipsilateral leg. These flaps were then placed into bivalved silicone rubber molds. Before the molds were closed, 18 were injected with osteogenin, .2 μg, and coated with demineralized bone matrix, 25 mg. The control flaps were injected with vehicle only and were not coated with mineralized bone matrix. The molds were placed subcutaneously into the flanks of the animals and re-opened 10 days later.

Results.—The control flaps showed intact muscle but no evidence of tissue transformation; all were soft and essentially shapeless. The osteogenin-treated flaps appeared rigid, gritty, and bony and were shaped like the molds, including the fine contour details. Almost all of the tissue had been transformed into bone, mainly cancellous, but some was organized into compact lamellae with a central core of bone marrow.

Conclusions.—By using tissue transformation, it was possible to generate in vivo, autogenous, well-perfused bone of specific shapes in rats. This technique has potential for use in reconstruction. It is up to clinicians to take it into the surgical laboratory and later into clinical use.

▶ A stunning example of the possibility of inducing the formation of bone or cartilage in vivo. In this laboratory model, muscle flaps treated with osteogenin and demineralized bone matrix undergo metaplasia to bone. The implications of this study and this approach are obvious and may point the direction to the next era of biologic replacement of tissues.—R. Poss, M.D.

The Morphogenesis of Bone in Replicas of Porous Hydroxyapatite Obtained From Conversion of Calcium Carbonate Exoskeletons of Coral

Ripamonti U (Univ of the Witwatersrand, Johannesburg, South Africa)
J Bone Joint Surg 73-A:692–703, 1991   4–43

Background.—There is increasing interest in the osteoconductive potential of porous hydroxyapatite obtained by hydrothermal conversion of the calcium carbonate exoskeleton of reef-building corals. Hydroxyapatite exhibits a uniform network of interconnected channels and pores resembling the inorganic supporting structure of living bone.

Methods.—Bone formation in a porous hydroxyapatite substratum was examined after intramuscular implantation into adult baboons. Replicas of porous hydroxyapatite were placed in 24 animals, and the implants were sampled at intervals up to 9 months.

Findings.—Initially fibrous connective tissue formed with collagen fibers condensing at the interface and later differentiating. Bone formed without an endochondral phase, sometimes extensively, to fill large parts of the porous spaces. Bone formed about one fifth of the total volume of the specimens on average. The hydroxyapatite framework itself exhibited moderate degradation over time. Bone formation was not enhanced by coating the hydroxyapatite substratum with a fibrin–fibronectin protein concentrate prepared from baboon plasma.

Conclusions.—Coralline replicas of hydroxyapatite can be used as an alternative to autogenous bone grafts to initiate bone formation in the clincial setting. The hydroxyapatite substratum probably acts as a solid-phase anchorage for osteogenin and related bone morphogenetic proteins.

▶ Porous hydroxyapatite acts as an excellent scaffold for the invasion of osteoblasts and bone formation. This type of approach may serve as a replacement for large contained bone defects where sufficient quantities of autogenous graft are impractical.— R. Poss, M.D.

Risk Factors for Falls as a Cause of Hip Fracture in Women
Grisso JA, Kelsey JL, Strom BL, Chiu GY, Maislin G, O'Brien LA, Hoffman S, Kaplan F, Northeast Hip Fracture Study Group (Univ of Pennsylvania, Philadelphia; Columbia Univ, New York; Hosp of the Univ of Pennsylvania, Philadelphia)
N Engl J Med 324:1326–1331, 1991   4–44

Background.—More than 90% of hip fractures are caused by falls, although only 1% to 14% of falls in women result in such an injury. A controlled trial was done to examine the importance of risk factors for falls in the epidemiology of hip fracture.

Methods.—Participants were 174 women (median age, 80 years), who were admitted with their first hip fracture to 1 of 30 hospitals. Controls were women from the general surgery and orthopedic surgery hospital services matched to study patients for age and hospital who had never fractured their hip or had a hip replacement. Patients were interviewed to obtain information on lower limb function before the fracture, on visual impairment, on neurologic disease and cognitive function, on alcohol and medications taken, on adjusted weight, and on the circumstances of the fall.

Results.—An increased risk of hip fracture was associated with lower limb dysfunction (odds ratio 1.7), visual impairment (odds ratio, 5.1), previous stroke (odds ratio 2), Parkinson's disease (odds ratio, 9.4), and use of long-acting barbiturates (odds ratio, 5.2) (table). There were no such associations with dizziness, limping, numbness, balance problems, or use of alcohol or long-acting benzodiazepines. A recent fall was sustained by 44 control patients (25%). Patients were more likely than controls to have fallen from a standing height or higher (odds ratio, 2.4). Patients with hip fracture who were younger than 75 years of age were more likely than those 75 years and older to have fallen on a hard surface (odds ratio, 1.9).

Conclusion.—Measures to prevent falls, as well as those to slow bone

Multivariate Adjusted Odds Ratios for the Major
Risk Factors or Hip Fracture

RISK FACTOR	ODDS RATIO	95 PERCENT CONFIDENCE INTERVALS
Lower-extremity dysfunction	1.9	0.9–3.8
Loss of distant vision	4.8	1.4–16.2
Previous stroke	4.5	1.5–13.5
Body-mass index† (in fifths of distribution)		
Lowest	1.0‡	
Second	0.6	0.3–1.2
Third	0.4	0.2–0.9
Fourth	0.2	0.1–0.4
Highest	0.2	0.1–0.5

Note: Ratios were based on conditional logistic regression models, with the patient's hospital as the conditional variable, and with control for age, estrogen use, use of thiazide diuretic agents, smoking, number of chronic illnesses, moderate cognitive impairment, and all these factors.
†Calculated as the weight in kilograms divided by the square of the height in meters.
‡Reference value.
(Courtesy of Grisso JA, Kelsey, JL, Strom BL, et al: *N Engl J Med* 324:1326–1331, 1991.)

loss, should be included in programs to prevent hip fracture in the elderly. Such measures may include aggressive treatment of ocular disease and visual impairment and physical therapy for patients with impaired mobility.

▶ There is increasing recognition that prevention of falls may play a major role in the prevention of hip fractures. Recognition of the numerous factors that contribute to traumatic falls in the elderly should decrease the incidence of hip fracture.—R. Ross, M.D.

The Predictive Value of Bone Loss for Fragility Fractures in Women: A Longitudinal Study Over 15 Years

Gärdsell P, Johnell O, Nilsson BE (Malmö Gen Hosp, Sweden)
Calcif Tissue Int 49:90–94, 1991   4–45

Background.—Forearm bone mineral content has predicted future fragility fractures only in women younger than 70 years; in older women, no factors could differentiate between those who would and would not have fractures.

Methods.—To determine whether the more important predictor of fragility fractures is initial bone mass or subsequent bone loss, forearm bone mineral content was measured by single photon absorptiometry in 1,076 women in 1970–1976. Using Swedish National Population Records, 519 women still living in the area were located. Of these, 366 responded to an invitation to have a repeated bone mineral content measurement using the same technique. All fractures that occurred after the initial measurement were recorded. The mean time between the first and second measurements was 14.6 years.

Results.—At least 1 fragility fracture had occurred since the first measurement in 96 women. Regardless of age, the women who had fragility fractures had lower initial bone mineral content than those who did not have such fractures. Trabecular bone mineral content was an earlier predictor than cortical bone mineral content. There was no correlation between fracture risk and rate of loss, with no significant difference in rate of loss between those who had fractures and those who did not.

Conclusions.—Initial bone mineral content is a better predictor of future fragility fracture than the subsequent rate of bone loss. In individuals, rate of loss may have predictive value in describing bone metabolic rate. Longitudinal study confirms that women have their peak bone value before age 40 years.

▶ The incidence of fracture in the elderly is in many ways determined by the peak bone mass reached before the age of 40. Those who attained a low peak bone mass had a higher incidence of fracture 15 years later than their counterparts with higher peak bone masses. The rate of bone loss does not seem to be as important as the initial reservoir of mineralized tissue attained during youth.—R. Poss, M.D.

Transient Osteoporosis of the Hip: Magnetic Resonance Imaging
Takatori Y, Kokubo T, Ninomiya S, Nakamura T, Okutsu I, Kamogawa M (Univ of Tokyo; Japanese Red Cross Med Ctr, Tokyo)
Clin Orthop 271:190–194, 1991   4–46

Background.—In transient osteoporosis of the hip MRI has been reported to provide considerable, if nonspecific, diagnostic evidence. This technique was used in studying 6 patients (7 hips) affected with transient osteoporosis.

Patients.—The 5 men and 1 woman were examined during a 5-year period. The mean age of the men was 38 years; the woman, who was diagnosed in the third trimester of pregnancy, was age 28 years. There was no definitive diagnosis for any patient at first examination. All had unilateral hip pain with no history of trauma or infection, full range of motion despite pain, and little discomfort at rest. A 1.5 T superconductive magnet system was used for MRI.

Findings.—Magnetic resonance imaging showed increased joint fluid and diffuse signal abnormalities in the marrow of the femoral head. These changes corresponded to decreased signal intensity on T1-weighted images and increased signal intensity on T2-weighted images, which also showed grade 3 joint effusion. There was considerable variation in the proximal femoral abnormalities. The diagnosis of transient osteoporosis was made, and patients were restricted to crutches for weight-bearing. At clinical improvement 3–5 months later MRI showed regression of the abnormalities.

Conclusions.—Magnetic resonance imaging can yield significant evidence to support the diagnosis of transient osteoporosis of the hip when used along with clinical history and laboratory findings. The abnormalities observed reflect the pathophysiology of the condition.

Hip Pain in Late Pregnancy
Brooks GG, Thomas BV, Wood MJ (Louisana State Univ, Shreveport)
J Reprod Med 35:969–970, 1990   4–47

Background.—Hip pain is a common complaint in late pregnancy. This symptom may be related to the rare and acute transient osteoporosis of the hip in late pregnancy that is a demineralization syndrome of unknown origin. The relationship between the hip pain of women in late pregnancy and bone mineral content was investigated.

Methods.—Twenty-six women (aged 20–44 years) were included. All patients rated hip pain subjectively and completed questionnaires about previous fractures, diet, calcium supplements, exercise, milk product allergies, and tobacco and alcohol use. Bone mineral content in all women was measured within 48 hours of delivery using dual photon absorptiometry.

Results.—Thirty-three percent of density measurements among women with severe pain were decreased, compared with 10% of the measurements of the remaining women. No marked reductions in the bone mineral content were seen, even in women with severe pain. No other variable could be correlated with hip pain or bone mineral content.

Conclusions.—A subacute form of acute osteoporotic syndrome may cause hip pain late in pregnancy. Further investigations measuring bone mineral content using sensitive methods should be undertaken.

Magnetic Resonance Imaging of Transient Osteoporosis of the Hip: A Case Report
Urbanski SR, De Lange EE, Eschenroeder HC Jr (Univ of Virginia, Charlottesville)
J Bone Joint Surg 73-A:451–455, 1991   4–48

Purpose.—The radiographic features of transient osteoporosis of the hip on MRI were examined in 1 woman.

Case Report.—Woman, 40, during her third trimester of pregnancy complained of progressive pain on the left hip, that was worse on weight-bearing and activity and absent at rest. Range of motion was limited by pain. Plain radiographs of the hip were normal. Magnetic resonance imaging showed that the normally high signal intensity of the bone marrow of the femoral head was replaced with relatively low signal intensity on T1-weighted spin-echo images and relatively high signal intensity on T2-weighted images. The abnormal signal extended into the femoral neck but did not involve the acetabulum. A joint effusion occurred, but there was no evidence of arthritic changes or soft tissue abnormalities. These abnormalities resolved as the patient improved with nonoperative treatment.

Conclusions.—Transient osteoporosis of the hip should be considered in the differential diagnosis of a painful hip. Magnetic resonance imaging is highly sensitive in the diagnosis of this condition, and it is helpful in the exclusion of other entities (e.g., avascular necrosis, osteomyelitis, and neoplasm).

▶ Transient osteoporosis of the hip is a common phenomenon, particularly in late pregnancy. Magnetic resonance imaging gives a characteristic picture and aids in the exclusion of other entities. Awareness of this diagnosis and recognition that it is transient and self-limiting should prevent other, more invasive diagnostic or therapeutic procedures.—R. Poss, M.D.

Prevention of Postmenopausal Osteoporosis: A Comparative Study of Exercise, Calcium Supplementation, and Hormone-Replacement Therapy
Prince RL, Smith M, Dick IM, Price RI, Webb PG, Henderson NK, Harris MM (Sir Charles Gairdner Hospital, Nedlands, Australia; King Edward Mem Hospital for Women, Subiaco, Australia)
N Engl J Med 325:1189–1195, 1991   4–49

Background.—There is a high prevalence of bone fractures among women with osteoporosis. This represents a major public health problem. A double-blind, placebo-controlled randomized trial was designed to compare the effects of 3 approaches to the prevention of osteoporosis: exercise, exercise plus calcium supplementation, and exercise plus hormone replacement therapy.

Methods.—Included were 120 postmenopausal women (mean age, 56 years) with distal forearm bone density values of less than 290 mg/cm^2. A group of 41 women was assigned to an exercise program; a group of 39 was assigned to exercise plus calcium lactate–gluconate, 1 g/day; and a group of 40 was assigned to exercise plus medroxyprogesterone acetate, 2.5 mg/day, and estropipate, .625 mg/day, for 1 month and then 1.25 mg/day for the rest of the 2-year trial period. Bone density at 3 forearm sites and indexes of calcium metabolism were measured periodically throughout the study, and symptom scores were recorded. For comparison, a control group of 42 women with normal bone density and a mean age of 55.5 years was observed.

Results.—The control group and the exercise group both lost significant bone at the distal forearm site: −2.7% and −2.6% of baseline per year, respectively. This compared to a decrease of −.5% in the exercise–calcium group and an increase of 2.7% in the exercise–estrogen group. At the median forearm site bone loss was significantly less in the exercise–calcium group than in the exercise group, and bone density increased significantly in the exercise–estrogen group. Forty-seven percent of women in the exercise–estrogen group experienced breast tenderness, compared to only 20% in the other 2 treatment groups. Among women in the exercise–estrogen group who had not had a hysterectomy 52% had vaginal bleeding at some point compared to 11% in the exercise group and 12.5% in the exercise–calcium group.

Conclusions.—Exercise and calcium supplementation or estrogen–progesterone replacement can slow or prevent bone loss in postmenopausal women with low bone density. Estrogen replacement is more effective in increasing bone mass than calcium supplementation, but it is also associated with more side effects. Osteoporosis may be prevented by bone-density screening and appropriate intervention.

▶ A comparison of many of the agents available to maintain bone mass demonstrates the advantages and relative disadvantages in their use. Physical exercise is advantageous in all people. Individual risk factors must be assessed when striking a balance between risks and benefits of these medications.—R. Poss, M.D.

5 Spine

Introduction

Few truly new insights have been reported for spinal disorders during the past year. The most exciting is the demonstration of enhanced post-traumatic neurologic recovery in spinal cord injury patients by a naturally occurring neural growth stimulator, monosialotetraherosylganglioside (GM-1) ganglioside. The implications of the study are far-reaching. The results are not only potentially applicable to traumatic neural injury but also possibly applicable to patients with longer standing compressive disorders. The need is apparent. For example, much of the enthusiasm for the surgical treatment of lumbar spinal stenosis is based on relatively short-term surveillance. Abstracts of articles presented later show that these early results give an incomplete picture and are overly optimistic because they do not register the later and ongoing deterioration in neurologic function. The reasons for this deterioration are complex and probably include intrinsic neural deterioration, co-morbid conditions, and later instability. Similarly, the results of extensive anterior cervical decompression are suboptimal when evidence of spinal cord atrophy accompanies the extrinsic compressive lesion. The hope of the future is that pharmacologic and physiologic manipulations will yield results that are greater than those produced by surgical decompressions and stabilizations alone.

Two other general themes emerge from this year's literature survey. First, there is a trend toward fusion accompanied by more aggressive and rigid fixation for the management of both traumatic and nontraumatic spinal conditions. For many years the debate has been waged over the need for decompression vs. decompression and fusion in patients with degenerative spondylolisthesis. A prospective study indicates that fusion has definite added benefit. Whether or not fusion is enhanced by internal fixation is yet to be proven conclusively, but a number of articles abstracted here continue to indicate a positive benefit. However, other studies underscore that there remains a price to be paid, including significant and unresolved complications of the devices.

The second general theme is the ongoing issue of disability as the greatest source of cost. Perhaps the most troubling, but not surprising, study reported here looks at the long-term results of patients with successful surgical procedures followed by prolonged return to work. Over time, significant reinjuries occurred that were related to the severity of job requirements. This type of information points out the complexity of disability as a balance between external physical factors, disease progression, and the complex psychosocial environment in which injury occurs.

John W. Frymoyer, M.D.

Cervical Spine

NEURAL COMPRESSION SYNDROMES

Chronic Nerve Compression Model for the Double Crush Hypothesis

Dellon AL, Mackinnon SE (Johns Hopkins Univ, Baltimore; University of Toronto, Ontario)

Ann Plast Surg 26:259–264, 1991   5–1

Background.—The double crush hypothesis proposes that a proximal source of nerve compression makes the distal nerve segment more vulnerable to compression at a second site. Although the hypothesis has been increasingly accepted, there is little experimental evidence to support it.

Methods.—Among 30 rats, 1 group had a single band of silastic tubing placed about the sciatic nerve 1.5 cm proximal to the sciatic trifurcation, another group had a single band placed just distal to the trifurcation, and a third group had bands placed simultaneously at both sites (Fig 5–1). Electrophysiologic data were recorded at monthly intervals. After 7 months the first group had a second band placed over the posterior tibial nerve and the second group had a second band placed at the proximal site. Follow-up was continued for 5 months longer.

Results.—The reduction in amplitude of the compound action potential was more marked in animals with a single band placed proximally, compared to those with distal placement. Both single-banded groups had a further significant decrease in potential amplitude after placement of the second band (Fig 5–2). Reduced conduction velocity was more marked in animals with a single band placed proximally than in those with a single band placed distally.

Conclusions.—These findings confirm the double crush hypothesis in this model of chronic nerve compression. Two concurrent sites of compression compromise nerve function more than compression at a single site.

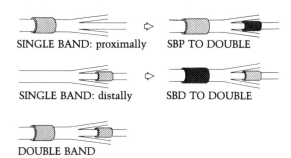

SINGLE BAND: proximally   SBP TO DOUBLE

SINGLE BAND: distally   SBD TO DOUBLE

DOUBLE BAND

Fig 5–1.—Schema of experimental design. Initially, 3 groups of rats were created: single-banded proximal, single-banded distal, and simultaneously double banded. Proximal band was around sciatic nerve and distal band was around posterior tibial nerve. Seven months after initial banding, 2 single-banded groups of rats were made double-banded by adding second band in appropriate location. (Courtesy of Dellon AL, Mackinnon SE: *Ann Plast Surg* 26:259–264, 1991.)

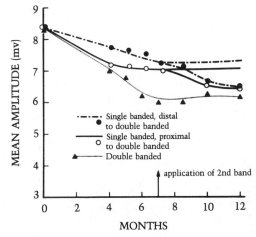

Fig 5–2.—Additional effect on amplitude of compound action potential by adding second, minimally compressive band. There is rapid loss of electrophysiologic function so that within 3 months, initially single-banded groups of rats reached level of simultaneously double-banded group. (Courtesy of Dellon AL, Mackinnon SE: *Ann Plast Surg* 26:259–264, 1991.)

▶ This elegant animal study confirms the clinical hypothesis that nerve compression at 2 sites has an additive adverse effect on neural function. In particular, it suggests that there is a strong neurophysiologic rationale for examining patients carefully to eliminate dual sites of compression such as cervical radiculopathy in combination with peripheral compression—for example, the ulnar nerve at the elbow. Further, it indicates the importance of relieving both compressive sites if optimal neurophysiologic recovery is to be anticipated.—J.W. Frymoyer, M.D.

Treatment of Cervical Spondylotic Myelopathy by Enlargement of the Spinal Canal Anteriorly, Followed by Arthrodesis
Okada K, Shirasaki N, Hayashi H, Oka S, Hosoya T (Kagawa Medical School, Japan; Himeji Red Cross Hospital, Hyogo, Japan)
J Bone Joint Surg 73-A:352–364, 1991   5–2

Background.—The appropriate surgical treatment for patients with multilevel involvement of cervical spondylotic myelopathy, often associated with stenosis, is controversial. Surgery involving enlargement of the narrowed spinal canal anteriorly and stabilization of the cervical spine was performed on patients who had myelopathy associated with spondylosis.

Patients.—Patients with any disease of the CNS, ossification of the posterior longitudinal ligament, previous surgery for the condition, or major trauma, were excluded. Included were 23 men and 14 women (average age, 58 years). Preoperatively, 32 patients had only myelopathy without radiculopathy and 5 had radiculomyelopathy (table). All 37 had hyperreflexia of the lower extremities, a disturbance in gait, and sensory

Preoperative and Postoperative Neurologic Status of the 37 Patients, Assessed by the Scoring System of the Japanese Orthopaedic Association

Motor function	Grade	Score (Points)	No. of Patients Preop.	At Interim Examination	At Final Examination
Upper extremity					
Normal	0	4	1	25	27
Able to eat with chopsticks, with slight difficulty	1	3	11	7	5
Able to eat with chopsticks, with much difficulty	2	2	13	3	4
Able to eat with a spoon but not with chopsticks	3	1	10	2	1
Unable to feed self	4	0	2	0	0
Lower extremity					
Normal	0	4	0	17	17
Able to walk without walking aid but has mild spasticity	1	3	2	9 (1)*	9
Needs handrail on stairs	2	2	18	8 (3)*	7 (3)*
Needs walking aid on flat surface	3	1	10 (3)*	3 (3)*	4 (4)*
Unable to walk	4	0	7 (4)*	0	0

loss in the upper extremities; 25 patients had a bladder disturbance. The 4 morphological types of myelopathy were classified as central in 9 patients, lateral in 6 patients, diffuse in 16 patients, and atrophic in 6 patients.

Technique.—The spinal canal was enlarged by diskectomy, by subtotal corpectomy and removal of the anteromedial parts of the pedicles, or by removal of os-

Sensory					
Upper extremity					
Normal	0	2	0	7	7
Minimum sensory loss	1	1	10	21	22
Apparent sensory loss	2	0	27	9	8
Lower extremity					
Normal	0	2	4	23	22
Minimum sensory loss	1	1	9	12	12
Apparent sensory loss	2	0	24	2	3
Trunk					
Normal	0	2	11	36	37
Minimum sensory loss	1	1	13	0	0
Apparent sensory loss	2	0	13	1	0
Bladder function					
Normal	0	3	12	30	31
Mild dysfunction	1	2	22	6	6
Severe dysfunction	2	1	3	1	0
Complete retention of urine	3	0	0	0	0
Total score and averages, with standard deviation		17	7.4 ± 2.4	13.8 ± 2.6	14.0 ± 2.6

*The numbers in parentheses are the numbers of patients who had motor weakness in the peroneal muscles with muscle strength of less than 3 (of 5). The patients are the same in each column.
(Courtesy of Okada K, Shirasaki N, Hayashi H, et al: *J Bone Joint Surg* 73-A;352–364, 1991.)

teophytes or of the posterior longitudinal ligament. Preoperative myelograms and CT myelograms were used to determine the extent of the levels to be decompressed and the number of levels to be fused. Three types of anterior procedures were performed: partial corpectomy cephalad and caudad to the level of the involved disk and interbody arthrodesis; subtotal corpectomy, including removal of the posterior parts of the vertebral bodies and of the posterior longitudinal ligament, and strut bone-grafting; and subtotal corpectomy, with detachment of the remaining posterior parts of the vertebral bodies and of the posterior longitudinal ligament, and strut bone-grafting. Arthrodesis was performed at 1–4 levels. Postoperatively, the patients who had an arthrodesis at more than 1 level used a halo vest, and patients with single-level arthrodesis used a Philadelphia collar.

Results.—Postoperatively all patients were improved neurologically and could walk. Forty-nine percent of patients had an excellent result, 30% had a good result, and 22% had a fair result. After initial improvement, 3 patients had deterioration in the ability to walk. Older patients had worse results than younger patients. There was a significant correlation between the preoperative and postoperative total scores. The duration of symptoms and signs of myelopathy correlated negatively with the postoperative score. Patients with arthrodesis at a single level had superior results compared to patients with multiple-level arthrodesis. Patients with the atrophic type of myelopathy had poorer results. Twelve complications in 8 patients included 4 patients with complications attributable to the bone graft. The radiculopathy worsened in 5 patients and was apparent immediately postoperatively in 4. One patient with severe myelopathy and 2 with less severe myelopathy had neurologic worsening after surgery.

Conclusions.—Anterior decompression followed by a secure arthrodesis should be an extensive procedure for patients who have cervical spondylotic myelopathy.

▶ This prospective study does not prove or disprove the superiority of their method, which involves extensive anterior decompression in patients with single or multilevel cervical spinal stenosis. It does give a careful analysis of the factors that influence the results obtained and correlates success and failure with the preoperative and later postoperative imaging studies. The predictive factors that are associated with failure (age, disease severity, spinal cord atrophy) are not surprising.—J.W. Frymoyer, M.D.

Artificial Ceramic Intervertebral Disc Replacement in Cervical Disc Lesion
Tsuji H, Itoh T, Yamada H, Morita I, Ichimura K, Ishihara H (Toyama Medical and Pharmaceutical University, Japan
J West Pacific Orthop Assoc 27:101–106, 1990   5–3

Introduction.—Among 110 patients who had anterior diskectomy for cervical disk degeneration between October 1979 and December 1987, 2 simultaneously received anterior interbody fusion with an autologous iliac bone graft and artificial disk replacement at a separate site. One of the 2 patients had herniated nucleus pulposus at skipped levels with mo-

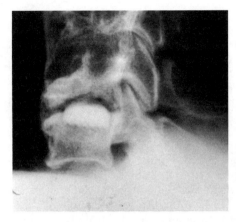

Fig 5–3.—Extension radiograph demonstrating 4-degree range of segmental motion. (Courtesy of Tsuji H, Itoh T, Yamada H, et al: *J West Pacific Orthop Assoc* 27:101–106, 1990.)

tor loss. The other had symptomatic disk degeneration at 2 levels adjacent to a long fused segment secondary to ankylosing spinal hyperostosis.

Technique.—The artificial disk, of alumina ceramic has a multicentric convex upper surface and a "blunt-toothed" lower surface. After completely removing the disk by an anterior approach with the cartilaginous plates left intact, a disk space-spreading system is set and the artificial disk is placed in the emptied space. The anterior longitudinal ligament then is resutured as the ceramic disk is covered.

Results.—The artificial disk remained a good spacer 3 months after operation and maintained a normal range of segmental mobility. Nevertheless, the disk had migrated into the C7 vertebra a year after operation; migration was evident 6 months after operation and progressed. Anterior spur formation was noted, and the space between the upper artificial disk surface and the distal border of the upper vertebra gradually widened (Fig 5–3).

Conclusions.—This experience shows the importance of an accurate design when using an artificial disk to replace a diseased conical disk. The replacement must conform to the upper disk space, and the material used should be sufficiently elastic.

▶ Why include this clinical report based on 2 cases? Currently, there is a growing interest in "artificial disks." Some of these devices attempt to re-create the normal kinematic and mechanical behavior of the intervertebral disc; others are simply spacers; and others are fusion substitutes. The device described here appears to be in the second category, despite the authors' attempts to recreate normal mechanical behavior. The results are evident; the devices failed by progressive intrusion into adjacent vertebral bodies. The postoperative radiography makes one wonder what additional risks will be incurred by these patients in the long term. The more crucial question is, is there any patient group for which artificial disks might be appropriate?—J.W. Frymoyer, M.D.

TRAUMA

Recovery of Motor Function After Spinal-Cord Injury: A Randomized, Placebo-Controlled Trial With GM-1 Ganglioside
Geisler FH, Dorsey FC, Coleman WP (Maryland Inst for Emergency Med Services Systems, Baltimore; Fidia Pharmaceutical Corp, Washington, DC)
N Engl J Med 324:1829–1838, 1991   5–4

Background.—Treatment of spinal cord injuries in specialized centers has decreased morbidity and mortality, but only some patients have major neurologic recovery, and recovery is rarely complete. In recent animal studies, monosialotetrahexosylganglioside (GM-1) ganglioside enhanced the functional recovery of damaged neurons. An investigation was conducted to determine whether the neurologic recovery in humans after a spinal cord injury can be altered by adding GM-1 ganglioside to the protocol of medical and surgical care used initially.

Methods.—In a prospective, randomized, placebo-controlled, double-blind drug trial of GM-1 ganglioside, 34 of 37 patients completed the protocol. The 34 patients included 23 patients with cervical injuries and 11 with thoracic injuries who were randomly assigned to a treatment group (16 patients) or placebo (18 patients) group. Nine GM-1–treatment patients and 9 placebo-treatment patients underwent surgery within 72 hours after the injury. The protocol for acute management of spinal cord injury consisted of 6 phases: (1) initial assessment and spinal immobilization, (2) medical treatment to correct neurogenic shock and optimize tissue perfusion and oxygenation, (3) prompt anatomic alignment of the spinal bony elements, (4) radiologic diagnostic examination, (5) prompt surgical decompression of neural elements if the closed spinal alignment failed to relieve the compression, and (6) stabilization of any bony instability. Medical management included administration of methylprednisolone sodium succinate. The Frankel scale and the American Spinal Injury Association motor score were used to measure the severity of spinal cord injury and its subsequent recovery. Patients were monitored for 12 months.

Results.—The treated patients' Frankel grade improved more than that of controls. The overall number of patients (8 of 34) whose scores improved by 2 or more Frankel grades was larger than historical data would have predicted. Seven of the 8 patients with this considerable neurologic recovery were in the GM-1–treated group. In the placebo group, the recovery of 1 to 18 patients was similar to that predicted on the basis of historical data. Despite randomization, the American Spinal Injury Association motor scores at entry were imbalanced, with 25.9 in the GM-1–treated group and 39.8 for the placebo group. Mean motor recovery from entry score to the score after 1 year for the GM-1–treated patients was 36.9 points, compared with 21.6 points for the placebo-treated patients.

Conclusions.—The drug effect of GM-1 ganglioside dramatically increased neurologic function, with most recipients changing from paralyzed to ambulatory status. These findings suggest that GM-1 is safe to administer in spinal cord injury and enhances the recovery of neurologic function after 1 year. A larger trial is needed to confirm its clinical benefit and safety.

▶ Gangliosides have experimentally been shown to induce neural regeneration and cause neuronal sprouting. This study demonstrates that neurologic function is improved in patients receiving gangliosides. Although the authors are quick to point out that the results should be considered preliminary, the potential to stimulate regrowth of damaged neural structures is exciting.—J.W. Frymoyer, M.D.

Immediate Closed Reduction of Cervical Spine Dislocations Using Traction

Star AM, Jones AA, Cotler JM, Balderston RA, Sinha R (Thomas Jefferson Univ, Philadelphia)
Spine 15:1068–1072, 1990   5–5

Background.—Cervical facet dislocations can be reduced rapidly and effectively using gradual application of traction through skull tongs, but there is no consensus on the maximum applied traction weight. A rapid method of reducing cervical spine facet dislocations using larger amounts of longitudinal traction than previously reported was examined.

Methods.—Reduction was attempted in all 57 patients using axial cervical traction through Gardner-Wells tongs. To reduce the dislocation as soon as it was recognized, a team applied cervical tongs and gradually added weights in increments never exceeding 10 lb, beginning with 10–20 lb. A neurologic examination and a roentgenogram was taken between each addition of weight. The end point was either reduction of the dislocation, evidence of excessive distraction, or a maximum weight between 60 and 160 lb. In a study of 4 cadavers, Gardner-Wells cervical tongs were applied and weight was gradually increased until tong pullout occurred or until 300 lb was reached.

Results.—The 39 male and 14 female patients who achieved reduction through closed traction (average age, 36 years were most commonly injured in motor vehicle accidents and falls. The most common levels of injury were C5 to C6 in 19 and C6 to C7 in 17. Twenty patients had unilateral dislocations, and 33 had bilateral dislocations. Initially, 49% were seen with Frankel A lesions with no neurologic function distal to the level of injury; 26% had Frankel B lesions; 4% had Frankel C lesions; 17% had Frankel D lesions; and 4% had Frankel E lesions. None of the patients lost a Frankel grade after reduction or at the time of discharge, and 45% improved at least 1 Frankel grade by discharge. The median time from injury to reduction was 8 hours for unilateral dislocations and 11 hours for bilateral dislocations. Fourteen patients required less than 45 lb of traction, and 39 required 50–160 lb of traction. In the cadaver studies, failure of the tongs occurred at 160 lb in 2 attempts, 250 lb in 2 attempts, and 280 lb in 1 attempt. Two attempts in 2 cadavers successfully held 300 lb without failure.

Conclusions.—Most cervical spine dislocations can be reduced rapidly and safely using axial traction with higher weights than are commonly used. Careful application of as much as 100 lb of traction had a low risk of neurologic compromise or tong failure and resulted in effective reduction of dislocations.

▶ The results obtained are self-explanatory. In patients with unilateral or bilateral facet dislocations with or without neurologic injury reduction can be accomplished in the majority by large traction forces applied sequentially. The authors are very specific about the surveillance required during application of traction forces, including clinical and radiographic examinations.—J.W. Frymoyer, M.D.

Posterior Wiring Without Bony Fusion in Traumatic Distractive Flexion Injuries of the Mid to Lower Cervical Spine: Long-Term Follow-Up in 30 Patients
Nielsen CF, Annertz M, Persson L, Wingstrand H, Saveland H, Brandt L (University Hospital, Lund, Sweden)
Spine 16:467–472, 1991   5–6

Background.—Distractive flexion injuries in the mid to lower cervical spine tend not to unite, and bony fusion usually is recommended in addition to stabilization to ensure long-term stability. A posterior wiring technique was used to treat 34 patients.

Patients.—All 34 patients had traumatic distractive flexion injuries in the mid to lower cervical spine. The average age of the 24 male and 10 female patients was 40 years (range, 10–86 years). Fifteen patients had signs of cord involvement and 9 had root involvement; 10 were neurologically intact. Mean follow-up was 38 months.

Technique.—If there substantial ligament injury the patient is placed in a Stryker bed with skull traction. If necessary, traction is increased to unlock the facet joints. A posterior incision is made and an unreduced dislocation, if present, is reduced by manual traction. With single-level instability, a hole is made through the base of the upper spinous process and a 2-mm Rissler pin inserted. One or 2 wires are looped about the upper and spinous process ventral to the pin and tightened until motion is absent in the damaged segment (Fig 5–4). No bone graft is used. The patient is mobilized with a semirigid collar for 6–8 weeks after operation.

Results.—One patient died of pulmonary embolism and another had reoperation for redislocation after a fracture of the spinous process. In 2 patients a root deficit occurred after operation. No patient, had late neurologic deterioration. All of those with incomplete cord injuries or root symptoms improved neurologically. The mean loss of lordosis was 7.5

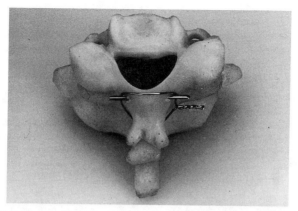

Fig 5–4.—Pin and wire relation of spinal canal. (Courtesy of Nielsen CF, Annertz M, Persson L, et al: *Spine* 16:467–472, 1991.)

degrees. Sixteen patients had evidence of spontaneous anterior interbody fusion at follow-up, and 11 had evidence of spontaneous posterior fusion. Mobility in the affected segment precluded fusion. No patient experienced late instability. Most patients had late pain, which usually was minor. All patients except for 6 who were tetraplegic resumed working. In 8 patients a wire broke.

Conclusions.—Simple posterior wiring is a reliable means of achieving a stable cervical spine in patients with traumatic distractive flexion injuries. Adding bony fusion may lessen late pain.

▶ The abstract published at the beginning of the paper concludes, "These results indicate that simple posterior wiring without bony fusion is a reliable method to obtain good immediate stability in traumatic distraction flexion injuries to the mid to lower cervical spine." The authors' results call into question the validity of their conclusion. In fact, the final sentence of the article tells the story: "Long-term results regarding late pain might be improved by adding bony fusion to the stabilization procedure." It is not clear why they chose NOT to include such fusion in the stabilization. A careful analysis of their results confirms that the best results were obtained when spontaneous bony fusion occurred. Why not guarantee that result by adding the graft in the first place?—J.W. Frymoyer, M.D.

Normal Cervical Spine Morphometry and Cervical Spinal Stenosis in Asymptomatic Professional Football Players: Plain Film Radiography, Multiplanar Computed Tomography, and Magnetic Resonance Imaging
Herzog RJ, Wiens JJ, Dillingham MF, Sontag MJ (San Francisco Neuro Skeletal Imaging Ctr, Daly City, Calif)
Spine 16:S178–S186, 1991   5–7

Background.—In 1986, Torg et al. defined a syndrome of neurapraxia of the cervical cord with transient quadriplegia. Developmental spinal

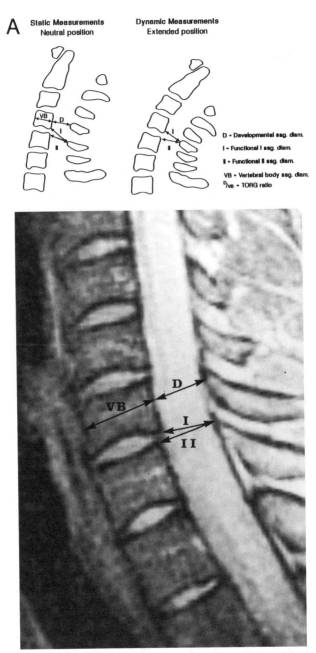

Fig 5–5.—A, measurements of cervical spine with neck in neutral and extended positions. **B,** plain film sagittal measurements. (Courtesy of Herzog RJ, Wiens JJ, Dillingham MF, et al: *Spine* 16:S178–S186, 1991.)

stenosis was shown to be an important factor disposing to cord contusion. To establish normal values for spinal morphometry, plain film measurements of the cervical spine were obtained for 80 athletes without symptoms. These were compared with measurements made by high-resolution multiplanar CT and MRI.

Methods.—Anteroposterior and lateral radiographs of the cervical spine were made, the latter at a tube–film distance of 72 in. Exposures were made with the neck in neutral position and with the neck fully flexed and extended. Vertebral alignment was determined by Gore's method, and 3 sagittal diameters of the spinal canal were recorded (Fig 5–5). Angular excursion and horizontal translation were measured at each motion segment on flexion and extension radiographs. Sixteen subjects also were examined by CT and MRI (Fig 5–6).

Results.—The error rate in CT measurements was less than 2%. The mean sagittal diameter of the cervical vertebral bodies varied 7% from

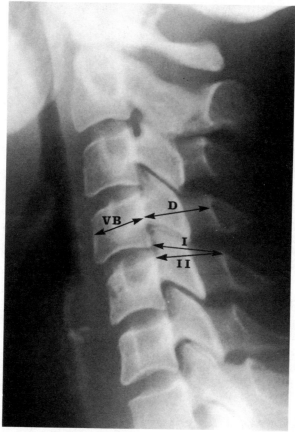

Fig 5–6.—Sagittal measurements at MR imaging. (Courtesy of Herzog RJ, Wiens JJ, Dillingham MF, et al: *Spine* 16:S178–S186, 1991.)

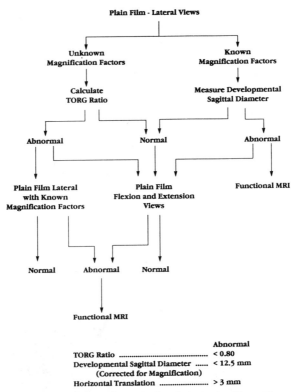

Fig 5–7.—Algorithm for assessment of stenosis of cervical spine in athletes. (Courtesy of Herzog RJ, Wiens JJ, Dillingham MF, et al: *Spine* 16:S178–S186, 1991.)

C3 to C7. Plain film and midline sagittal CT images correlated at a level of .87. Axial estimates correlated slightly less closely (.84). The developmental sagittal diameter was the most accurate midline sagittal dimension. An abnormal Torg ratio of less than .8 was found at 100 of 454 cervical vertebral levels and in 49% of the athletes. No subject had more than 3 mm of horizontal translation on flexion or extension.

Conclusions.—Use of the Torg ratio (the developmental sagittal diameter of the cervical spinal canal divided by the sagittal diameter of the corresponding vertebral body) precludes the need to know the exact magnification factors. If significance spinal stenosis was a developmental sagittal diameter of more than 1 SD below the mean, an abnormal Torg ratio had a positive predictive value of 33%. Use of the Torg ratio to screen athletes may label as stenotic many persons who have a normal spinal canal but large vertebral bodies. An algorithm for evaluating the cervical spine in athletes is presented in Figure 5–7.

▶ If one believes that the San Francisco Forty-Niners are representative of the population at large, then this study gives important insights into the usefulness of various radiologic methods in determining the player "at risk" for cervical injury because of an underlying developmental stenosis. Although you might quarrel with the selection procedure that determined who did and did not have MRI and CT, the calculations of sensitivity and positive predictive values are important. Particularly helpful is the algorithm that outlines a utilitarian method for screening players in potentially high-risk sports. A little sidelight of this paper is that 7 of 16 of the toughest athletes in the world could not complete the MRIs because of claustrophobia. Apparently tough dudes have the same phobias as "wimpy couch potatoes."—J.W. Frymoyer, M.D.

Thoracic Spine

Asymptomatic Versus Symptomatic Herniated Thoracic Discs: Their Frequency and Characteristics as Detected by Computed Tomography After Myelography

Awwad EE, Martin DS, Smith KR Jr, Baker BK (St Louis Univ, Mo)
Neurosurgery 28:180–186, 1991   5–8

Background.—The introduction of MRI of the spine has increased the identification of thoracic herniated disks. There is approximating a 15% to 20% frequency of incidental detection of thoracic herniated disks in the MRI literature; therefore when this diagnosis is made in a patient with confusing findings or without thoracic symptoms, the physician must decide on the significance of the finding and whether or not to operate on a possible asymptomatic disk. This retrospective analysis was undertaken to define the frequency of asymptomatic thoracic herniated disks (ATHDs) as determined by a CT scan done after myelography and to identify any imaging attributes that might differentiate them from symptomatic thoracic herniated disks (STHDs).

Methods.—The myelograms of 433 patients were retrospectively reviewed and were evaluated for focal posterior disk protrusion indicative of thoracic disk herniation. Water-soluble contrast studies were performed as an extension of indicated cervical or lumbar myelograms. When extradural defects were detected, the patients underwent postmyelography CT scanning, except when the defects were clearly caused by osteophytes.

Results.—The patients' charts revealed no clinical evidence predictive of the presence of thoracic herniated disks. Evaluation of 433 myelograms found a total of 54 ATHDs in 40 patients (9.2%). A 13% frequency was calculated by summing the frequency of detection at each individual interspace and then using the incidence of multiplicity of ATHDs detected in these patients. Eighty-eight percent of the ATHDs demonstrated some deformity of the spinal cord with diffuse deformity in 28% and focal deformity in 72% (Fig 5–8). Sixty percent of the deformities were detected at levels T6 to T7, T7 to T8, and T8 to T9; 23.5% of the ATHDs had calcified fragments.

Conclusions.—No single feature or combination of features clearly separated ATHDs from STHDs. Spinal cord deformity often was associated with ATHDs, and spinal cord flattening was marked in some pa-

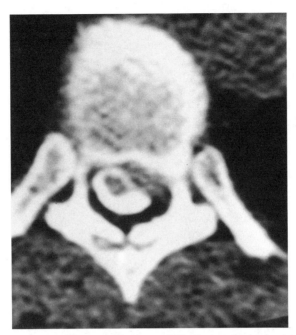

Fig 5–8.—A woman, aged 40 years, with symptoms secondary to a lumbar herniated nuclei pulposus with a lateral herniated nuclei pulposus at T-7 to T-8 with focal spinal cord deformity. (Courtesy of Awwad EE, Martin DS, Smith KR Jr, et al: *Neurosurgery* 28:180–186, 1991.)

tients. Imaging can identify disks but cannot distinguish between ATHDs and STHDs.

▶ This is not a truly rigorous retrospective study. However, it shows that thoracic disk protrusions in individuals who have no evidence of thoracic compression are far more common than the literature would suggest. At least 10% of their participants had a lesion. Some were impressive and were associated with evident spinal cord flattening. Because these participants had other degenerative pathology, they may not represent a truly random sample of the population. However, the study does parallel other more rigorous studies of imaging in the lumbar spine. In aggregate, a reasonable conclusion is that imaging abnormalities usually are only meaningful when they confirm a clinical diagnosis.—J.W. Frymoyer, M.D.

Vertebral Alterations in Scheuermann's Kyphosis
Scoles PV, Latimer BM, DiGiovanni BF, Vargo E, Bauza S, Jellema LM (Case Western Reserve Univ, Cleveland; Cleveland Museum of Natural History; Univ of Michigan, Ann Arbor)
Spine 16:509–515, 1991   5–9

Background.—Scheuermann's kyphosis has never been investigated by extensive review of cadaver material. The bony features of this physicians condition were examined directly in a large collection of human skeletons. In addition, single-photon absorptiometry was used to evaluate the possible role of osteoporosis.

Methods.—A group of 1,384 thoracolumbar spinal columns from a museum collection of more than 3,000 cadaver-derived human skeletons were examined. Postmortem data, including probable cause of death,

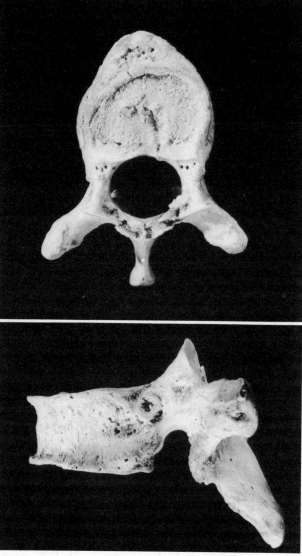

Fig 5–9.—Superior and lateral views of thoracic vertebrae (T-8) showing anterior extensions. *Arrows* are directed toward external margin of the ring apophysis. (Courtesy of Scoles PV, Latimer BM, DiGiovanni BF, et al: *Spine* 16:509–515, 1991.)

were available for each specimen. Seventy-one percent of the skeletons were male. When wedging was seen, 3 additional vertebrae were also analyzed. Affected specimens had consistent, clearly demarcated anterior extensions to the vertebral bodies (Fig 5–9).

Results.—Criteria for Scheuermann's kyphosis were met in 103 skeletons (7.4%). Of these individuals, 91% were males, of whom 82% were white. Incidence was 11% in white males, 6% in black males, and 2% in females. At every level except T12, L3, and L4, the affected skeletons had significantly greater vertebral wedging in the thoracolumbar spine. In L3–L5, wedging was posteriorly directed, resulting in a lordotic rather than a kyphotic curvature. Ninety-three percent of affected spines and 36% of control spines had Schmorl's nodes. Ninety-four percent of affected specimens had distinct anterior extension of thoracic vertebral bodies compared to none of the controls. There was no significant difference in bone mineral content between the affected and unaffected specimens.

Conclusions.—The cause of Scheuermann's kyphosis appears to be defective anterior endochondral ossification. It appears that either anterior extension occurs after the completion of posterior growth or the forces that produce abnormal anterior growth were not active in the posterior direction. This origin is further supported by the presence of the condition in the earliest known bipedal hominid species, *Australopithecus afarensis.*

▶ The author's examination of 1,384 cadaveric thoracolumbar spinal columns confirms a higher prevalence of Scheuermann's kyphosis in males, particularly white males. The notable finding was the prevalence of "a distinct anterior extension of the thoracic vertebral bodies in 94%," which looks to me like nothing more than a large osteophyte. An interesting sidelight is their comment about a similar finding in the hominid, "Lucy." Osteoporosis was not identified in these adult specimens. The authors conclude that there is a mechanical cause for Scheuermann's kyphosis, strengthening the argument that the condition is osteochondrosis affecting the ring apophyses (1).

The authors retrospectively compare their results with the ISSI and Harrington instrumentation. The hypothesis is that the enhanced rigidity of the ISSI leads to reduced hospitalization, costs, complications, and pseudoarthroses, and to enhanced functional results. Their data suggest confirmation of that hypothesis.—J.W. Frymoyer, M.D.

Reference

1. Noel SH, et al: *Spine* 16:32–136, 1991.

Pathophysiology of Degeneration

Mechanism of Disc Rupture: A Preliminary Report
Gordon SJ, Yang KH, Mayer PJ, Mace AH Jr, Kish VL, Radin EL (West Virginia Univ, Morgantown; Wayne State Univ, Detroit)
Spine 16:450–456, 1991

5–10

Background.—Senescent changes in the nucleus pulposus are the cause of lumbar intervertebral disk herniation, except in the rare case of trauma. The first in vitro model of disk prolapse was developed in which disks rupture reliably under reasonable physiologic stress.

Methods.—The model used blocks specimens of human spine from the lower thoracic to the sacral regions. After plain radiographs and MRI scans were taken of the blocks, vertebral motion segments, consisting of the intervertebral disk and the entire superior and inferior vertebra, were

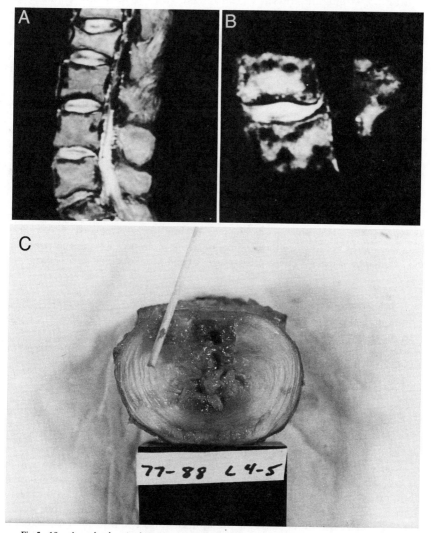

Fig 5–10.—A, preload sagittal T2-weighted image. Note intact posterior annulus. **B,** postload. Note nuclear extrusion with annular disruption. This sagittal plane is in the midline. **C,** gross examination. Note central extrusion with disrupted posterior annulus. (Courtesy of Gordon SJ, Yang KH, Mayer PJ, et al: *Spine* 16:450–456, 1991.)

formed. Posterior elements were left intact. The segments were potted and placed on a materials testing machine; they were loaded repetitively at 1.5 Hz in a combination of 7 degrees of flexion, less than 3 degrees of rotation, and 1,334 N of compression. When reaction force leveled off for more than 1 hour loading was terminated. Magnetic resonance imaging and gross examination were used to assess disk prolapse; nuclear extrusion was shown by a complete radial fissure between the central nucleus and an intact or disrupted annulus (Fig 5–10).

Results.—Imaging criteria were fulfilled by 14 disks from 9 spines; all specimens were from white men (average age, 57 years). Annular protrusion was seen grossly in 10 disks, and nuclear extrusion was found in 4. All of the specimens had posterolateral annular tears in association with annular protrusion or adjacent to the radial fissure of a nuclear extrusion. Rotation was always applied in a counterclockwise direction and averaged 1.9 degrees. Average duration of testing was 6.9 hours.

Conclusions.—Annular separation and disk rupture will predictably occur with the appropriate combination of flexion, rotation, and compression during a sufficient length of time. Annular disruption appears to be the primary cause of prolapse, and the load on the disk, rather than its inherent qualities, is what leads to prolapse.

▶ Vertebral specimens were subjected to cyclic loads where compression was accompanied by modest torsional deformation. The forces were within the range experienced by the lumbar spine in conditions such as lifting in twisted postures. The result was annular failures, protrusions, and, in some specimens, nuclear extrusion. The authors conclude that their study supports the hypothesis that intervertebral disk prolapse is peripheral in origin.—J.W. Frymoyer, M.D.

Anulus Tears and Intervertebral Disc Degeneration: An Experimental Study Using an Animal Model
Osti OL, Vernon-Roberts B, Fraser RD (Institute of Medical and Veterinary Science; Royal Adelaide Hospital; University of Adelaide, Australia)
Spine 15:762–767, 1990   5–11

Background.—There is controversy as to the causes of intervertebral disk degeneration and its relationship with low back pain. A trial was performed in sheep to test whether discrete peripheral annular tears cause secondary degenerative changes in other parts of the disk.

Methods.—The animals were 21 adult Merino wethers sheep in which a cut was made in the left anterolateral annulus of 3 randomly selected lumbar disks. Cuts were 5-mm deep and 5-mm wide, and they were made parallel and adjacent to the inferior end-plate of the upper vertebra. This left the inner third of the annulus and the nucleus pulposus intact. Animals were randomized to be killed between 1 and 18 months after creation of the defect. The lumbar spines were then placed into individual joint units and decalcified, after which each disk was sectioned into 6 parasagittal slabs. Each slab was examined under the dissecting microscope, and 2 of them—the slab with the anular lesion and the contralateral slab—were examined histologically.

Results.—At 1–2 months postoperatively 12 disks with rim lesions were seen. Only 1 had failure of the inner annulus, which was associated with nuclear displacement to the outer annulus. All disks showed granulation tissue, which was markedly vascularized in 10 disks. At 4–12 months postoperatively, 39 disks with rim lesions were found. Thirty-six had failure of the inner annulus lamellae near the transverse anular cut (Fig 5–11). Marked disk degeneration was seen in 10 of 12 disks from sheep killed at 12 months, and moderate intervertebral disk narrowing was noted in all but 1 of 24 disks from sheep killed between 8 and 12 months. Early osteophytes were seen in most disks from animals killed between 4 and 6 months. Animals killed in this intermediate phase showed marked degeneration of the nucleus pulposus, including areas of chondroid metaplasia, especially in the displaced tissue. Twelve disks with rim lesions were found 18 months postoperatively. All disks showed inner annulus failure with nuclear displacement toward the site of the original cut, and all showed marked nuclear degeneration. All disks showed osteophytes, and both end-plates had symmetric new bone formation.

Conclusions.—Peripheral annulus fibrosus tears appear to play a major part in degeneration of the intervertebral joint complex. In the study model, despite the care taken to leave the inner annulus intact, it progressively failed in all animals. Although new, ordered collagen can develop

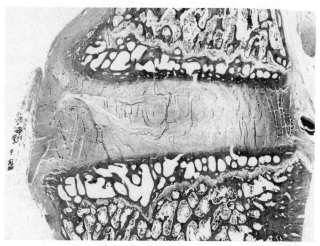

Fig 5–11.—Low-power micrograph of intervertebral disk of sheep killed 12 months after operation. Although the overall height is only moderately reduced, nuclear material is displaced toward the site of the original lesion, with cleft extending from the initial cut toward the central portion of the disk. The outer anulus has healed, but the collagen bundles of the outer anulus appear distorted in relation to the anulus cut. (Courtesy of Osti OL, Vernon-Roberts B, Fraser RD: *Spine* 15:762–767, 1990.)

in response to such an injury, this process cannot prevent and may accelerate degeneration of the disk.

▶ This experimental model created peripheral annular defects in sheep. Morphologic and histologic analyses demonstrated time-dependent alterations within the disk, including extension of the defects, nuclear migration and degeneration, and, later, osteophyte formation. Combined with the article by Gordon (Abstract 5–10), it adds further credence to the agument for a peripheral mechanism of mechanical failure creating the later nuclear extrusion. Both studies are compatible with a mechanical cause, as suggested by Farfan (1), namely, that torsion adversely affects the disk. It is also compatible with the epidemiologic data demonstrating increased risk for disk herniation in those who lift repetitively in twisted postures.—J.W. Frymoyer, M.D.

Reference

1. Farfan HF: *Mechanical Disorders of the Low Back*. Philadelphia, Lea and Febiger, 1973, pp 63–92.

Occupation Injury and Epidemiology

Lumbar Spinal Pathology in Cadaveric Material in Relation to History of Back Pain, Occupation, and Physical Loading

Videman T, Nurminen M, Troup JDG (Institute of Occupational Health, Helsinki)
Spine 15:728–740, 1990   5–12

Background.—Investigations of the association between occupational exposures and lumbar spine degeneration have been complicated by the absence of firm diagnoses and objective pathologic criteria. Cadaver material was examined to determine whether pathologic changes could be found in individuals whose exposure to physical loading fell between overexertion and inactivity. Histories of back pain were related to spinal pathologic findings and physical loading.

Methods.—The lumbar spines from L1 to S1 in 149 cadavers of men who died after a short illness before the age of 64 years were examined. Information from the family was available in 86 cases. Diskography was performed using barium sulfate contrast medium to evaluate symmetric disk degeneration, annular rupture, and end-plate defects. Radiography was done to assess osteophytosis, and osteologic examination was performed to assess facet osteoarthrosis. Intraobserver reliability was good. Subjects were classified as to occupation, and the family was asked about any history of back pain, disability, and physical loading.

Results.—Subjects who had heavy occupations or occupations involving driving had the greatest incidence of back pain, sciatica, and disability or injury (Fig 5–12). Bar graphs for back pain and sciatica showed a J-shaped relationship with heaviness of work as opposed to a linear relationship for disability. The clearest differences in incidence of back pain and sciatica were seen with annular ruptures. Significant changes were more likely to be located in the lower rather than the upper vertebral lev-

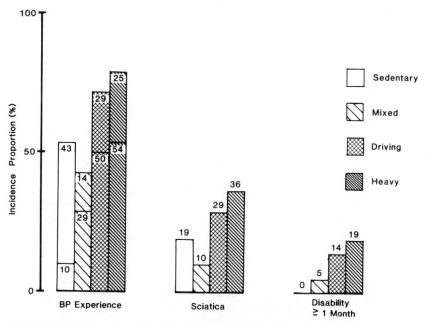

Fig 5–12.—Incidence proportion of back pain (BP) experience in the 4 occupational groups. The lower part of each column represents the answer "often" and the upper represents the answer "sometimes." The P-value for occupational differences was .01 for BP experience, <.07 for sciatica, and <.05 for disability. (Courtesy of Videman T, Nurminen M, Troup JDG: *Spine* 15:728–740, 1990.)

els. Among subjects who performed heavy work, pathologic progression was faster for mixed work for each outcome variate except annular rupture. Severe symmetric disk degeneration was more clearly related to sedentary and heavy work than to mixed and driving work. Significant factors for severe degeneration were aging, sedentary work, and history of back injury. Incidence of severe annular rupture was unrelated to age, physical exercise, and heaviness of occupation; it was seen most often with driving work. Heavy work was more closely related to osteophytosis than was driving. The only significant factor in facet joint osteoarthrosis was aging.

Conclusions.—There is a relationship between pathologic findings in the spine and back injuries and sedentary or heavy work. Heaviness of work affects the severity of back pain. Confirmation of these findings is most likely to come from some application of MRI.

▶ This is an extraordinary study. To present all of the authors' material in an abstract is impossible. What are the highlights? The authors suggest that there are 2 extremes of physical activity associated with back pain and spinal degeneration, namely, sedentary lifestyle and heavy physical labor. In general, they proved this hypothesis. Predictive factors for disk degeneration were heavy work, aging, and history of back injury. Back injury also was significant in predicting annular ruptures.—J.W. Frymoyer, M.D.

Risk for Occupational Low-Back Injury After Lumbar Laminectomy for Degenerative Disc Disease

Ryan J, Zwerling C (Boston Postal Service Med Unit)
Spine 15:500–503, 1990   5–13

Background.—In evaluating the work capability of patients who have undergone back surgery, orthopedic consultants often cite a symptom-free period of several years as a good prognostic factor, although this is not addressed in the medical literature. Risk of occupational low-back injury was evaluated in patients who had made a good recovery from lumbar laminectomy and were employed in positions involving heavy physical labor.

Methods.—Data on preplacement medical evaluations, employment status, and occupational injuries maintained by the United States Postal Service were evaluated. Each employee completed a medical history questionnaire and physical examination addressing back problems. For applicants with a history of back surgery, a detailed medical and occupational history was obtained. Generally, applicants who were asymptomatic after working in a job demanding physical exertion or who were free of symptoms for 1–2 years received favorable reports. Forty-seven participants had undergone a simple lumbar laminectomy for a herniated disk; 33 of these were hired, 29 without limitations. Thirty-two participants were each matched to 6 controls for sex, hiring date, age, and job classification. Records were then examined for all occupational injuries reported by the participants. Mean duration of employment was the same for both groups, and those who had undergone surgery before employment were a mean of 7 months older than controls.

Results.—Overall, those who had undergone surgery had an estimated odds ratio for occupational low-back injury of 5.9 compared to controls. By job classification, odds ratio was 9.1 for letter carriers, 2.8 for clerks, and 3.1 for mailhandlers. Of patients who had laminectomy, 25% had disabling low-back injuries compared to 6% of controls. Of letter carriers who had undergone laminectomy, 44% had an injury compared to 5% of controls. For postal clerks, the injury rate was 13% in the operated group and 5% in controls.

Conclusions.—Materials-handling workers who had undergone lumbar laminectomy for disk disease appear to have an increased incidence of occupational low-back injury. The findings indicate that letter carriers have a somewhat greater risk than those in other job classifications. This may be because, although letter carriers occasionally perform some heavy lifting, they do so too infrequently to become well conditioned to it.

▶ The subjects were individuals who had recovered from lumbar laminectomy, who had successfully returned to work (often for a period of many years), and who had no demonstrated consequential residuals from their surgery. Their risk of sustaining back injury was compared to that of individuals who had no history of back surgery. The results are impressive: a 25% re-injury rate compared with a 6% rate for controls. The risk of re-injury was related to the physical loads lifted on the job.—J.W. Frymoyer, M.D.

Comparison of Eight Psychometric Instruments in Unselected Patients With Back Pain
Greenough CG, Fraser RD (Middlesbrough Gen Hospital, England; Royal Adelaide Hospital, Australia)
Spine 16:1068–1074, 1991   5–14

Background.—Many patients who have had back injuries have psychological disturbances. However, it is difficult to assess psychometric instruments in patients with pain or illness. Several such instruments were compared in patients with low back pain, and the influence of pain and other factors on the instruments was assessed.

Methods.—Patients were new referrals to a single practice with a complaint of back pain during a 5-year period. For each year, eligible patients were classified according to sex and compensation status. Two hundred seventy-four patients were interviewed and examined by an unbiased observer. Each patient completed 8 psychometric instruments; in addition, the Zung Depression Scale was assessed in combination with the Modified Somatic Perception Questionnaire, and the Hospital Anxiety Scale was assessed with the Hospital Depression Scale. If a patient had a positive result in 3 or more scales, he or she was classified as disturbed. Specificity and sensitivity of each test were assessed for a number of cutoff values, and scores of disturbed and nondisturbed patients were compared.

Results.—Twenty-three percent of patients were classified as disturbed including 36% of compensation patients and 9.2% of noncompensation patients. There were no other significant differences in the incidence of disturbance between sexes or social groups. Specificities and sensitivities of the psychometric instruments varied, but the best results were seen with the Modified Somatic Perception Questionnaire, Hospital Anxiety Scale, Hospital Depression Scale, and Zung Depression Scale (Fig 5–13). For these, a large part of their variance was explained by the other instruments.

Conclusions.—For patients with back pain, the combination of the Modified Somatic Perception Questionnaire and the Zung Depression Scale is a useful psychological assessment tool that is not greatly affected by such factors as pain, social group, and compensation status. To avoid misclassification, the suggested cutoff scores for unemployment should be used when appropriate.

▶ I debated the relevance of this article for orthopedists treating spinal disorders. Periodically, we all face patients who we believe have a significant psychological component contributing to severity of symptoms and disability as

SENSITIVITY

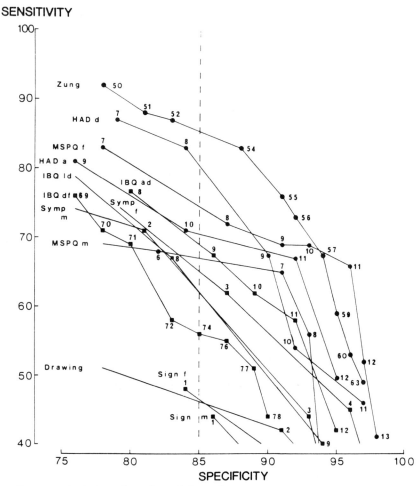

Fig 5–13.—Sensitivity and specificity of the psychometric instruments plotted for a number of cutoff scores. The 4 most discriminating tests are represented by *circles,* the others are represented by *squares. Abbreviations: Drawing,* pain drawing; *Symp m,* inappropriate symptoms, men; *Symp f,* inappropriate symptoms, women; *Sign m,* inappropriate signs, men; *Sign f,* inappropriate signs, women; *IBQ df,* Illness Behavior Questionnaire, discriminant function; *MSPQ m,* Modified Somatic Perception Questionnaire, men; *MSPQ f,* Modified Somatic Perception Questionnaire, women; *HAD a,* Hospital Anxiety Scale; *HAD d,* Hospital Depression Scale; *Zung,* Zung Depression Scale; *IBQ ad,* Illness Behavior Questionnaire, affective and hypochondriacal disturbance; *IBQ ld,* Illness Behavior Questionnaire, life disruption. (Courtesy of Greenough CG, Fraser RD: *Spine* 16:1068–1074, 1991.).

well as predicting treatment response. This article will tell you that pain drawings and Waddell's signs are not too helpful, whereas the combination of the Modified Somatic Perception Questionnaire and the Zung Depression Scale has a high degree of sensitivity and specificity. The article's usefulness is to help you guide consulting psychologists in choosing tests relevant to low-back disability.—J.W. Frymoyer, M.D.

A Longitudinal Study of Back Pain and Radiological Changes in the Lumbar Spines of Middle Aged Women. I. Clinical Findings

Symmons DPM, van Hemert AM, Vandenbrouke JP, Valkenburg HA (University Hospital, Leiden, The Netherlands; Erasmus Univ, Rotterdam, The Netherlands)

Ann Rheum Dis 50:158–161, 1991   5–15

Background.—There are many unanswered questions about the fate of patients with back pain, including whether they simply continue to have pain and whether there is any way of predicting who will have it. Few reports have addressed the long-term prognosis of this problem in the general population. A longitudinal investigation of back pain was done in middle-aged women, who have a particularly high incidence of the problem.

Methods.—The sample was drawn from respondents to a population survey of rheumatic and cardiovascular diseases. The main goal was to investigate risk factors for postmenopausal osteoporosis. The original survey included 1,167 women (aged 45–64 years) for a response rate of 78%. Nine years later, 1,009 of those women were invited to participate in a follow-up survey; 742 did so, for a response rate of 74%. In the original survey, 241 reported that they had never had back pain and 236 that they had recurrent back pain.

Results.—In the original survey, the 2 groups were comparable in mean age, height, weight, body mass index, blood pressure, and postmenopausal status. The group with back pain was more likely to have taken oral contraceptives, but there were no differences in menstrual irregularity and pain. Women with back pain were more likely to smoke,

TABLE 1.—Predictors of Continuing Pain in the
Group With Recurrent Back Pain

Univariate analysis	*RR* *(95% CI)*
Joint pains	1·33 (1·05 to 1·68)
Hip/knee pain on standing	1·28 (1·09 to 1·50)
Falls 1978–1985	1·23 (1·05 to 1·45)
Weekly headaches	1·19 (1·01 to 1·40)
Hip/knee gelling	1·17 (1·01 to 1·37)
Limited flexion	1·06 (0·92 to 1·23)
Deterioration of disc degeneration 1978–85	1·03 (0·86 to 1·23)
Smoker	1·03 (0·85 to 1·25)
Hormone replacement therapy	1·01 (0·91 to 1·13)
Limited rotation	0·98 (0·76 to 1·27)
Osteoporotic fracture	0·91 (0·72 to 1·15)
Disc degeneration	0·88 (0·76 to 1·02)
Kyphosis	0·88 (0·68 to 1·14)

Note: Except where otherwise stated the figures refer to factors detected by the first questionnaire (1975–1978).
Abbreviations: RR, relative risk; CI, confidence interval.
(Courtesy of Symmons DPM, van Hemert AM, Vandenbrouke JP, et al: *Ann Rheum Dis* 50:158–161, 1991.)

TABLE 2.—Predictors of Incident Pain in the Group
With no Previous Back Pain

Univariate analysis	RR (95% C.
Hip/knee gelling	2·65 (1·62 to 4·33)
Joint pains	2·56 (1·64 to 4·00)
Hip/knee pain on standing	2·07 (1·16 to 3·69)
Limited rotation	1·93 (0·83 to 3·79)
Hormone replacement therapy	1·54 (0·97 to 2·45)
Incident osteoporotic fracture	1·52 (0·82 to 2·81)
Osteoporotic fracture 1975–8	1·42 (0·87 to 2·32)
Kyphosis	1·42 (0·64 to 3·14)
Deterioration of disc degeneration 1978–85	1·03 (0·63 to 1·69)
Weekly headaches	1·00
Limited flexion	0·99 (0·50 to 1·96)
Smoker	0·78 (0·47 to 1·30)

Note: Except where otherwise stated, the figures refer to factors detected by the first questionnaire (1975–1978).
Abbreviations: RR, relative risk; *CI,* confidence interval.
(Courtesy of Symmons DPM, van Hemert AM, Vandenbrouke JP, et al: *Ann Rheum Dis* 50:158–161, 1991.)

to have a history of cystitis or frequent headaches, and to have pain in other joints. A mean of 8.7 years later, all participants were postmenopausal. Women with back pain were now more likely to use estrogen, and fewer of them smoked. Seventy-two percent of the group with back pain still had pain, and 24% of the pain-free group had some back pain. Thus recurrent back pain in the first survey carried a 2.99 relative risk of back pain at follow-up. Continuing pain was not associated with age, body mass index, or other factors (Table 1) but was associated with pain in other joints, hip or knee pain on standing, gelling of the hip or knee on sitting, and a history of falls. The only significant independent predictor was hip or knee pain on standing. This pattern was similar in both groups (Table 2).

Conclusions.—The long-term follow-up of back pain in the general population suggests that past symptoms are the strongest predictor of future pain. Radiography appears to be of little prognostic help; thus there is little indication for repeat radiographs.

▶ The Dutch are way ahead in defining the natural history of spinal disorders. Despite the wide range of variables that they analayzed in the spine equivalent of the Framingham study of heart disease, few predictors are identified. Their studies also demonstrate that radiographs have little merit. The depressing, albeit not surprising, feature is that those who had pain continue to have pain, whereas those who did not have pain have symptoms develop with some frequency. What this paper does not tell us is the severity of symptoms. If the symptoms are fairly mild, then the consequences are minimal. If the symptoms are significant and associated with increasing disability, then the implications of their study are far-reaching.—J.W. Frymoyer, M.D.

Lumbar Spine

▶ ↓ One of the major issues in the research of chronic back pain relates to the relative contributions of mechanical factors vs. psychosocial factors. These issues are of particular importance in patients who are disabled by their symptoms and who do not have clearly demonstrable pathology such as tumors and infections. The first group of articles further defines some of the possible mechanical causes of back pain, whereas the latter evaluate the psychosocial factors.—J.W. Frymoyer, M.D.

TREATMENT: DEGENERATIVE CONDITIONS

▶ ↓ The following 3 papers present important insights to guide our surgical treatment of the spine as well as helping us to inform our patients of those factors that will favorably or adversely influence the outcome of treatment.—J.W. Frymoyer, M.D.

The Outcome of Decompressive Laminectomy for Degenerative Lumbar Stenosis
Katz JN, Lipson SJ, Larson MG, McInnes JM, Fossel AH, Liang MH (Brigham and Women's Hosp; Robert B Brigham Multipurpose Arthritis Ctr; Harvard Med School, Boston)
J Bone Joint Surg 73-A:809–816, 1991   5–16

Background.—Many patients with degenerative lumbar stenosis do not respond to conservative treatment and are candidates for decompressive laminectomy, with or without arthrodesis. Despite the frequency of laminectomies for lumbar stenosis, few data are available on the indications for the procedure or its long-term outcome.

TABLE 1.—Intervertebral Levels That Were Decompressed
at Operation

No. of Levels Included at Operation	No. of Patients	Levels Decompressed (No. of Patients)
1	16	Third to fourth lumbar (3), fourth to fifth lumbar (10), fourth lumbar to first sacral (3)
2	33	Second to fourth lumbar (1), third to fifth lumbar (30), fourth lumbar to first sacral (2)
3	29	Second to fifth lumbar (11), third lumbar to first sacral (18)
4	10	First to fifth lumbar (1), second lumbar to first sacral (9)

(Courtesy of Katz JN, Lipson SJ, Larson MG, et al: *J Bone Joint Surg* 73-A:809–816, 1991.)

Methods.—A group of 88 patients (Table 1) had a laminectomy for degenerative lumbar stenoses between 1983 and 1986. Eight had concomitant arthrodesis. Excluded were persons younger than 55 years of age (to rule out congenital or developmental causes of lumbar stenosis) and patients who had previously undergone laminectomy or spinal arthrodesis, or both, for spinal stenosis. The patients' mean age at the time of the operation was 69 years. Variables examined at baseline and postoperatively included pain, walking ability, and comorbid illnesses.

Results.—Seventy patients available for outcome analysis (Table 2) were followed for a median of 4.2 years. Of the original 88 patients, 16 had undergone a repeat operation, 5 in the first postoperative year (Fig 5–14). Of the 70 patients who completed questionnaires in 1989, 21 had very severe or severe pain, 32 were unable to walk at least 2 blocks, and 15 could not walk a distance of 50 ft (Table 3). Yet about half of the patients (48%) reported being satisfied with the results of laminectomy. Predictors of poor outcome were the comorbidity score, duration of follow-up, and an initial laminectomy involving a single interspace (Table 4).

TABLE 2.—Principal Questions from the Outcome Questionnaire

In the past month, how would you describe the back pain you have had, on average?
1. Very severe (6 patients)
2. Severe (15 patients)
3. Moderate (22 patients)
4. Mild (6 patients)
5. Very mild (10 patients)
6. None (11 patients)

During the past month, how far have you been able to walk?
1. More than 2 miles (3 kilometers) (8 patients)
2. More than 1 mile (2 kilometers) but less than 2 miles (3 kilometers) (11 patients)
3. More than 2 blocks but less than 1 mile (2 kilometers) (19 patients)
4. Less than 2 blocks but more than 50 feet (15 meters) (17 patients)
5. Less than 50 feet (15 meters) (15 patients)

In the past month, have you gone shopping for groceries or other items?
1. Yes, comfortably (16 patients)
2. Yes, but sometimes with pain (21 patients)
3. Yes, but always with pain (17 patients)
4. No (15 patients)

How satisfied are you with the over-all results of the operation on your back?
1. Very satisfied (33 patients)
2. Somewhat satisfied (15 patients)
3. Somewhat dissatisfied (8 patients)
4. Very dissatisfied (13 patients)

Note: Numbers in parentheses indicate the number of patients who gave each response at the most recent follow-up. Seventy patients answered the first 2 questions, and 69 answered the last 2 questions.
(Courtesy of Katz JN, Lipson SJ, Larson MG, et al: *J Bone Joint Surg* 73-A:809–816, 1991.)

TABLE 3.—Outcomes of Decompression at the 1-Year Follow-Up
and at the Latest Follow-Up in 1989

	No. of Patients Who Had Outcome/ No. of Patients Who Were Evaluated	
	One-Year Follow-up*	Follow-up in 1989†
Poor outcome	8/74 (11%)	31/72 (43%)
Severe pain	5/74 (7%)	21/70 (30%)
Reoperation for stenosis or instability	5/88 (6%)	15/88 (17%)‡
Limited physical function	6/74 (8%)	26/74 (35%)
Unable to walk 15 meters (50 feet)	6/74 (8%)	15/70 (21%)
Unable to shop	NA	15/69 (22%)
Lived in a nursing home	0/74 (0)	5/74 (7%)

*Fourteen patients were lost to follow-up; however, all charts (88 patients) were available to determine whether re-operation had been done.

†All charts (88 patients) were available to determine whether repeat operation had been done.

‡One additional patient had re-operation for osteomyelitis and was not included in this category because no relationship between the original operation and the osteomyelitis could be established difinitively.

(Courtesy of Katz JN, Lipson SJ, Larson MG, et al: *J Bone Joint Surg* 73-A:809–816, 1991.)

TABLE 4.—Predictors of Poor Outcome at the Latest Follow-Up
(in 1989): Proportion of Poor Outcomes in Each Stratum and
Adjusted Odds Ratios from Logistic Regression (72 Patients)

Predictor Variable	Poor Outcomes/No. of Patients Evaluated	Adjusted Odds Ratio*	P Value
Co-morbidity score			0.004
0-2 points	6/24 (25%)	1	
3-5 points	16/33 (48%)	10.9 (2.0, 58.4)	
≥6 points	9/15 (60%)	26.6 (3.4, 207)	
Year of operation			0.01
1983	7/12 (58%)	13.7 (2.1, 90.3)	
1984	10/15 (67%)	23.3 (3.0, 183)	
1985	8/19 (42%)	4.6 (0.9, 24.6)	
1986	6/26 (23%)	1	
No. of levels decompressed			0.040
One	10/15 (67%)	12.1 (1.8, 83.4)	
Two	10/25 (40%)	1.8 (0.5, 7.0)	
Three or four	11/32 (34%)	1	
Motor deficit	15/32 (47%)	3.8 (0.9, 15.3)	0.059
Female sex	24/52 (46%)	4.3 (0.9, 20.9)	0.067

*Adjusted odds ratios estimate the effect of each stratum on outcomes, accounting for other variables in the regression; higher odds ratios are associated with worse outcomes.

†The adjusted critical P value to account for multiple comparisons is .006.

(Courtesy of Katz JN, Lipson SJ, Larson MG, et al: *J Bone Joint Surg* 73-A:809–816, 1991.)

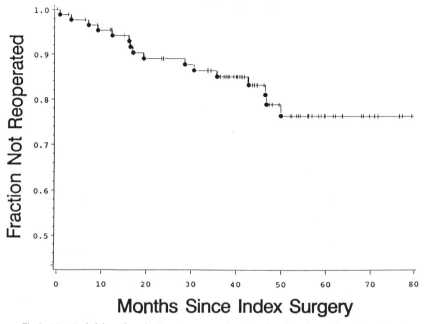

Months Since Index Surgery

Fig 5–14.—Probability of not having repeat operation plotted against the number of months of follow-up, made with the use of the Kaplan-Meier technique. The 16 *circles* represent repeat operations. The *vertical lines* indicate the times when patients were last contacted and were censored from the analysis. One operation, performed at 50 months, was for vertebral osteomyelitis; the remainder for stenosis or instability. (Courtesy of Katz JN, Lipson SJ, Larson MG, et al: *J Bone Joint Surg* 73-A:809–816, 1991.)

Conclusion.—The therapeutic benefits of laminectomy for degenerative lumbar stenosis tend to deteriorate with time. The operation appears to be most successful in patients without substantial comorbidity, such as cardiovascular disease or arthritic conditions.

▶ This study presents the outcome after decompression in degenerative lumbar spinal stenosis. Although the design is retrospective, the message is bleak. The initial results obtained do not appear to endure. Concurrent illnesses are unfavorable prognosticators, and, surprisingly, so is single-level decompression. Age is not. Reoperations are common (17%), most often for recurrent stenosis or instability. Walking incapacity secondary to neurologic claudication recurred and progressed with the passage of time.—J.W. Frymoyer, M.D.

Long-Term Roentgenographic and Functional Changes in Patients Who Were Treated With Wide Fenestration for Central Lumbar Stenosis
Nakai O, Ookawa A, Yamaura I (Kudanzaka Hospital, Tokyo)
J Bone Joint Surg 73-A:1184–1191, 1991   5–17

Background.—Clinicians currently believe that in patients with stenosis of the lumbar spinal canal the medial parts of the superior facets of

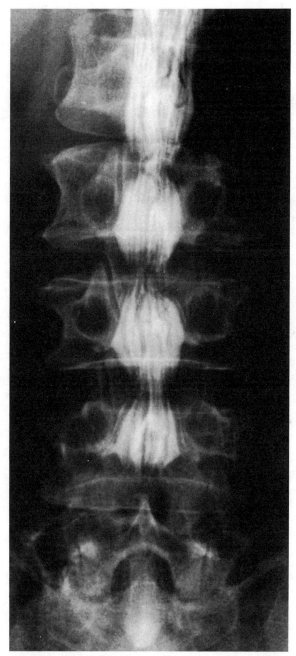

Fig 5–15.—Metrizamide myelogram of man age 51 years who had intermittent claudication, showing convergence of nerve roots (medial deviation) at level of disk. (Courtesy of Nakai O, Ookawa A, Yamaura I: *J Bone Joint Surg* 73-A:1184–1191, 1991.)

the zygapophyseal joints are responsible for trapping the nerve roots. Long-term radiographic and functional changes in patients treated with wide fenestration for central lumbar stenosis were investigated.

Methods.—Wide fenestration, which is illustrated in Figure 5–15 was done in 41 patients seen between April 1980 and December 1983 with signs and symptoms that suggested spinal stenosis. Patients with degenerative spondylolisthesis were excluded. Thirty-four patients were available for follow-up, which averaged 5½ years. Before operation 24 patients had signs and symptoms of intermittent claudication (Fig 5–16), 7 had unilateral sciatica, and 3 had paraparesis.

Results.—At early follow-up, 28 patients had an excellent or good result, but 4 years later only 24 patients did. Eight patients had deteriorating conditions, although 1 recovered spontaneously. Three of the 8 had recurrent central stenosis at 1 of the treated segments, and 2 patients reported disabling low-back pain. In 5 patients the persistence of symptoms was thought to be related to segmental instability, which was confirmed radiographically. Two of the 8 patients had signs of central spinal stenosis at a segment adjacent to the treated segment, and they underwent a second operation. In the remaining patient a cervical myelopathy occurred after operation that prevented him from walking. Roentgenograms showed bone regeneration in 28 patients. The transverse diameter of the fenestrated region was reduced by more than 5 mm in 8 patients, but the degree of bone regeneration was not commensurate with the severity of clinical symptoms. There appeared to be no association between clinical symptoms and the postoperative increase in degree of lordosis. In 9 patients the vertical height of the disk was reduced. Two of those who had a clinically poor result had signs of disk resorption, which resulted in segmental instability. At 3–5 years after surgery the horizontal translation of the affected vertebra was increased in 8 patients, with anterior slipping in 5 and posterior slipping in 3. Two of the 5 with anterior slip-

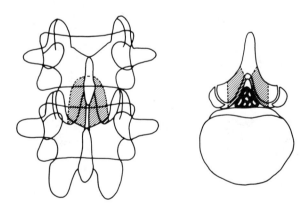

Fig 5–16.—Diagram illustrating operative procedure of wide fenestration. Medial parts of inferior facets and ligamentum flavum are removed, with preservation of lamina, superior facets, spinous process with interspinous ligament, and zygapophyseal joints. (Courtesy of Nakai O, Ookawa A, Yamaura I: *J Bone Joint Surg* 73-A:1184–1191, 1991.)

ping had severe pain in the lower extremities, possibly caused by recurrent central stenosis.

Conclusions.—In these patients wide fenestration successfully relieved symptoms. New bone laid down in the segments treated at operation appeared to stabilize those segments rather than to reproduce the symptoms of spinal stenosis.

▶ The Japanese experience somewhat mimics the United States experience reported by Katz. Initial relief was followed in some patients by recurrent symptoms, usually after 2 years of follow-up. The authors' conclusion is that "the current treatment of stenosis of the spinal canal is not completely satisfactory." Instability appears to be part of the source for failure.—J.W. Frymoyer, M.D.

Degenerative Lumbar Spondylolisthesis With Spinal Stenosis: A Prospective Study Comparing Decompression With Decompression and Intertransverse Process Arthrodesis
Herkowitz HN, Kurz LT (William Beaumont Hosp, Royal Oak, Mich)
J Bone Joint Surg 73-A:802–808, 1991   5–18

Background.—Orthopedic surgeons remain divided on the optimal management of degenerative lumbar spondylolisthesis. Some have had success with decompressive laminectomy alone, whereas others stress the need for concomitant spinal arthrodesis. To determine the indications for these procedures, prospectively studies were made of 50 consecutive patients who had spinal stenosis associated with degenerative lumbar spondylolisthesis.

Methods.—All of the patients had a single level of degenerative lumbar spondylolisthesis without a transitional fifth lumbar segment (Fig 5–17) and were unresponsive to an adequate trial of nonoperative treatment. The group included 36 women and 14 men. Half of the patients were randomly assigned to decompressive laminectomy and half to decompressive laminectomy and bilateral-lateral intertransverse process arthrodesis. The level of the operation was between the fourth and fifth lumbar vertebrae in 41 patients and between the third and fourth lumbar vertebrae in 9.

Results.—At a mean follow-up of 3 years, results in the arthrodesis group were excellent in 11 patients (unrestricted activity and complete relief of pain), good in 13, and fair in 1; there were no poor results. Without arthrodesis, treatment was significantly less effective; decompressive laminectomy alone yielded 2 excellent results, 9 good, 12 fair, and 2 poor. Patients who had not had an arthrodesis had significantly more residual pain in the back and lower limbs. The outcome was not influenced by the age and sex of the patient or height of the disk space.

Conclusion.—Findings clearly indicate the use of concomitant arthrodesis for patients who have spinal stenosis associated with degenerative lumbar spondylolisthesis at a single level. The poorer results in patients

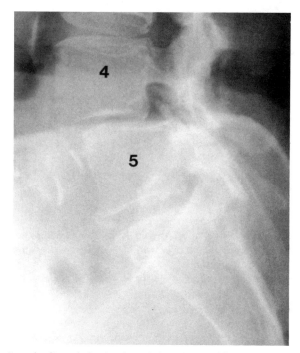

Fig 5–17.—Lateral radiograph showing the typical appearance of degenerative spondylolisthesis (the fourth on the fifth lumbar vertebrae). (Courtesy of Herkowitz HN, Kurz LT: *J Bone Joint Surg* 73-A:802–808, 1991.)

without an arthrodesis is related to the postoperative increase in olisthesis in 96% of these patients (vs. 28% of the arthrodesis group).

▶ Read this article in its entirety! It answers with considerable certainty the important clinical question, "does fusion improve the clinical success in the subset of spinal stenosis patients with degenerative lumbar spondylolisthesis?" Although the patients were not randomized by strict criteria, the authors have conducted a careful prospective analysis using clinical and radiologic criteria. The results quite convincingly demonstrate that fusion has added benefit, as measured by relief of back and leg pain over time. However, a solid arthrodesis did not always occur, and a pseudarthrosis did not necessarily predict failure. Although this study gives a sound basis for fusion in degenerative spondylolisthesis, it should not be generalized to the treatment of all forms of lumbar spinal stenosis.—J.W. Frymoyer, M.D.

CT Five Years After Myelographic Diagnosis of Lumbar Disk Herniation
Hurme M, Katevuo K, Nykvist F, Aalto T, Alaranta H, Einola S (Turku City Hosp; Turku University Central Hospital; Rehabilitation Research Centre of the Social Insurance Institute, Turku, Finland)
Acta Radiol 32:286–289, 1991

Background.—Lumbar disk disease is usually evaluated by CT. Post-operatively, these patients may have degenerative changes of the erector spinae muscles, but it is unknown whether herniation-induced denervation plays a part in this.

Methods.—Fifty-seven patients with low-back pain and sciatica were assessed by CT 5 years after primary myelography. The patients were drawn from a prospective study of 342 patients, 220 operated on for herniated nucleus pulposus in the lumbar spine and 122 treated conservatively. In each group, every fifth patient with a good and poor outcome was selected, for a total of 40 surgically treated and 17 conservatively treated patients. Follow-up CT examination included measurements of anterior disk height, posterior disk height, interpedicular distance, interarticular distance, midsagittal distance, anteroposterior diameter of the intervertebral foramen, and pedicular length. A scale of 0 to 3 was used to grade central and lateral spinal canal stenosis, degeneration of the intervertebral disk and scar tissue around the nerve root, and degenerative changes in the erector spinae muscles at 3 levels. Ligamentum flavum thickness was also measured.

Results.—Patients treated operatively had a significantly shorter anterior disk height at level L4, anteroposterior diameter of the intervertebral foramen at levels L3–L5, and pedicular length at level S1 than the conservatively treated patients. In neither group was there any difference in correlation of mean diameters in patients with good and poor outcomes. Among the operatively treated patients, those with good results had less scarring at L4 but more scarring at L5 than those with poor results. Central stenosis at L4 was negatively correlated with clinical result for conservatively treated patients. Among patients with poor outcomes, those treated operatively had more lateral stenosis and scarring at L4 than those treated conservatively. Operatively treated patients with good results had significantly more degeneration of erector spinae muscle than conservatively treated patients with good results. All but 9% of operatively treated patients had some muscle degeneration.

Conclusions.—Follow-up with CT of patients with lumbar disk herniation suggests that, although operation does not stop disk degeneration, there is no correlation between clinical outcome and changes in the dimensions of the spinal canal. In operatively and conservatively treated patients there was no difference in recurrence of herniations, but surgically treated patients tended to have a better outcome. Computed tomography is recommended as the examination of first choice in patients with so-called failed back syndrome.

▶ The take-home message for this important study is that scar and lateral recess stenosis are associated with poorer clinical results over a 5-year interval after spinal decompression. A secondary important observation was the high percentage of patients with paraspinal muscle degeneration in the operated patient subset. Although this finding had little correlation with the clinical result, it does raise the question, "will muscle degeneration lead to muscle weakness, making operated patients more susceptible to reinjury.—J.W. Frymoyer, M.D.

Effects of Sodium Hyaluronate on Peridural Fibrosis After Lumbar Laminotomy and Discectomy

Songer MN, Ghosh L, Spencer DL (Univ of Illinois, Chicago)
Spine 15:550–554, 1990   5–20

Background.—Recurrent radicular or low-back pain after lumbar laminectomy and diskectomy has been ascribed to peridural fibrosis that occurs after surgery. Scar tissue can restrict nerve root mobility and make the root vulnerable to recurrent disk protrusion and stenosis. The value of sodium hyaluronate, 1.9% solution, for retarding peridural fibrosis was examined in dogs.

Methods.—The dogs underwent unilateral lumbar hemilaminotomy, annular fenestration, and nucleotomy. Either hyaluronate, a fat graft, or gelfoam was placed at the time of surgery, and the animals were killed at intervals up to 26 weeks after operation.

Results.—Hyaluronate inhibited fibrosis more than the other materials (Fig 5–18). Adhesions were much less tenacious in animals treated with sodium hyaluronate than in those receiving other treatment (Fig 5–19). Neither the area of fibrosis nor the tenacity of adhesions differed significantly in the animals given gelfoam and fat and in control animals given no treatment.

Conclusion.—Sodium hyaluronate meets many of the criteria for an ideal material with which to prevent perineural adhesions. It is semifluid and biologically inert and is absorbed slowly over time. The material acts as a spacer to retard clot formation, the first stage in the development of peridural fibrosis.

▶ Convincing evidence is presented for the effectiveness of sodium hyaluronate in preventing postoperative scar formation. The authors' experimental

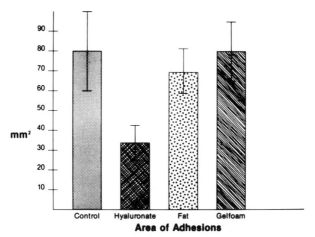

Fig 5–18.—Area of fibrosis was carefully measured and was notably smaller in sodium hyaluronate group. All time periods were averaged for each group. (Courtesy of Songer MN, Ghosh L, Spencer DL: *Spine* 15:550–554, 1990.)

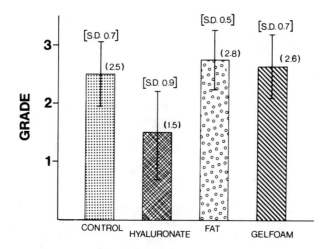

TENACITY OF ADHESIONS

Fig 5–19.—Grade of tenacity of lesions was significantly less in sodium hyaluronate group and not significantly different among other groups. Time periods were averaged for each group. (Courtesy of Songer MN, Ghosh L, Spencer DL: *Spine* 15:550–554, 1990.)

model is also of note. Deliberate invasion of the disk was added to the laminotomy; this technique has not been used by previous investigators, who have performed only the laminotomy. Unproven by this study is whether the diskectomy may have been the source of substantial scar, as opposed to the traditional view that scar invades from the muscle adjacent to dura. In view of the clear association of scar with poorer clinical results, as reported in Abstract 5–19 by Hurme et al., the authors' technique merits further clinical investigation.—J.W. Frymoyer, M.D.

A Controlled Trial of Corticosteroid Injections into Facet Joints for Chronic Low Back Pain

Carette S, Marcoux S, Truchon R, Grondin C, Gagnon J, Allard Y, Latulippe M (Laval University, Quebec City, Canada)
N Engl J Med 325:1002–1007, 1991
5–21

Background.—Chronic low-back pain is a common problem. Many treatments exist for this condition, few of which have been assessed rigorously. A randomized, placebo-controlled trial was done to evaluate the efficacy of corticosteroid injections into facet joints to treat chronic low-back pain.

Methods.—Ninety-seven patients were enrolled in the trial. All had chronic low-back pain and experienced immediate relief of the pain after injections of local anesthetic into the facet joints between the fourth and fifth lumbar vertebrae and the fifth lumbar and first sacral vertebrae. By random assignment, 49 received 20-mg injections of methylprednisolone acetate and 48 received injections of isotonic saline in the same facet joints. Injections were done under fluoroscopic guidance. Ninety-five patients were available for follow-up for 6 months.

Results.—At 1 month, there were no clinical or statistical differences between the groups in any of the outcome measures assessing pain, functional status, and back flexion. Forty-two percent of those receiving treatment and 33% of those receiving placebo reported marked or very marked improvement. At 3 months the results were similar. At 6 months patients treated with methylprednisolone reported more improvement, less pain on the visual analog scale, and less physical disability. However, the between-group differences were reduced when concurrent interventions were considered. Only 22% of those receiving treatment group and 10% of those receiving placebo had sustained improvement from the first to the sixth month.

Conclusions.—Methylprednisolone injection into facet joints appears to be of little benefit in the treatment of chronic low-back pain. Even though the patients in this series were selected for their positive response to facet-joint injections with a local anesthetic, only 1 in 5 had sustained improvement 6 months after the injection of steroids compared with 1 in 10 after injection of placebo.

▶ Facet injections, whether steroids are used or not, appear to have minimal therapeutic efficacy, as determined during a 6-month interval in this randomized, prospective analysis. The selection of their patients was interesting. All had initial relief (phase I of study) with single- or multiple-joint injection with lidocaine, controlled by a facet arthrogram. It is on this basis that they selected patients who might have a facet causation for their pain. The underlying issue is whether "Facet Syndrome" exists or can be diagnosed with certainty. Jackson and Jacobs' meticulous study (1) suggests that the "syndrome," if it exists, cannot be diagnosed by today's technology. In this light, the results of the current study are predictable.—J.W. Frymoyer, M.D.

Reference

1. Jackson RP, et al: *Spine* 13:966–971, 1988.

A Community-Based Study of the Use of Chiropractic Services
Shekelle PG, Brook RH (Univ of California, Los Angeles; RAND Corp)
Am J Public Health 81:439–442, 1991   5–22

Introduction.—Investigations of the use of chiropractic services have relied on data obtained from selected chiropractors' offices or clinics. To determine population-based use rates and demographic information on persons seeking chiropractic care, data from a prospective, large-scale, community-based population were analyzed.

Methods.—The source of the study data was the RAND Health Insurance Experiment (HIE) conducted between 1974 and 1982. Six sites chosen for the HIE represented the 4 major census regions, including both

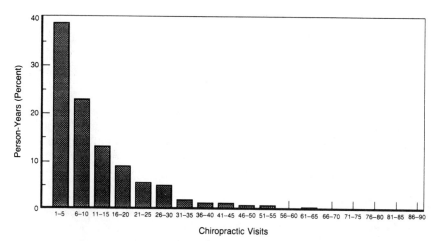

Fig 5–20.—Number of chiropractic visits per person-year. (Courtesy of Shekelle PG, Brook RH: *Am J Public Health* 81:439–442, 1991.)

urban and rural areas. The enrolled population was representative of the United States population younger than age 65 years. Insurance claim forms for all fee-for-service patients who completed the investigation were examined for all visits coded as visits to a chiropractor.

Results.—During the 9-year period, 395 of 5,279 persons (7.5%) made at least 1 visit to a chiropractor. There were 7,873 visits in all, with repeat visits accounting for 82% of the total. The median number of visits per year was 7 (Fig 5–20). Fewer than 1% of the visits resulted from a referral by another health-care provider. Chiropractic users, compared with nonusers, tended to be white, middle-aged, married, and high-

Comparison of Selected Demographic Characteristics of Chiropractic Users and Nonusers in the RAND Health Insurance Experiment

Characteristic	Chiropractic Users (%)	Nonusers (%)	Difference (95% Confidence Interval)
Male*	49	48	1 (-4, 6)
White*	96	84	12 (9, 15)
Age			
< 18	16	36	-20 (-24, -16)
18–50	70	50	20 (15, 25)
51+	14	13	1 (-3, 5)
Education*			
< High school	26	31	-5 (-10, 0)
High School graduate	47	36	11 (5, 17)
>High school	27	33	-6 (-11, -1)
Married*	74	45	29 (24, 34)
Working* (not homemaker)	67	64	3 (-2, 8)
Median family income* (1973 dollars)	$11,078	$11,192	114 (-666, 894)

*For adults aged 18 years and older.
(Courtesy of Shekelle PG, Brook RH: *Am J Public Health* 81:439–442, 1991.)

school educated. The median family income was similar for users and nonusers (table). The most common reason for seeking chiropractic care was back pain (42%). Sixty-six percent of repeat-visit services provided consisted of spinal manipulation. The number of persons seeking care per 100 person-years ranged from .6 in the Charleston, SC area to 3.1 in the Seattle area.

Conclusion.—The symptoms for which patients seek chiropractic care are similar across the United States, although the rate and intensity of use vary considerably in different geographic regions. Demographic findings confirm those of previous reports and document the fact that a substantial amount of health care is delivered by chiropractors.

▶ For many years, many orthopedists have found the nonoperative treatment of low-back pain to be less than a favored pastime. If the increasing enrollment of orthopedists in courses that stress nonoperative treatment is any indication, this attitude may be changing. In the meantime, practitioners who engage in manipulative therapy have filled at least part of the void. This study gives additional data on how often patients choose a chiropractor, how many treatments are given, and what type are given. The article will not necessarily answer any questions, but you may be surprised by the information that it contains.—J.W. Frymoyer, M.D.

Percutaneous Posterolateral Lumbar Discectomy and Decompression With a 6.9-Millimeter Cannula: Analysis of Operative Failures and Complications
Schaffer JL, Kambin P (Graduate Hosp, Philadelphia; Univ of Pennsylvania, Philadelphia)
J Bone Joint Surg 73-A:822–831, 1991   5–23

Introduction.—Protrusion of a lumbar disk with associated persistent radiculopathy can be treated by several operative means. Posterolateral diskectomy, accomplished through a 7-mm incision, spares patients the pain and morbidity of an open operative procedure and permits rapid rehabilitation. Whether percutaneous posterolateral diskectomy compares favorably with laminectomy in the rate of operative failures and complications was investigated.

Methods.—Conservative treatment had failed in the 100 patients eligible for posterolateral lumbar diskectomy; all had neurologic impairment and positive tension signs. The operative procedure was performed under local anesthesia and involved a sheath with an internal diameter of 4.9 mm (Fig 5–21). Follow-up was at least 2 years.

Results.—Four patients could not be located and 3 died during the follow-up period. The cause of death in the latter patients was unrelated to the diskectomy; all 3 were judged to have had excellent results at a minimumn of 15 months postoperatively. Of 93 patients available for review, 81 (83 herniated disks) had a successful result. There were no major complications or instances of postoperative neurologic or muscular

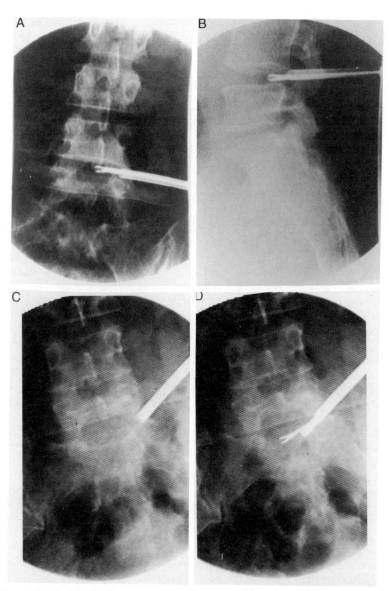

Fig 5–21.—Intraoperative radiographs made during percutaneous posterolateral lumbar disectomy and decompression. **A,** anteroposterior view showing the 6.9-mm cannula and forceps in the disk space between the fourth and fifth lumbar vertebrae. **B,** corresponding lateral view. **C,** the 6.9-mm cannula in the disk space between the fifth lumbar and first sacral vertabrae. **D,** deflector tube and flexible forceps inserted into the disk space between the fifth lumbar and first sacral vertebrae. (Courtesy of Schaffer JL, Kambin P: *J Bone Joint Surg* 73-A:822–831, 1991.)

deficits. Eleven of the 12 in whom the procedure failed underwent a subsequent laminectomy, which was successful in 8 patients. Causes of failure included lateral-recess stenosis and a history of multiple unsuccessful operations.

Conclusions.—The technique described is effective and safe for treatment of a herniated disk in selected patients. Operative failures are few and can be improved by a subsequent laminectomy. Use of a modified arthroscopic instrument and intermittent uniportal diskoscopic control are recommended.

▶ Dr. Kambin has pioneered the percutaneous diskectomy. His technique is somewhat more invasive than suction percutaneous diskectomy but also seems to involve the removal of a larger amount of disk material. Although this study does not have controls, it does suggest a role for this technique in a small group of patients. Dr. Kambin is quite clear about his patient selection and who should not have the operation. Key points are that are technique is contraindicated for patients with free fragments, caudal symptoms, or any degree of lateral stenosis. He also emphasizes the importance of the patient being awake—a lesson learned the hard way in the catastrophic failures of chymopapain. His results overall are surprisingly good. Although the hospitalization was short, the period before return to work seems long. For the 13 patients with a successful result and workers' compensation, the average duration was 262 days! For the 72 patients who had a successful result and no compensation, the figure was 92 days. Apparently, the decreased invasiveness of the procedure has little to do with the rapidity with which patients return to work. Overall, his technique merits consideration. My only problem is that the number of patients I see who would fulfill his criteria are not large in number.—J.W. Frymoyer, M.D.

Nucleolysis of the Rabbit Intervertebral Disc Using Chondroitinase ABC
Henderson N, Stanescu V, Cauchoix J (Institut de Recherche sur les Maladies du Squelette, Berke-sur-Mer, France; Hôpital des Enfants Malades, Paris)
Spine 16:203–208, 1991   5–24

Background.—Chondroitinase ABC has a specific action on the proteoglycans of the nucleus pulposus. It almost totally degrades chondroitin-4-sulfate, chondroitin-6-sulfate, and dermatan sulfate, which form the main part of the molecule. Chymopapain, by contrast, is less specific. It cleaves the central protein chain of the proteoglycans. The effect of intradiskal injection of chondroitinase ABC in the rabbit lumbar spine was assessed.

Methods.—Twenty-five white Bouska rabbits aged 10–13.5 months were used. A 29-gauge needle was used to inject 1 unit of chondroitinase ABC in .02 mL of phosphate-buffered saline directly into the center of the nucleus pulposus at a depth of 3 mm. In each rabbit 2 disks at various levels between L1–2 and L6–7 were injected with enzyme. One or 2 disks were injected with buffer alone. The disks were then studied radiographically, histologically, and biochemically.

Results.—Injection of chondroitinase ABC resulted in no increase in surface area at 2 days. At 6 days there was significant reduction. When a

Bonnferroni correction was applied, the statistical significance of these results was doubtful. Histologically, disk narrowing with condensation of the nucleus was not seen consistently at 2 days. It was observed more clearly at 6 days. Necrosis of cells in the nucleus was apparent consistently at 2 days. The nucleus pulposus took up Safranin O to give a punctate appearance with stronger, more even staining in the stroma than in the cells. Nuclei injected with enzyme had loss of staining within and around the cells at 2 days, with the changes becoming more obvious and widespread at 6 days. There was also some loss of color from the inner layer of the annulus at 6 days. Biochemically, there was no significant treatment-related difference in the proportion of wet weight to dry weight. At 2 days there was a significant diminution of hexuronic acid content. At 6 days enzyme treatment resulted in a highly significant decrease in all parameters.

Conclusions.—The enzyme chondroitinase ABC is able to degrade the major glycosaminoglycan component of the nucleus pulposus proteoglycans. It significantly reduces nucleus volume and proteoglycan content at 6 days. The characteristics and advantages of chondroitinase ABC compared with those of chymopapain have yet to be defined.

▶ This basic investigation analyzes the effects of a newer chemonucleolytic agent, as measured by radiologic, histologic, and chemical changes. The presumed benefits of this enzyme compared to chymopapain are its selective action on chondroitin rather than a more general effect on the proteoglycans of the disk. It reminds me that the basic appeal of chemonucleolysis has not died; its recrudescence awaits a safe and effective agent. To determine whether chondroitinase will be that drug, further investigation is needed.—J.W. Frymoyer, M.D.

Segmental Instability

▶ ↓ Segmental instability continues to be one of the common indications for lumbar spinal fusion. The following 3 articles represent the latest attempts to rigorously define the radiologic criteria of instability. The encapsulation of these 3 articles is captured in Shaffer's article (Abstract 5–25): "Lumbar fusions have been and continue to be performed because of this radiographic abnormality when accompanied by chronic pain, despite the fact that there is no universally accepted definition of instability." These 3 investigational efforts suggest that we have made little headway in that definition.—J.W. Frymoyer, M.D.

The Consistency and Accuracy of Roentgenograms for Measuring Sagittal Translation in the Lumbar Vertebral Motion Segment: An Experimental Model

Shaffer WO, Spratt KF, Weinstein J, Lehmann TR, Goel V (Ventura County Med Ctr–Univ of California, Los Angeles; Univ of Iowa, Iowa City; Louisville Orthopedic Clinic, Ky)
Spine 15:741–750, 1990   5–25

Background.—Despite long experience with lumbar spinal instability the condition still lacks the definition needed for meaningful epidemiologic studies. Lumbar fusions continue to be done on the grounds of radiographic abnormality when chronic pain is present. The accuracy and consistency of sagittal translation estimates were determined in roentgenograms of varying quality.

Methods.—A model of the L4–5 lumbar motion segment was developed that allows precise manipulation of sagittal translation, rotation of L5 relative to L4, tilt of L4 on L5, and control of image clarity by placing a water bath between the tube and the vertebra. A series of experiments was designed to systematically assess the consistency and accuracy of sagittal translation measurements from roentgenograms of varying quality.

Results.—Considerable reliability was evident independent of the particular rater, the measurement used, and the quality of the roentgenograms. However, there were high rates of false positive and false negative studies. Higher quality films were more accurately evaluated, regardless of the method of measurement used. Within-rater consistency and accuracy were remarkably high with all methods of measurement and with all degrees of concomitant motion. Less consistency was noted when clinical roentgenograms were analyzed than when the model was used.

Implications.—Errors in classification will occur if roentgenograms are used as a basis for diagnosing lumbar spinal instability. False positive findings are especially likely to occur with lower quality films, if there is substantial obliquity, and if concomitant motion is present.

Lumbosacral Segmental Motion in Normal Individuals: Have We Been Measuring Instability Properly?
Boden SD, Wiesel SW (George Washington Univ)
Spine 15:571–576, 1990   5–26

Background.—Great controversy surrounds the concept of lumbar spine segmental instability, but most reports agree that instability includes excessive motion beyond normal constraints. Weight-bearing lateral flexion–extension radiographs of volunteers were examined in an attempt to define normal lumbosacral segmental motion in vivo.

Methods.—The 40 male volunteers had no history of back pain or sciatica. They ranged in age from 19 to 43 years. The relative positions of the lumbar vertebral motion segments were determined by standard weight-bearing lateral flexion–extension radiographs. For each segment, anteroposterior displacement and sagittal angular rotation were determined. Angulation between vertebrae and the relative slip were measured (Fig 5–22). Reproducibility of measurements was assessed by calculating the coefficient of variation between 2 sets of measurements made by the same observer on 50 vertebral levels 3 months apart.

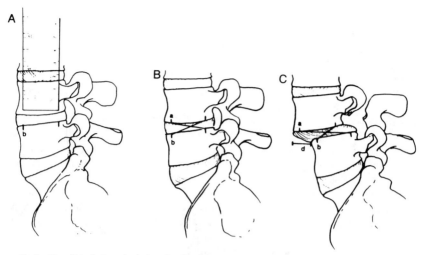

Fig 5–22.—Calculation of relative slip *(d)* of superior on inferior vertebral body. **A,** a ruler of any diameter slightly less than the vertebral body width is vertically positioned parallel to and centered between the anterior and posterior vertebral cortices. The intersection of the sides of the ruler with the end-plate is marked. **B,** diagonal lines *a* and *b* are drawn to connect the end-plate; marks and their dimensions are measured. **C,** static slip *(d)* is calculated as one half *(a-b)*. Dynamic translation is the relative difference of the static slip calculated in flexion and the static slip in extension. (Courtesy of Boden SD, Wiesel SW: *Spine* 15:571–576, 1990.)

Results.—At each lumbar level, the mean dynamic sagittal angular rotation from flexion to extension ranged from 7.7 degrees to 9.4 degrees, with the greatest motion at L4–L5 and L5–S1. The lumbar spine had an intervertebral angle of 9 degrees and L5–S1 had an angle of 12 degrees. More than 90% of participants had 1–3 degrees of dynamic anteroposterior translation; at all levels, mean anteroposterior translation was 1.3 mm or 3.2% of the superior vertebral body width. Measurements were highly reproducible, with a nonsignificant .7% coefficient of variation; interobserver variation was insignificant.

Conclusions.—In normal persons, measurement of dynamic motion as opposed to static slip increases the frequency of radiographic instability by 8 times. The finding of static anteroposterior slip on a single lateral radiograph does not mean that the same amount of motion is present; instead, it may reflect abnormal relative position of 2 vertebrae. The findings can serve as a basis for a normal database, but the significance of the dynamic instability described must be clarified.

Compression–Traction Radiography of Lumbar Segmental Instability
Kälebo P, Kadziolka R, Swärd L (University of Gothenburg; Västra Frölunda Hospital, Gothenburg, Sweden)
Spine 15:351–355, 1990

Background.—In patients with spondylolisthesis symptoms may result in part from segmental instability. It is important to have some objective means of confirming pathologic segmental movements so as to select proper treatment and clarify the indications for surgical stabilization. Compression–traction provocation was used to study movements in the sagittal plane of the lumbosacral joint, both in asymptomatic participants and patients with lytic spondylolisthesis.

Methods.—The series included 15 healthy males (mean age, 23 years) and 29 patients (20 males, 9 females; mean age, 35 years) with symptomatic lateral true lytic spondylolisthesis, mostly at L5–S1 and of grade I. For such participant, lateral spot radiographs were taken in the recumbent, compression, and traction positions. Compression views were taken with patients in standing position and a 20-kg weight on their shoulders, which provided an extra axial compression force. For traction views, patients hung by their hands from a bar. Degree of slip was measured by the difference in slip between the compression and traction views. Degree of sagittal rotation also was determined.

Results.—In the control group, compression and traction views showed no significant difference in translatory movement. There was a mean displacement of .8%. A small sagittal backward rotation was noted, but there was no significant correlation between translation and rotation values. In the patient group, there was a significant difference in slip, with an average displacement of 5.2%. The mean difference in analysis of compression–recumbent radiographs was 3.7% (Fig 5–23). Sixty-nine percent of the patients had a translatory displacement greater than the limit of detectability, i.e., 2.5%. Most had anterior translation as their main cause of displacement. There was also a small but signifi-

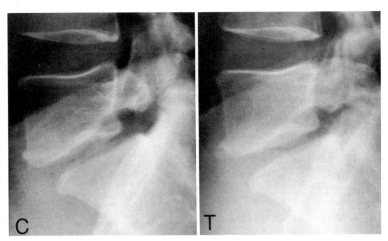

Fig 5–23.—Compression (C) and traction (T) examination of a 53-year-old man with a symptomatic spondylolisthesis. Compression view shows an anterior translatory displacement, spondylolysis, malalignment of the isthmic pedicles, and disk degeneration. Traction view results in reduction of slip, alignment of the pars interarticularis, and a manifestation of an intervertebral "vacuum phenomenon." (Courtesy of Kälebo P, Kadziolka R, Swärd L: *Spine* 15:351–355, 1990.)

cant difference in sagittal angulatory motion between compression–traction views. Sixty-two percent of patients had greater translations of the lytic vertebra than the largest displacement exhibited by controls. The patients had predominant anterior displacement on the compression view with a smaller posterior movement in the traction view. There was no significant difference in angulatory movements of the L5–S1 segment between the 2 groups.

Conclusions.—Compression–traction radiography appears to be a useful and practical method of assessing segmental movements of the lower lumbar spine. About two thirds of patients with spondylolisthesis so evaluated had pathologic translatory movements suggesting lumbar spine instability.

▶ These 3 articles taken in aggregate point out the major problems in the radiographic diagnosis of instability. Although films can be interpreted with some degree of reliability in the controlled laboratory environment, the realities of the clinical setting make the everyday experience less certain.—J.W. Frymoyer, M.D.

INTERNAL FIXATION

▶ ↓ In earlier editions of the YEAR BOOK OF ORTHOPEDICS I have commented on the growing interest in pedicle fixation. Longer-term studies are becoming available that put this technique in perspective and detail some of the expected results and complications.—J.W. Frymoyer, M.D.

Results of Spinal Arthrodesis With Pedicle Screw-Plate Fixation
West JL III, Bradford DS, Ogilvie JW (Univ of Minnesota)
J Bone Joint Surg 73-A:1179–1184, 1991   5–28

Background.—The popularity of screw-plate systems for pedicle fixation in patients with spinal arthrodesis is increasing. However, there have been no long-term investigations of this procedure.

Methods.—Sixty-one patients were followed for 24–35 months (mean, 30 months) after arthrodesis of the lumbar or lumbosacral spine with pedicle screw-plate fixation for painful degenerative arthritis, spondylolisthesis, or pseudarthrosis. The series included 21 men and 40 women aged 22–63 years. The patients rated the clinical result by using an analog scale. The surgical result was considered a clinical failure if the patient believed it was, if an additional operation was needed, or if the functional and pain scores were not good.

Results.—Most patients reported a marked reduction in pain and an increase in function. Two thirds were able to work full time. Clinical failure occurred in 28%, with the lowest rate (20%) in patients with painful degenerative arthritis and the highest rate (47%) in those who had a pseudarthrosis before surgery. The fusion rate was 90% in patients with painful degenerative disease, 93% in those with spondylolisthesis, and 65% in those with a pseudarthrosis before surgery.

Conclusions.—In this series a successful arthrodesis did not always yield a reduction in symptoms. The rate of clinical failure was about 10% greater than that of pseudarthrosis. Treatment of patients who have had a successful arthrodesis that failed to provide a good clinical result remains a perplexing problem.

▶ This study involves a complex group of patients whose primary disorder is degenerative, spondylolisthesis, or a pseudoarthrosis. Twenty-eight percent had clinical failure; the worst results were in patients with a previous pseudoarthrosis (47% failure). Fusion rates were 90% overall but only 65% in repair of pseudoarthrosis. Complications occurred in 25% of the patients, including a 7% risk of neurologic compromise of which 3 of 4 related to the fixation device. My interpretation of these results suggests pedicle fixation is not a panacea; it does not guarantee success as measured by symptomatic relief or fusion. The results are obtained at a small but significant price, even in the hands of very experienced surgeons.—J.W. Frymoyer, M.D.

Survivorship Analysis of Pedicle Spinal Instrumentation
McAfee PC, Weiland DJ, Carlow JJ (Johns Hopkins Univ; St Joseph Hosp, Baltimore)
Spine 16:S422–S427, 1991   5–29

Background.—Pedicular spinal instrumentation is a recent development designed to increase spinal stability in spinal reconstructive procedures. Survivorship analysis was applied to the first 120 consecutive patients having pedicle instrumentation in an attempt to predict long-term outcomes at 5 years and 10 years.

Methods.—The procedures were performed between 1985 and 1989; 78 involved the Steffee Variable Slotted Plate (VSP) instrumentation technique, and 42 used Cotrel–Dubousset (CD) spinal instrumentation. All procedures were performed in conjunction with posterolateral fusions. The patients' mean age was 43 years. Spondylolisthesis accounted for 72 of the cases of spinal deformity. The second most common cause (in 23 patients) was iatrogenic or postlaminectomy instability. Twenty-five reductions were considered to be major.

Results.—The procedures employed 175 CD screws and 351 VSP screws. There were 22 (4.18%) problem screws—6 bent and 16 broken. The problem-screw events occurred in 12 patients, 7 with solid posterolateral fusion and 5 with pseudarthrosis. None of the screws was infected or loose. All failed screws were located at the junction of the uppermost thread and the collar of the pedicle screw. Survivorship of solid posterolateral fusion at 10 years' follow-up was predicted by actuarial analysis to be 90%. Life-table calculations for the same period predicted an 80% survivorship of instrumentation without complications. Cumulative survival function estimates for all hardware problems showed the probability of avoiding instrumentation difficulty to be 80% at 5 years and 10 years postoperatively (Fig 5–24).

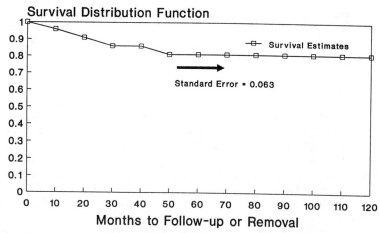

Fig 5–24.—Kaplan-Meier survival curve for no hardware problems: absence of screw, rod or plate breakage, loosening, or bending. If an implant was removed because of neurologic complications or infection, then this would have been included; however, this did not occur in this series. The *ordinate axis* is probability, and the *curve* denotes the cumulative probability of survival up to the specific number of postoperative months after pedicular instrumentation. (Courtesy of McAfee PC, Weiland DJ, Carlow JJ: *Spine* 16:S422–S427, 1991.)

Conclusions.—The survivorship rate predicted for pedicle spinal instrumentation is similar to that of other more widely used orthopedic surgical implants. In the absence of spinal pseudarthrosis, hardware breakage is not associated with a bad result.

▶ How often does a pedicle screw fail? Can we predict the risk for the future? In a diverse group of patients, 4.18% of screws failed during the actual period of clinical and radiologic observation. The survivorship analysis suggests, but does not prove conclusively, that 20% will ultimately fail. Five patients had pseudoarthrosis. Although neurologic complications occurred, the authors felt that these events were independent of the fixation system.—J.W. Frymoyer, M.D.

A Comparison of Single-Level Fusions With and Without Hardware
Lorenz M, Zindrick M, Schwaegler P, Vrbos L, Collatz MA, Behal R, Cram R
(Loyola Univ; Maywood, Ill; Hinsdale Orthopaedic Associates, Ill)
Spine 16:S455–S458, 1991   5–30

Introduction.—The use of MRI and the development of pedicle screw internal fixation systems have advanced lumbar spine care in the past decade. With the combination of MRI and diskography, symptomatic degenerative disks can be identified with increased accuracy. Whether adjunctive pedicular fixation enhances the clinical outcome was investigated in 68 patients undergoing single-level spinal fusion between January 1985 and December 1988.

Methods.—All 68 patients had experienced disabling back pain for at least 6 months and were unable to work. Conservative treatment had failed in all patients. A group of 29 patients underwent fusion without hardware, and a group of 39 underwent fusion with the Variable Slotted Plate (VSP) system; the fusion procedure was otherwise identical. Patients were evaluated according to fusion success, perceived pain, and return to the same or similar employment.

Results.—Follow-up averaged 26 months in the non-hardware group and 31 months in the hardware group. Pseudarthrosis occurred in 59% of the non-hardware group but was not apparent in the instrumented group. Significant improvement of pain was reported by 77% of patients with the VSP system, but by only 41.4% of those in the non-hardware group. Whereas 72% of those receiving hardware returned to work, only 31% of the non-hardware group did so. Patients without hardware but with a solid fusion had a higher rate (75%) of reemployment. Fusion was less successful in smokers.

Conclusion.—The use of internal fixation is associated with a higher rate of success in single-level lumbar fusion. In addition, the use of hardware moderately increases the probability of obtaining a solid spinal fusion.

▶ Although this clinical analysis is not randomized, it presents fairly strong evidence that single-level fusion is enhanced by the addition of pedicle fixation. Pseudarthrosis occurred in 59% of those without fixation and in no patient with fixation. Pseudarthrosis in turn was associated with a poor clinical result. What surprises me is the extraordinarily high level of fusion failure compared with the literature, particularly when the study was limited to single-level fusions. In light of the preceding 2 abstracts, the issue is, are the risks of the pedicle screw worth the increased rate of fusion? Also, underlying the main objective of this study remains the lingering question as to who should be selected for the operation. Their population was a group of patients with primary back pain, MRI evidence of disk degeneration, and diskographic abnormalities and reproduction of pain symptoms. Not all would agree that these constitute indications for surgical intervention, but some would.—J.W. Frymoyer, M.D.

6 Foot and Ankle

Introduction

Interest in medical and surgical care of the foot and ankle continues to expand. The number of scientifically correct and diverse articles increases yearly, making the selection of papers a stimulating challenge.

The following abstracts highlight the literature of the past year and are grouped into the following sections:

1. Trauma and Its Sequelae: Osseous Injuries
2. Trauma and Its Sequelae: Soft Tissue Injuries
3. Problems of the Forefoot
4. Miscellaneous Topics

Trauma continues to be an area of great interest, and we have abstracted a number of papers on this subject. One paper assesses the long-term follow-up of tibia plafond fractures treated with open reduction and internal fixation. The operative results of intra-articular fractures of the calcaneus are discussed, as is the importance of the timely treatment of ankle fractures in 2 separate papers. The management of Weber C ankle fracture subluxation remains a challenge. A paper selected analyzes the indications for syndesmotic screws, and the authors conclude than when rigid medial and lateral osteosyntheses can be achieved a syndesmotic screw is probably not indicated. Compartment syndromes continue to baffle physicians because their symptoms are diverse and occasionally subtle. This topic continues to be extremely important, and 2 articles deal with compartment syndromes of the foot.

Orthopedic imaging has made enormous strides in the past few years and is well represented in this YEAR BOOK. Papers on this topic point out the use of 3-dimensional analysis of calcaneal fractures. Likewise, MRI is useful in the diagnosis of injuries to the tibialis posterior, flexor hallucis longus, and flexor digitorum longus tendons.

Bunions and bunionettes are the common fare of the foot surgeon. Two studies show that the Akin procedure and the Keller arthroplasty can be used with success when performed within certain guidelines. New surgical procedures for correction of a bunionette deformity are described. One study uses a distal Chevron procedure of the fifth metatarsal, and another employs a longitudinal diaphyseal osteotomy.

A biomechanical study once again provides evidence of the detrimental effects of wearing high-heeled shoes. This study eloquently shows that, among other biomechanical abnormalities, wearing high-heeled shoes causes the forces at the first metatarsophalangeal joint to be twice normal values.

The best method for treating ruptured lateral ankle ligaments is still a matter of debate. Early immobilization has been shown to result in a better early functional result, and nonoperative measures remain the preferred treatment.

Indeed, it was another excellent year for the orthopedic subspecialty of foot and ankle. The interest and enthusiasm in this area continues to grow. No doubt, as our understanding of the foot and ankle continues to evolve, improved care of all patients with foot and ankle problems will result.

Kenneth A. Johnson, M.D.
Robert D. Teasedall, M.D.

Trauma and Its Sequelae: Osseous Injuries

Long-Term Results of Tibial Plafond Fractures Treated With Open Reduction and Internal Fixation

Etter C, Ganz R (University of Bern, Switzerland)
Arch Orthop Trauma Surg 110:277–283, 1991   6–1

Background.—Tibial plafond fractures have the potential for severe functional deficit, but improved results have been reported with open reduction and internal fixation. However, not all reports have matched the 70% to 90% good functional results of the initial reports. Fifty-five patients with tibial plafond fractures were treated with open reduction and internal fixation over a 6-year period.

Patients.—Forty-one of the 55 patients were clinically and radiographically reviewed an average of 10 years postoperatively. There were 30 men and 11 women (mean age, 41.9 years). Most of the injuries occurred during sports activity. According to Rüedi's classification, 9.75% of the fractures were type I; 41.5%, type II; and 48.75%, type III.

Results.—Objective results at follow-up (average, 10 years) were good in 66% of patients and fair in 24%. Subjective results were good in 75.6%. In type I and II fractures, which are essentially low-velocity injuries, results were satisfactory in 86% of patients. For type III injuries, results were good or fair in 95% of patients, better than in most other reports; this was probably because only half of those injuries were high-velocity injuries and because of technical methods used to stabilize the injury during surgery. There was a direct correlation between development of severe arthrosis and initial fracture type, but no correlation between radiographic signs of arthrosis and subjective results. No systemic complications were noted, but 3 patients required reoperation.

Conclusion.—Severe tibial plafond fractures can be satisfactorily managed by adequate open reduction and internal fixation. Quality of reduction is related to later arthrosis, although arthrosis can result from articular cartilage damage. The surgeon must use meticulous soft tissue care, and fixation devices may be needed to insure the best soft tissue status for fracture healing.

▶ A tibial plafond fracture can be a surgical challenge. On occasion it is tempting just to go straight to an arthrodesis procedure. This article cautions against such an approach, because a fracture configuration that initially appears hopeless may actually achieve a satisfactory result. Also, arthrosis at late follow-up in itself does not mean a poor subjective result. Again, anatomical reduction, rigid fixation, meticulous soft tissue handling, and early range of motion seem to be the answer.— K.A. Johnson, M.D.

Compartment Syndrome of the Foot After Intraarticular Calcaneal Fracture
Mittlmeier T, Mächler G, Lob G, Mutschler W, Bauer G, Vogl T (University of Munich; University of Ulm, Germany)
Clin Orthop 269:241–248, 1991   6–2

Introduction.—Patients with intra-articular calcaneal fracture may be left with permanent disability. A central plantar ecchymosis may be a specific sign of calcaneal compression fracture. There has been surprisingly little attention to the consequences of fracture hematoma, specifically the formation of compartment syndrome leading to ischemic neuromuscular structural damage despite fracture reconstruction. A prospective analysis of plantar tissue after intra-articular calcaneal fracture was conducted.

Methods.—Twenty-one fractures in 17 consecutive patients were examined. Tissue pressure was measured before and after treatment, beginning from 3 hours to 30 days after injury. Pressures also were measured in 16 patients being treated for acute knee or ankle trauma. Eighteen fractures were reconstructed a mean of 13 days after the injuries. Three patients were treated conservatively because of their severe concomitant injuries.

Results.—A significant increase in tissue pressure was noted in 12 patients. Pressures reached values of more than 30 mm Hg as a result of primary fracture hematoma or interstitial fluid accumulation. The greatest values were noted 2 days after injury and persisted for 3–5 days. After a mean of 18 months, 7 of the 12 patients had plantar contractures or claw toe, or both, which interfered with walking. Those complications did not occur in patients with tissue pressures consistently less than 30 mm Hg.

Conclusions.—In patients with intra-articular calcaneal fracture, regular measurement of plantar compartmental pressure can help to avoid functional deficit. This compartment syndrome results from the plantar aponeurosis, which forms the constricting fascial envelope of the plantar muscles. If pressures exceed 30 mm Hg, the plantar aponeurosis should be longitudinally incised, preferably by a plantar incision as soon as the diagnosis is made.

Management of Compartment Syndromes of the Foot
Myerson MS (Union Mem Hosp, Baltimore)
Clin Orthop 271:239–248, 1991   6–3

Background.—Compartment syndromes of the foot, in contrast to those in other locations in the extremities, are not well understood and are frequently missed. If untreated the injury may result in pain and dysfunction, with sensory disturbance, stiffness, forefoot contracture, and clawing of the toes. Fourteen foot compartment syndromes in 12 patients with isolated extremity injuries seen during an 18-month period were reviewed.

Methods.—Patients were 10 men and 2 women (average age, 35

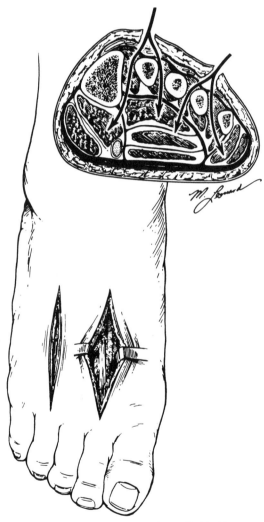

Fig 6–1.—The dorsal approach to fasciotomy uses 2 longitudinal incisions centered over the second and fourth metatarsals. No subcutaneous dissection is performed in the horizontal plane. The interosseous and central compartments are entered through each web space and the medial and lateral compartments using curved clamps. (From Myerson MS: *Clin Orthop* 271:239–248, 1991. Courtesy of Myerson MS: *Foot Ankle* 8:308, 1988.)

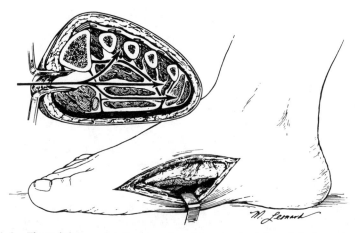

Fig 6–2.—The medial approach to fasciotomy is made between the abductor hallucis muscle and the inferior base of the first metatarsal. Through the medial incision, the central compartment may be decompressed with a curved clamp. (From Myerson MS: *Clin Orthop* 271:239–248, 1991. Courtesy of Myerson MS: *Foot Ankle* 8:308, 1988.)

years); 5 had been injured in industrial accidents. In 9 feet a fracture dislocation of the Lisfranc joint complex was present. Circulation pressures were measured according to the appearance of the foot. Interstitial pressure greater than 30 mm Hg in either the central or interosseous compartment was considered pathologic and was treated by fasciotomy. Nine feet underwent dorsal fasciotomy incisions (Fig 6–1) and 5 had medial incisions (Fig 6–2), after which open reduction and internal fixation of fractures was done in most cases. Delayed split-thickness skin grafting was used in 8 feet, and primary split-thickness skin incision and delayed primary wound closure were each used in 3 cases. A mean of 22 months after injury, patients were examined specifically for myoneural ischemia.

Outcome.—Four patients resumed their normal work and exercise activities; 6 had occasional discomfort with walking, standing, or shoe wear. One patient with calcaneus fracture had mildly symptomatic claw toes with fixed extension of the metatarsophalangeal joint and mild numbness over the toes. None of the other patients had any signs of myoneural ischemia.

Conclusions.—Compartment syndromes of the foot are best diagnosed by absolute compartment pressure measurements rather than clinical findings. Treatment is with medial or dorsal fasciotomy, depending on the fracture or dislocation pattern. All compartments should be decompressed and all pressures measured again after fasciotomy is done.

▶ Awareness of the possibility of a compartment syndrome of the foot needs reemphasis. Pain on passive dorsiflexion of the toes was the most reliable clinical finding in patients with elevated compartment pressure. Early decompression should eliminate the occurrence of a contracted painful foot associated with a nicely healed fracture (Figs 6–1 and 6–2).—K.A. Johnson, M.D.

Results of Operative Treatment for Intra-Articular Fractures of the Calcaneus

Melcher G, Bereiter H, Leutenegger A, Rüedi T (Rätisches Kantons-und Regional-spital, Chur, Switzerland)
J Trauma 31:234–238, 1991   6–4

Background.—Intra-articular fractures of the calcaneus are difficult to treat. Conservative treatment may result in disability, and surgical treatment is technically demanding.

Methods.—Seventeen displaced intra-articular fractures of the calcaneus were operatively treated during a 6-year period. The patients were 13 men and 3 women (average age, 35), 9 of whom had additional fractures of the lower extremities. Open reduction was performed generally through a posterolateral approach with a distractor (Fig 6–3), bone grafting, and internal fixation. With this technique, splints were unnecessary and early postoperative motion was possible. Computed tomography was used for precise preoperative planning. Sixteen patients, 14 with depression-type and 2 with tongue-type fractures, were reassessed an average of 36 months postoperatively.

Results.—Clinical and radiologic results were good in 50% of patients, satisfactory in 25%, and poor in 25%. All but 3 patients were able to return to work with in an average of 5 months. The remaining 3 received 33% disability compensations, results that compared favorably with those of nonoperative treatment.

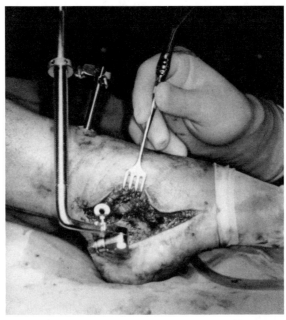

Fig 6–3.—Early intraoperative view with skin incision and position of the distractor. (Courtesy of Melcher G, Bereiter H, Leutenegger A, et al: *J Trauma* 31:234–238, 1991.)

Conclusions.—Most patients with comminuted intra-articular calcaneal fractures benefit from open reduction and internal fixation. Functional results are more reliable than with conservative treatment. Assessment of surgical indications, precise anatomical knowledge, and careful technique are essential for good results of osteosynthesis.

▶ Surgical treatment of a calcaneal fracture can be worthwhile when the fragments are of a size that can be reduced and fixated. It seems reasonable that grafting of the defect beneath the posterior facet after fracture reduction was helpful. Saving arthrodesis as a secondary treatment as with tibial plafond fractures again may be the reasonable approach. It certainly is tempting, however, to consider a primary subtalar arthrodesis for a comminuted fracture of the calcaneus with marked posterior facet depression and a blowout of the lateral wall into the subfibular region for a person who is a manual laborer with a Worker's Compensation injury. This article cautions to avoid such a temptation (Fig 6–3).—K.A. Johnson, M.D.

Early Complications in the Operative Treatment of Ankle Fractures: Influence of Delay Before Operation

Carragee EJ, Csongradi JJ, Bleck EE (Stanford Univ)
J Bone Joint Surg 73-B:79–82, 1991   6–5

Background.—Ankle fractures often are considered low priority cases, and patients with these injuries are frequently transferred to a second hospital for definitive care. Although the reported complication rate for operative treatment of ankle fractures varies widely, no analysis of what factors affect this rate has been done. The early complications of 121 surgically treated closed ankle fractures were reviewed to identify risk factors for postoperative complications.

Methods.—All patients were 16 years old or older, with closed distal, tibial, and fibular physes. Many were transferred for treatment to this facility, which serves the medically indigent. All received operations performed by residents under the direction of attending surgeons, using the anterior oblique method for reduction and fixation of the fractures in 119 of the 121 cases. Operations were not performed through damaged skin; prophylactic antibiotics were always administered. Follow-up occurred 4–120 weeks after fracture (average, 24 weeks).

Results.—Fourteen major and 22 minor complications occurred. Significantly more patients with breach of skin integrity had infection or reduction complications than those with intact skin. Patients with fracture–dislocations had significantly more major and minor complications than those with simple fractures. Delay in operation and transfer from another facility were associated with increased complication rates, especially with fracture–dislocations. Preexisting conditions and associated injuries were also significant risk factors for complications.

Conclusions.—Transfer of patients with serious ankle fractures before the completion of definitive care increases the risk of major and minor complications. Patients with these injuries should receive timely operative treatment.

▶ The ankle joint is such a close tolerance joint that it would be expected that surgical reduction would markedly improve the functional outcome. The need to pay particular attention to those situations where the skin has been broken and to provide early rather than late operative care is worthwhile information.— K.A. Johnson, M.D.

Ankle Mortise Stability in Weber C Fractures: Indications for Syndesmotic Fixation
Solari J, Benjamin J, Wilson J, Lee R, Pitt M (Univ of Arizona)
J Orthop Trauma 5:190–195, 1991   6–6

Introduction.—Weber type C ankle fractures are fairly common injuries seen in association with lateral talar subluxation. Current manage-

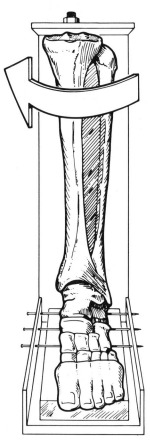

Fig 6–4.—Experimental setup of cadaver limb. (Courtesy of Solari J, Benjamin J, Wilson J, et al: *J Orthop Trauma* 5:190–195, 1991.)

TABLE 1.—Rotational Stability

Osteotomy performed	Mean rotation	% Increase from baseline	% Total instability
Intact ankle	7.7°	0	0
Medial malleolus fracture	13.8°	79	25
Medial malleolus fracture; anterior inferior tibiofibular ligament sectioned	18.9°	145	46
Medial malleolus fracture; anterior and posterior inferior tibiofibular ligament, interosseous membrane sectioned	23.8°	209	67
Medial and lateral malleolus fractures anterior and posterior inferior tibiofibular ligament sectioned	31.8°	313	100

Note: P < .05.
(Courtesy of Solari J, Benjamin J, Wilson J, et al: *J Orthop Trauma* 5:190–195, 1991.)

ment is initial fixation of the lateral malleolus and then treatment of the lateral side. Controversy remains as to whether a screw should be used to restore stability to the ankle syndesmosis. Cadaver limbs were studied to better define the use of syndesmotic fixation in Weber C fractures.

Methods.—Twelve cadaver lower extremities with the ankle joint left intact (Fig 6–4) were mounted in a specially designed frame. A Weber C or pronation external rotation injury was reproduced by sequential transection of the medial malleolus, anterior and posterior distal tibiofibular ligaments, and distal fibula, with external rotation torque applied at each point. The fractures were then repaired in staged fashion while the rotational stability of the ankle mortise was evaluated.

Results.—In the intact ankle, average maximum external talar rotation was 7.7 degrees. After creation of the Weber C injury, rotation increased by 311% to 31.8 degrees (Table 1). Thirty-two percent of the rotational stability was restored by rigid fixation of the fibular fracture, compared

TABLE 2.—Rotation Stability Postrepair

Structure	Mean rotation	% Increase in stability
Weber C	31.8°	0
Fibular plate	24°	32
Fibular plate, syndesmotic screw	19.6°	51
Fibular plate, medial malleolus screw	14.3°	73
Fibular plate, syndesmotic screw, medial malleolar screw	7.6°	100
Medial malleolar screw	18.2°	56

Note: P < .05.
(Courtesy of Solari J, Benjamin J, Wilson J, et al: *J Orthop Trauma* 5:190–195, 1991.)

with 57% by isolated fixation of the medial malleolus. When fibular fixation was combined with a syndesmotic screw 51% of stability was restored, and when medial malleolar fixation was added stability improved to 101%. Without a syndesmotic screw, bimalleolar fixation provided 73% of original stability (Table 2).

Conclusions.—In Weber type C ankle fractures, although lateral malleolar reduction is critical, the medial site provides stability of the mortise. Syndesmotic fixation may be unnecessary when rigid medial and lateral osteosynthesis can be achieved. Significant rotational displacement of the talus within the mortise probably cannot be detected by routine radiography.

▶ The management of Weber C ankle fracture subluxation remains a challenge. Based on this biomechanical study the authors conclude that, although reduction of the lateral malleolus is critical in reconstituting the ankle mortise and reducing the talus, it is the medial side, composed of the deltoid and medial malleolus, that provides mortise stability. Furthermore, syndesmotic fixation is indicated in Weber C ankle fractures in which the deltoid is disrupted or the medial malleolus cannot be rigidly fixed. When rigid medial and lateral osteosynthesis can be achieved, a syndesmotic screw is probably not indicated (Fig 6–4, Tables 1 and 2).—K.A. Johnson, M.D.

Three Dimensional Analysis of Calcaneal Fractures
Allon SM, Mears DC (Holy Redeemer Hosp and Med Ctr, Meadowbrook, Pa; Pittsburgh)
Foot Ankle 11:254–263, 1991   6–7

Background.—The treatment of calcaneal fractures is difficult, in part because of incomplete visualization of the 3-dimensional geometry of the bone. A specific 3-dimensional imaging protocol based on CT scans was developed and compared with conventional radiography and 2-dimensional CT scans in the evaluation of calcaneal fractures.

Methods.—Thirty calcaneal fractures in 22 patients were evaluated with conventional radiographs, 2-dimensional CT scans, and 3-dimensional CT reformations. The 2-dimensional CT scans were performed with the patient supine and the lower extremity in a bulky dressing or splint. The x-ray beam was positioned perpendicular or substantially oblique to the subtalar and calcaneocuboid articular and fracture surfaces.

Results.—Conventional radiographs led to underestimation of the degree of comminution, the magnitude of rotational displacement of the fracture surface, and the extent of subtalar facetal depression. The 2-dimensional CT coronal views provided the best views of intra-articular comminution, and CT scans yielded the best 3-dimensional CT images when a soft tissue algorithm, contiguous 3-mm cuts, an immobilized limb at the appropriate alignment, and a minimized field size were used. The 3-dimensional CT reformations thus obtained enhanced evaluation of the magnitude of joint depression, the extent of comminution, and the vector of rotational malalignment.

Conclusions.—Three-dimensional CT scans can reproducibly visualize a calcaneal fracture. The appropriate reformations can provide more information than 2-dimensional images, especially highlighting the rotational displacement of major fracture fragments.

▶ This study is the first of its kind to demonstrate reproducibly the usefulness of 3-dimensional CT scans in visualizing a calcaneal fracture. This information highlights the rotational displacement of major fracture fragments (multiplanar malrotation) and can facilitate the preparation of the appropriate surgical approach and reconstruction.— K.A. Johnson, M.D.

Ankle Arthrodesis Using Internal Screw Fixation
Holt ES, Hansen ST, Mayo KA, Sangeorzan BJ (Harborview Med Ctr, Seattle)
Clin Orthop 268:21–28, 1991   6–8

Background.—Good mechanical and biologic characteristics are essential to achieving precise ankle arthrodesis. External fixation often results in complications such as pin tract infection, loss of position, nonunion, and malunion. Based on extensive experience with internal fixation for traumatic injuries, a method of internal fixation with screws was developed for ankle arthrodesis.

Technique.—The arthrodesis is performed through an anterior or lateral approach. The anterior approach is used for medial or lateral talar displacement (Fig 6–5), and the posterior approach is used when the talus is displaced anteriorly. The primary fixation hardware is 6.5-mm cancellous screws. The most important screw is placed from the posterior malleolus into the talar neck and head. This screw is difficult to place; inside-out drilling is used through the anterior incision. Fixation is secured by lateral and medial malleolar screws. Because little or no bone is moved, the procedure maintains near normal anatomy.

Patients.—The anterior approach was used to perform 23 arthrodeses in 22 patients during a 9-year period. There were 15 men and 7 women (average age, 29 years). Traumatic arthrosis was present in 17 patients, and degenerative joint disease was present in 5. The fusion rate was 74%; avascular talus, pyarthrosis, and spasticity were associated with a high failure rate. Excluding this high-risk group, fusion rate was 93%, with only 1 patient having a delayed union. After this experience, special techniques were developed for screw placement and strain-relieving bone grafts to promote union.

Conclusions.—Internal screw fixation is a useful technique of ankle arthrodesis for the low-risk patient. The described technique provides a solid fusion and gives an aesthetically pleasing result. Patients in high-risk categories need other procedures.

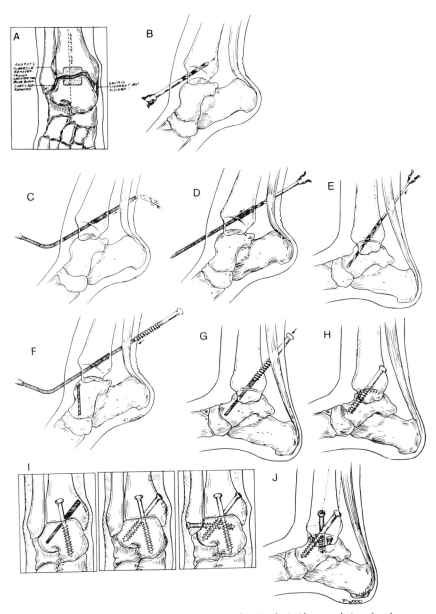

Fig 6–5.—Ankle fusion through an anterior approach using the inside-out technique for placement of the posterior malleolar screw. **A,** the deltoid ligament must be left sufficiently intact to maintain a blood supply to the medial talus. **B,** the drill bit is inserted slightly anterior to the center of the plafond and angled up approximately 50 degrees through the posterior malleolus. **C,** a Frazier suction tip is advanced to the heel cord. **D,** The Frazier tip guides a 3.5-mm drill bit into the ankle joint. **E,** after the foot is positioned for fusion, a 3.5-mm drill bit is advanced into the dome of the talus. **F,** the procedure is repeated through a posterior stab wound. **G,** a 6.5-mm screw is advanced into the talus. **H,** the threads of the screw are tightened into the talus across the fusion site. **I,** 2 additional screws are placed. **J,** the trough *(shaded area),* where a strain-relieving bone graft will be placed, is seen in front of the ankle. (Courtesy of Holt ES, Hansen ST, Mayo KA et al: *Clin Orthop* 268:21–28, 1991.)

Ankle Arthrodesis With the Calandruccio Frame and Bimalleolar Onlay Grafting

Malarkey RF, Binski JC (Miami Valley Hosp, Dayton, Ohio)
Clin Orthop 268:44–58, 1991   6–9

Background.—Compression arthrodesis has evolved into one of the main treatments for pain and disability resulting from arthritis of the ankle. A new technique using external triangular compression and a 2-incision technique was developed for bimalleolar onlay grafting.

Patients.—Twelve arthrodeses were performed during a 4-year period. All patients but 1 had posttraumatic arthritis. The average time from injury to arthrodesis was 7.5 years.

Technique.—The surgical technique of Stewart et al., with an anteromedial and an anterolateral incision, was used. Four-cm wedges are resected from the medial fibula and medial malleolus to create cancellous onlay grafts. The outer tibial cortex and tibiotalar joints are resected to facilitate neutral flexion and mild external rotation and valgus. After position is confirmed, a lag screw is placed across each malleolar graft, and the Calandruccio frame is applied. The external fixator was left on for 8 weeks with crutch weight-bearing.

Results.—Solid bony fusion was achieved in all patients but 1 who was noncompliant. Nine patients (mean age, 49 years) were reevaluated an average of 1.7 years postoperatively. The ankle was rated as good or excellent in 6 of these 9 and poor in 2; the remaining patient was not rated because of underlying disease that weakened ambulatory status. The patients with a poor result had pain but acceptable function. Of 4 nonretired patients, 3 were able to return to work.

Conclusions.—Bimalleolar onlay grafting and triangular compression give good results in patients with complex deformities of the ankle. Fusion rate and patient satisfaction are good. The main strength of this technique is its versatility.

▶ Abstracts 6–8 and 6–9 discuss ankle arthrodeses. In Abstract 6–8, a clever method of ankle arthrodesis using 6.5-mm cancellous screws as the primary fixation hardware was developed. The most important screw is placed from the posterior malleolus into the head and neck of the talus, and medial and lateral malleolar screws are added to secure fixation (Fig 6–5). The arthrodesis may be performed through an anterior or lateral approach, as necessitated by the type of deformity and by the presence of a previous incision or retained hardware. Abstract 6–9 emphasizes that there is still a place for external fixation in ankle arthrodesis. The most important advantage of the technique in this study is that it can be extremely versatile and capable of accommodating an ankle that is grossly deformed. The external fixator should remain as a possible stabilizer for ankle arthrodesis.—K.A. Johnson, M.D.

Triple Arthrodesis in Adults
Bennett GL, Graham CE, Mauldin DM (Univ of Texas, Dallas; Orthopaedic Foot Surgery, Dallas; Southwest Orthopaedic Inst, Dallas)
Foot Ankle 12:138–143, 1991   6–10

Background.—In triple arthrodesis, the talocalcaneal, talonavicular, and calcaneocuboid joints are fused. The procedure can be used to treat painful disorders and deformities of the hindfoot.

Methods.—Records of 22 adults who underwent a triple arthrodesis for hindfoot pain or deformity, or both, were reviewed retrospectively. Minimum follow-up was 3 years. The same surgeon performed all of the procedures using a 2-incision technique and internal fixation.

Results.—Objective results were good in 36% of patients, fair in 59%, and poor in 5%. Two asymptomatic nonunions of the talonavicular joint occurred. There were no infections or neuromas. Eleven patients had radiographic evidence of tibiotalar arthritis. Eleven had midfoot arthritic changes that had progressed after surgery. Patient satisfaction was high; 95% felt that they were improved overall and would have the operation again if needed.

Conclusions.—Triple arthrodesis is a technically demanding procedure. However, patient satisfaction appears to be high, and, with proper surgical technique, complications can be kept to a minimum.

▶ This study evaluates the results of triple arthrodesis in adult patients. Progression of degenerative arthritis occurred in 50% of the patients at the ankle and midfoot joints. The arthritis was quite minimal in most of the cases and was either asymptomatic or minimally symptomatic. It would be interesting to see whether deterioration of the ankle and midfoot joints continues to progress with time. In the future, it would also be necessary to compare the results of triple arthrodesis with the results of single-joint arthrodesis procedures in the hindfoot. Whether or not limited arthrodesis procedures can obtain good results and "protect" the ankle and midfoot joints from increased stress remains to be determined.—K.A. Johnson, M.D.

Trauma and Its Sequelae: Soft Tissue Injuries

Long-Term Results of the Evans Procedure for Lateral Instability of the Ankle
Korkala O, Tanskanen P, Mäkijärvi J, Sorvali T, Ylikoski M, Haapala J (Lahti City Hospital, Finland)
J Bone Joint Surg 73-B:96–99, 1991   6–11

Background.—Severe ankle sprains left untreated or treated inadequately are commonly complicated by persistent lateral instability. The long-term results of the Evans procedure for treatment of lateral instability of the ankle in 40 patients were evaluated.

Methods.—Forty-two ankles were treated consecutively with a modified Evans procedure. A static tenodesis was fashioned using the peroneus

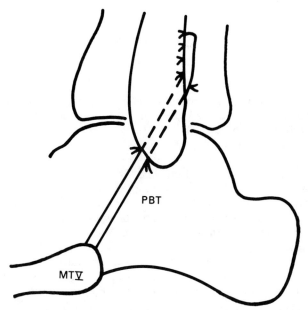

Fig 6–6.—The modified Evans operation. *Abbreviations: PBT*, peroneus brevis tendon; *MTV*, fifth metatarsal. (Courtesy of Korkala O, Tanskanen P, Mäkijärvi J, et al: *J Bone Joint Surg* 73-B:96–99, 1991.)

brevis tendon (Fig 6–6). Follow-up was 9–12 years; 40 ankles were available for review.

Results.—Results in 33 ankles (82.5%) were excellent or good. Results were fair in 3 ankles and poor in 4. These clinical findings were matched by the radiographic findings, which showed significant talar tilt or anterior talar translation in only 3 ankles. Functional results were not correlated with the stress-radiographic analysis.

Conclusion.—The modified Evans procedure appears to be simple and safe. It can be done through 2 small incisions. There is no damage to the talus. The tendon is not vulnerable to rupture at the sharp edges of the bony tunnel because it is not acutely angulated.

▶ Excellent and good results were achieved in 33 ankles (82.5%) treated by a modified Evans procedure with a follow-up period between 9 and 12 years. These results contrast with the disappointing long-term results of Karlsson et al. (1988) who used a method of Evans reconstruction that had dynamic characteristics, with the possibility of the tendon sliding inside the bone tunnel (1). The modification of the Evans operation used in this study by Korlaka et al. is a static reconstruction and, thus, a real tenodesis. Because the tendon is not acutely angulated, it is not vulnerable to rupture at the sharp edges of the bony tunnel (Fig 6–6). Eventually, I suspect that these lateral weaving–tethering procedures will be supplanted by limited procedures that use local tissues such as the inferior peroneal retinaculum, as advocated by Gould (2).—K.A. Johnson, M.D.

References

1. Karlsson J, et al: *J Bone Joint Surg* 70-B:476, 1988.
2. Gould N, et al: *Foot Ankle* 1:84, 1980.

Arthroscopic Treatment of Anterolateral Impingement of the Ankle
Ferkel RD, Karzel RP, Del Pizzo W, Friedman MJ, Fischer SP (Southern California Orthopedic Inst, Van Nuys, Calif)
Am J Sports Med 19:440–446, 1991   6–12

Background.—The cause of chronic lateral ankle pain after inversion injury often is difficult to establish, especially when the ankle is stable. This condition has been called "anterolateral impingement of the ankle."

Clinical Features.—Thirty-one patients with this diagnosis who did not have fractures had an average age of 34 years. All had sustained a "sprain" injury, and 6 patients had multiple sprains before the most recent major event. Most often, after a sprain patients experienced persistent ankle pain on walking, weakness, and, often, a sensation of giving way. Localized tenderness was present at the anterolateral gutter of the ankle.

Management.—All patients received conservative treatment for a prolonged period. Arthroscopic surgery was done an average of 2 years after injury. A distractor was used only if necessary. Abnormalities were confined primarily to the lateral side and included synovitis and scar tissue. Hypertrophic soft tissue was débrided and, if necessary, chondroplasty of the talus was carried out.

Results.—Synovial hyperplasia and subsynovial capillary proliferation were constant findings; many patients also had hyaline cartilage degeneration and fibrosis. Follow-up an average of 33 months postoperatively revealed excellent results in 15 patients, good results in 11, and fair results in 4. One patient had a poor outcome.

Conclusion.—Arthroscopic surgery relieves pain and disability from anterolateral impingement of the ankle in a high proportion of patients who fail to respond to conservative treatment.

▶ Will the ankle arthroscopic diagnosis and treatment of the anterolateral impingement syndrome become an expression of faith akin to synovial plica of the knee? Controlled studies are necessary, but who is to do them? Probably not the heathens.—K.A. Johnson, M.D.

Early Mobilizing Treatment for Grade III Ankle Ligament Injuries
Konradsen L, Hølmer P, Søndergaard L (Hørsholm Hospital, Denmark; Hillerød County Hospital, Denmark)
Foot Ankle 12:69–73, 1991   6–13

Background.—Clinicians still debate the best treatment for ruptured lateral ankle ligaments. The results of a functional approach in patients in whom grade III lateral ligament and capsule injury had produced gross mechanical instability were assessed.

Methods.—The 80 patients were treated with total immobilization in a walking plaster cast or early mobilization using a stabilizing orthosis. Entry criteria were a talar tilt of more than 9 degrees and an anterior translation of more than 10 mm at stress radiography, a previously stable ankle, and normal stress radiographic values in the other ankle. Ninety-one percent of the patients were assessed at 7 weeks, 3 months, and 1 year after injury.

Results.—Patients treated with a functional approach reached normal mobility and returned to work and sports sooner than immobilized patients. There were no differences between treatment groups in ankle stability or symptoms during activity after 1 year. In both groups, 95% of the ankles were mechanically stable after treatment. Residual symptoms were noted at 1 year in 13% of the functionally treated ankles and in 9% of the cast-mobilized ankles.

Conclusions.—Early mobilization using an orthosis that reduces inversion movement of the foot–ankle complex results in satisfactory mechanical stability and a functional end result in patients with severe grade III ligament lesions. Patients treated functionally are able to return early to work and sports.

▶ The best method for treating ruptured lateral ankle ligaments is still a matter of debate. This study nicely shows that for a lateral ankle ligament injury causing gross mechanical instability, early mobilization results in a better early functional result. However, at 1 year after injury, there was no statistically significant difference in outcome as compared to ankles treated by cast immobilization. Injuries of the lateral ligaments of the ankle are very common. Nonoperative measures remain the mainstay of treatment and produce satisfactory results in most patients.—K.A. Johnson, M.D.

Magnetic Resonance Imaging of the Foot and Ankle: Correlation of Normal Anatomy With Pathologic Conditions
Ferkel RD, Flannigan BD, Elkins BS (Southern California Orthopedic Inst, Van Nuys, Calif; Valley Presbyterian Hosp, Van Nuys Calif; Univ of California, San Francisco)
Foot Ankle 11:289–305, 1991   6–14

Background.—Magnetic resonance imaging offers a possible alternative to conventional radiography in diagnosing abnormalities of the foot and ankle.

Methods.—One hundred ten normal feet and ankles were to define the normal MR anatomy, and 150 scans were obtained to characterize various abnormalities. Slices 3-mm thick were acquired with a 1-mm interslice gap.

The Ankle.—Medially, a retracted tendon can be identified in patients with rupture. Tenosynovitis is recognized as fluid within a tendon or sheath. A range of Achilles tendon abnormalities is seen on MRI. Insertional tendinitis presents as focal high-signal intensity at the site of insertion of the distal Achilles tendon into the calcaneous. Laterally, ligament disruption can be recognized. Accumulation of fibrous debris and a meniscoid type lesion in the anterolateral gutter, producing anterolateral impingement syndrome, can also be recognized. Centrally, the commonest pathologic conditions include osteochondral lesions of the talus, loose bodies, and avascular necrosis of the talus.

The Foot.—Magnetic resonance imaging of the foot can demonstrate angiosarcoma, ganglion cysts, plantar fibromatosis, and osteomyelitis.

Discussion.—Oblique-angle imaging often allows a structure to be seen entirely on a single slice rather than having to piece slices together. It is necessary in examining this region to use thin slices with small gaps. Currently, head and knee coils provide good spatial resolution, but dedicated foot and ankle coils are expected to provide even better images.

▶ Clinical detection of foot and ankle abnormalities can be difficult because of swelling and pain. This study defines both normal and pathologic anatomy of the foot and ankle. Magnetic resonance imaging can assist in the evaluation of acute ruptures of the posterior tibialis tendon, and ligamentous injuries of the foot and ankle also can be diagnosed with greater accuracy. The future of MRI is exciting, as we have only touched the surface of this technology.—K.A. Johnson, M.D.

Longitudinal Attrition of the Peroneus Brevis Tendon in the Fibular Groove: An Anatomic Study
Sobel M, Bohne WHO, Levy ME (Hosp for Special Surgery, New York; Case Western Reserve Univ, Cleveland)
Foot Ankle 11:124–128, 1990   6–15

Background.—Little research has been done on the attrition of the peroneus brevis tendon since Meyers' report in 1924. A series of dissections was done to establish the incidence of attrition of the peroneus brevis tendon at the fibular groove and to document the anatomical relationship of the tendon attrition to the bony anatomy of the distal fibula.

Methods.—Dissections were done on 124 fresh human ankles obtained from 65 cadavers using loupe magnification. When peroneus brevis attrition was discovered, the extent of attrition was measured, and the anatomical proximity of the tendon to the distal fibular groove was noted.

Findings.—Peroneus brevis tendon attrition was found in 11.3% of the specimens. The attrition was limited to the peroneus brevis tendon. The peroneus longus was not involved in any specimen. The degree of attrition ranged from a simple splaying out of the peroneus brevis in the fibular groove to longitudinal splits in the peroneus brevis tendon with significant fraying of the remaining halves of the tendon. Longitudinal ruptures of the peroneus brevis tendon ranged from 1 cm to 4 cm (average, 1.9 cm). The central part of the longitudinal split was centered over the distal tip of the fibula in the fibular groove in all cases. There were no cases of complete rupture. Ankles with attrition had gross evidence of chronic inflammation and synovitis.

Conclusions.—The incidence of peroneus brevis tendon in the fibular groove has not previously been documented. Chronic ankle pain disability may be related to attrition of the peroneus brevis tendon in the fibular groove.

▶ The significance of this article is that attrition of the peroneus brevis tendon should be considered in patients with chronic ankle pain, swelling, and instability, as well as in those patients with symptoms suggesting stenosis in the lateral compartment of the ankle. There has been little research concerning the attrition of the peroneus brevis tendon since Meyers' observation in 1924 (1).—K.A. Johnson, M.D.

Reference

1. Meyers AW: *Am J Anat* 34:241, 1924.

Problems of the Forefoot

The Akin Procedure: An Analysis of Results
Frey C, Jahss M, Kummer FJ (Univ of Southern California, Los Angeles; Hosp for Joint Diseases, New York)
Foot Ankle 12:1–6, 1991   6–16

Background.—In 1925 Akin described an operation for hallux valgus entailing resection of the medial prominence of the first metatarsal head and a medial wedge osteotomy of the proximal phalanx of the great toe. If necessary, bone is removed from the medial aspect of the base of the proximal phalanx, and a lateral capsular release is done.

Methods.—Forty-five Akin procedures were done in 1966–1985, 36 of which were for a great toe valgus deformity producing symptoms in the second toe. Nine other feet had residual hallux valgus after operative treatment. Follow-up for the 38 patients averaged 54 months. The mean patient age was 46 years. Most of the feet had additional surgery at the same session—most often correction of hammer toe deformity.

Results.—Almost 90% of the patients had excellent or good results. The most common technical problem—in one fifth of the patients—was plantar angulation at the osteotomy site. Deficient bony apposition may have produced 1 nonunion and 1 recurrence. Shortening of the hallux was invariable as a result of the osteotomy. In only 2 patients, motion was severely restricted. Most excellent results occurred when the intermetatarsal angle remained normal or increased only slightly.

Conclusions.—In most patients, the Akin procedure must be combined with other surgery to correct all aspects of hallux valgus deformity. The operation should be avoided if there is an abnormal intermetatarsal angle or if degenerative changes are seen in the metatarsophalangeal joint. Shortening of the hallux can be minimized by limiting the amount of bone removed from the proximal phalanx.

▶ In 1925 Akin described a procedure for correction of hallux valgus that involved resection of the medial prominence of the first metatarsal head and medial wedge osteotomy of the proximal phalanx of the great toe (1). In this study, the authors report excellent and good cosmetic and functional results in 89% of the feet. This contrasts with Goldberg's study, in which only 53% of the patients were satisfied with the procedure (2). The Akin procedure should be performed within certain guidelines. Rarely is an Akin procedure alone indicated for correction of hallux valgus deformity. In most patients the proximal phalangeal osteotomy needs to be performed in combination with some other procedure to correct other components of the hallux valgus deformity. One should avoid using the Akin procedure when the hallux deformity is associated with an uncorrected intermetatarsal 1–2 angle and when degenerative changes or instability are present at the first metatarsophalangeal joint. If instability is present, return of the hallux valgus with subluxation of the proximal phalanx base laterally may occur.—K.A. Johnson, M.D.

References

1. Akin OF: *Med Sentinel* 33:678, 1925.
2. Goldberg I, et al: *J Bone Joint Surg* 69-A:64, 1987.

The Keller Resection Arthroplasty: A 13-Year Experience
Vallier GT, Petersen SA, LaGrone MO (Letterman Army Med Ctr, San Francisco; Seattle)
Foot Ankle 11:187–194, 1991   6–17

Background.—The common condition of painful hallux valgus is caused by both intrinsic and extrinsic factors, leading to the development of many therapeutic surgical procedures. Keller arthroplasty has been one of the most common methods used to correct the hallux valgus, with a 96% patient satisfaction rate. However, complications with Keller resection have been identified so that it has fallen out of use. The long-term effectiveness of Keller arthroplasty was investigated by retrospective review of records and by surveying patients undergoing this procedure.

Methods.—Between 1976 and 1988, 59 patients had 70 Keller resection arthroplasties at 1 center. Forty-six of these 59 were contacted, including 40 who completed a questionnaire. Follow-up information was available for 44 patients (54 feet) with a mean age of 62 years. Seventy-five percent of these patients were female, and 23% of patients had bilateral operations. The surgical procedure used a standard dorsal approach in all patients. The general indication for the Keller operation was painful hallux valgus related to degeneration in the first metatarsophalangeal joint. The Bonney and MacNab 12-point grading system was used to analyze results.

Findings.—After resection, 72% of the patients had good or excellent results. The average anatomical grade before surgery was 2.18, whereas the average postsurgical score was 3.38, for a 55% improvement rating. The average metatarsophalangeal angle and the average preoperative intermetatarsal angle improved significantly after surgery. A significant correlation between patient dissatisfaction and excessive proximal phalanx resection was found. Before surgery, 96% of patients had foot pain; only 15% had this symptom after surgery. Lateral metatarsalgia and use of nonsteroidal anti-inflammatory medication decreased after surgery. A K-wire was inserted for postsurgical fixation in 34 feet that had a follow-up arc of motion of the great toe of 50.8 degrees. In the 14 feet treated without a K-wire, the average final arc of motion was 48.2 degrees. The difference in satisfaction rate between these 2 groups (K-wire and non–K-wire) was statistically significant. No major wound complications occurred in these patients, although 7 of the feet required further surgery. The 4 patients with rheumatoid arthritis also required other surgical procedures.

Conclusions.—Keller resection arthroplasty provides predictable patient satisfaction when used for certain indications, (e.g., hallux valgus accompanied by degenerative changes of the first metatarsophalangeal joint). Successful results appear to depend on the preservation of the proximal phalanx length and of the great toe plantarflexion.

▶ A resection arthroplasty for hallux valgus (Keller) has received short shift by orthopedic surgeons in the recent past. With proper indication, however, such a procedure may be useful. Silicone, either in breasts or great toes, has not been that rewarding. Maybe we should be satisfied with the less than perfect.—K.A. Johnson, M.D.

Distal Chevron Metatarsal Osteotomy for Bunionette
Kitaoka HB, Holiday AD Jr, Campbell DC II (Mayo Clinic and Found, Rochester, Minn)
Foot Ankle 12:80–85, 1991   6–18

Background.—Bunionette, or tailor's bunion, was first described in 1949. Since then, an assortment of operations have been found to decrease the lateral prominence. Chevron osteotomy of the first metatarsal has been successful in the treatment of hallux valgus.

Methods.—Thirteen patients with painful bunionette underwent 19 distal chevron metatarsal osteotomy procedures. The patients were 12 females and 1 male aged 20–67 years. Mean follow-up was 7.1 years.

Results.—Of a possible total of 75 points, the mean forefoot score improved from 35.8 to 73.9 points. Intermetatarsal 4–5 angle and metatarsophalangeal 5 angle improved significantly, as did forefoot width. Overall, results were judged to be good in 17 feet and fair in 2. None were considered treatment failures. Complications included transfer metatarsalgia in 1 foot and wound infection in 1 foot (Fig 6–7).

Conclusions.—The distal chevron fifth metatarsal osteotomy is an effective procedure for the treatment of symptomatic bunionette that is refractory to nonsurgical treatment. This procedure is associated with a

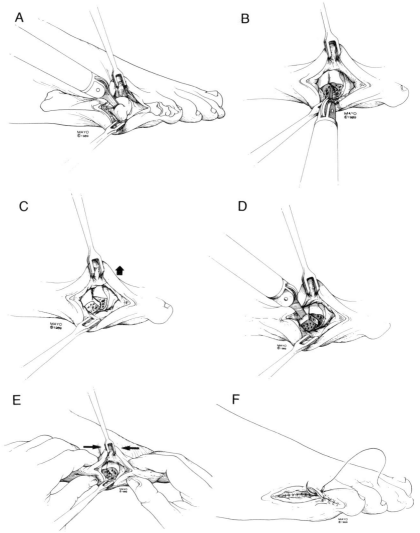

Fig 6–7.—Chevron osteotomy operation. **A**, through dorsolateral approach, lateral condylar process is resected. **B**, Chevron-shaped osteotomy made with microsagittal saw at 60-degree angle. **C**, displacement of distal fragment 3–4 mm. *Arrow* indicates displacement in medial direction. Care was taken to avoid any dorsal displacement. **D**, removal of remaining head and neck fragment. **E**, *arrows* denote impaction of osteotomy by longitudinal compression. Stability is then tested by metatarsophalangeal joint motion. **F**, closure of capsule and skin. (Courtesy of Kitaoka HB, Holiday AD Jr, Campbell DC II: *Foot Ankle* 12:80–85, 1991.)

high success rate based on clinical factors, improved alignment, a low complication rate, and high patient satisfaction.

Treatment of Bunionette Deformity With Longitudinal Diaphyseal Osteotomy With Distal Soft Tissue Repair
Coughlin MJ (St Alphonsus Regional Med Ctr, Boise, Idaho)
Foot Ankle 11:195–203, 1991   6–19

Introduction.—Twenty-one consecutive patients had symptomatic bunionette deformity corrected in 31 feet by longitudinal diaphyseal osteotomy, lateral condylectomy, and distal metatarsophalangeal realignment. All patients were resistant to conservative measures. The average postoperative follow-up was 31 months.

Technique.—The fifth metatarsophalangeal joint capsule is incised in an L-shaped manner (Fig 6–8, *A*), after which the fibular condyle of the metatarsal head is removed. The metatarsophalangeal joint then is distracted and the medial capsule of the fifth metatarsophalangeal joint is released so that the joint can be realigned later (Fig 6–8, *B*). An oblique diaphyseal osteotomy then is made (Fig 6–8, *C*). Rotation rather than translation of the osteotomy will maximize bony contact (Fig 6–8, *D*). The osteotomy site is fixed with a screw, a screw and K-wire, or multiple K-wires.

Results.—Good or excellent subjective results were achieved in 93% of the operated feet. The average degree of metatarsal shortening was .5 mm. No infections or incisional neuromas developed, but 2 of the wounds healed slowly.

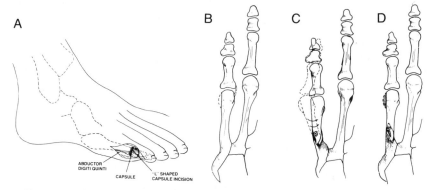

Fig 6–8.—**A,** the lateral fifth metatarsal capsule is released with an inverted L-shaped capsular incision releasing the dorsal and proximal capsule. **B,** the medial capsule is released and the lateral condyle is resected. **C,** an oblique diaphyseal osteotomy is created. The saw cut is directed from a lateral to medial direction, with the obliquity oriented from a dorsal-proximal to a plantar-distal direction. **D,** the osteotomy is rotated in the diaphyseal region until the distal fragment is parallel with the fourth metatarsal. (Courtesy of Coughlin MJ: *Foot Ankle* 11:195–203, 1991.)

Conclusion.—The longitudinal diaphyseal osteotomy, if carefully planned, is an effective means of correcting bunionette deformity.

▶ Abstracts 6–18 and 6–19 report on 2 separate surgical procedures for correction of a bunionette deformity. Abstract 6–18, describes the distal Chevron osteotomy of the fifth metatarsal for effective treatment of a symptomatic bunionette (Fig 6–7). In Abstract 6–19, painful bunionette deformity was treated with longitudinal diaphyseal osteotomy, lateral condylectomy, and distal metatarsophalangeal realignment (Fig 6–8). For those less severe deformities, a distal fifth metatarsal osteotomy requires less surgical dissection and may be appropriate. In the presence of a prominent callus associated with a metatarsal diaphyseal prominence or an increased intermetatarsal 4–5 angle, a diaphyseal osteotomy, lateral condylectomy, and distal soft tissue realignment affords a more extensive realignment.—K.A. Johnson, M.D.

First Metatarsophalangeal Joint Reaction Forces During High-Heel Gait
McBride ID, Wyss UP, Cooke TDV, Murphy L, Phillips J, Olney SJ (Kingston Gen Hosp, Canada)
Foot Ankle 11:282–288, 1991   6–20

Background.—Few reports have described the forces at the first metatarsophalangeal joint. The effect of heel height on the joint reaction forces at the first metatarsophalangeal joint and the metatarsal-sesamoid joint at toe-off during gait was examined.

Methods.—First metatarsophalangeal joint reaction forces were determined for 11 normal women during toe-off while walking barefoot and in high-heeled shoes. Kinematic, kinetic, footprint, and radiographic data were used in a biomechanical model to calculate these forces.

Results.—Compared with barefoot walking, the metatarsophalangeal joint reaction forces, metatarsal-sesamoid forces, and the resultant of these forces were twice as large in high heels. The average peak forces for barefoot and high-heeled walking were .8 and 1.58 times body weight for metatarsophalangeal joint reaction forces, .44 and 1.03 times body weight for metatarsal-sesamoid forces, and .93 and 1.88 times body weight for the resultant of these forces. Kinematics also changes during high-heeled walking, making angles of application of forces and sesamoidal articulation less favorable.

Conclusions.—This biomechanical study provides evidence of the detrimental effects of wearing high-heeled shoes. Both kinematic and kinetic changes occur at the first metatarsophalangeal joint and metatarsal-sesamoid joint during high-heeled gait.

▶ Heel height has a marked effect on foot pressures with walking. No wonder approximately 90% of patients with forefoot pain at a foot clinic are women. It is important to study the results of various shoe designs to, perhaps, provide a shoe that is socially acceptable yet not detrimental to the foot.—K.A. Johnson, M.D.

A Chevron-Akin Double Osteotomy for Correction of Hallux Valgus
Mitchell LA, Baxter DE (Southern Sports Medicine Orthopaedic Ctr, Nashville, Tenn; Univ of Texas, Houston)
Foot Ankle 12:7–14, 1991   6–21

Introduction.—The Chevron osteotomy of the first metatarsal was combined with an Akin osteotomy of the proximal phalanx to correct mild to moderate hallux valgus deformity in 16 patients (average age, 43 years). Eight of the patients had bilateral operations.

Technique.—The Chevron osteotomy is done using a single .045-in. smooth pin. The metatarsal head is displaced laterally for about 3 mm. No adductor tentotomy is done. The base of the proximal phalanx then is exposed subperiosteally, and a tibial closing wedge osteotomy is performed, removing a 1-mm wedge of bone. No attempt is made to remove the contiguous lip of the proximal phalanx. The pin is removed after 2 weeks.

Results.—Pain was relieved or improved in 95% of the operated feet. The mean follow-up was 29 months. More than half of the feet had a totally satisfactory appearance. All but 2 feet were back in regular shoewear within 3 months of surgery. All patients had solid union of both osteotomy sites. Metatarsophalangeal subluxation did not change significantly. Degenerative joint changes were found in 2 feet, but there was no radiographic evidence of avascular necrosis.
Conclusions.—The Chevron-Akin osteotomy has given satisfactory results in many patients having mild to moderate hallux valgus deformity. Advanced sesamoid subluxation with a wide intermetatarsal angle contraindicates this procedure.

▶ Combining 2 operative treatments for hallux valgus increases the possibility of complications such as joint stiffness. In this report, the compounding of complications did not seem to be a problem. It should be noted that the Akin procedure in this article involved a very small (a few millimeters) medially based phalangeal wedge osteotomy. It may be that the Chevron osteotomy alone would have given comparable results.—K.A. Johnson, M.D.

Miscellaneous Topics

Long-Term Followup of Physeal Injury to the Ankle
Caterini R, Farsetti P, Ippolito E (Univ of Reggio Calabria, Italy)
Foot Ankle 11:372–383, 1991   6–22

Background.—Although many reports on physeal injuries to the ankle have appeared in the literature, there have been no long-term follow-up reports. A long-term follow-up analysis was done to assess the possible late sequelae of the primitive injury.
Patients.—Sixty-eight patients with a distal physeal injury to the tibia or fistula, or both, were followed for an average of 27 years 4 months

from initial injury. Mean age at injury was 12 years 6 months. Average age at follow-up was 40 years. Salter-Harris injury type I was seen in 17 patients, type II in 27 patients, type III in 10, and type IV in 14. All but 6 patients were managed conservatively.

Results.—Forty-seven patients were judged to have a good result; 13, fair; and 8, poor. The 3 main factors determining the end result were type of Salter-Harris lesion, amount of initial displacement, and quality of reduction, Radiographic evidence of osteoarthritis was noted in 11.8% of patients, all of whom had a type III or type IV lesion, except for 1 who had a type II lesion.

Conclusions.—These findings suggest that the traumatic mechanism affects prognosis only in relationship to the type of lesion, based on the Salter-Harris classification. The risk of complications is much higher in Salter-Harris type III and type IV lesions. The severity of initial displacement also strongly influenced prognosis.

▶ Again, the quality of reduction is important in the long-term result of a physeal injury. When the fracture line traverses the physis, beware. These findings are in accordance with Cass and Peterson (1).— K.A. Johnson, M.D.

Reference

1. Cass JR, Peterson HA: *J Bone Joint Surg* 65-A:1059, 1983.

Valgus Deformities of the Feet and Characteristics of Gait in Patients Who Have Rheumatoid Arthritis
Keenan MAE, Peabody TD, Gronley JK, Perry J (Kaiser Found Hosp, Bellflower, Calif; Rancho Los Amigos Med Ctr, Downey, Calif)
J Bone Joint Surg 73-A:237–247, 1991   6–23

Background.—Many patients with rheumatoid arthritis will have the disabling problem of valgus deformity of the hindfoot. There is little information on the pathogenesis or implications for foot function of this defect. Patients who had rheumatoid arthritis with and without valgus deformity of the hindfoot were examined to determine the deformity's cause and effect on gait.

Patients.—The prospective trial included 17 patients with seropositive adult-onset rheumatoid arthritis. Group 1 consisted of 7 patients with normal alignment of the feet (mean age, 63 years; mean duration of disease, 14 years). Group 2 consisted of 10 patients with valgus deformity of the hindfoot, confirmed by lateral and dorsoplantar radiographs (mean age, 60 years; mean duration of disease, 25 years). Patients were evaluated by clinical and radiographic examination and laboratory gait analysis.

Results.—Both groups had significant pain in the feet, but group 2 had more pain. Group 2 patients had no muscular imbalance, equinus contracture, valgus deformity of the tibiotalar joint, or isolated tibialis posterior deficiency that could have led to valgus deformity. Quantitated electromyography showed that they had significantly increased intensity and duration of tibialis posterior activity. This seemed to reflect an effort to support the collapsing longitudinal arch. Both groups had decreased gait velocity, stride length, and single-limb support time and delayed heel rise, but the decreases were more pronounced in group 2.

Conclusions.—Patients with rheumatoid arthritis may have valgus deformity of the hindfoot as a result of exaggerated pronation forces on the subtalar joint that is in a weakened and inflamed condition. Symmetric muscle weakness and the patient's efforts to reduce pain lead to changes in gait, which result in the forces described. There may be an association between valgus deformity of the feet and knees in these patients.

▶ The cause for hindfoot valgus in patients with rheumatoid arthritis is apparently exaggerated pronation forces on an inflamed subtalar joint. These forces are the result of gait alterations brought about by symmetrical muscular weakness and the patient's spontaneous efforts to minimize foot pain. So it is not a rupture of the tibialis posterior tendon that causes the deformity in most instances. This study raises the possibility that preventive measures such as bracing or early talonavicular arthrodesis might prevent the late deformity.—K.A. Johnson, M.D.

Effect of Isolated Talocalcaneal Fusion on Contact in the Ankle and Talonavicular Joints
Beaudoin AJ, Fiore SM, Krause WR, Adelaar RS (Med College of Virginia, Richmond)
Foot Ankle 12:19–25, 1991   6–24

Background.—Isolated fusion of the talocalcaneal joint is a standard treatment for foot pain and deformity. However, there is disagreement about whether fusion of the talocalcaneal joint alone leads to secondary degenerative changes in other foot joints, particularly the midtarsal joint. An investigation was done to characterize articular contact and force distribution in the normal ankle, talocalcaneal posterior facet, and talonavicular joints with the foot in neutral, dorsiflexed, and plantarflexed positions. The influence of talocalcaneal fusion on articular contact in the ankle and talonavicular joints also was examined.

Methods.—A cadaveric model was used to establish the articular contact area and load distribution in the ankle joint, posterior facet of the talocalcaneal joint, and talonavicular joint. Pressure-sensitive film was used. Dorsiflexion, neutral, and plantarflexion positions were assessed.

Results.—Articular contact changes were most marked in the talonavicular joint. In this joint a significant reduction in contact area after fusion was noted when the foot was in the plantarflexed position. In most specimens, reductions in ankle joint articular contact area were seen in the dorsiflexed and plantarflexed positions. Lateral displacement of the region of articular contact was observed in some specimens.

Conclusions.—The most striking finding in this cadaveric model was the significant reduction and lateral isolation of articular contact area in the talonavicular joint after isolated talocalcaneal fusion. Talonavicular joint contact area reduction was found in the plantarflexed position in all cases.

▶ The reduction and displacement of talonavicular contact area, as well as altered ankle joint force transmission after talocalcaneal arthrodesis, brings into question the advisability of such a procedure. Of course, if a triple arthrodesis is done the joint changes will undoubtedly be present in fewer joints of the foot. Clinically, progressive hindfoot degeneration after an isolated talocalcaneal arthrodesis has not been a problem.—K.A. Johnson, M.D.

The Assessment of Dynamic Foot-to-Ground Contact Forces and Plantar Pressure Distribution: A Review of the Evolution of Current Techniques and Clinical Applications
Alexander IJ, Chao EYS, Johnson KA (Crystal Clinic, Akron, Ohio; Mayo Clinic and Found, Rochester, Minn; Mayo Clinic, Scottsdale, Ariz)
Foot Ankle 11:152–167, 1990   6–25

Background.—Physical examination and radiographic analysis are the mainstays of evaluating the results of therapeutic interventions of the foot. Some objective methods of evaluating foot function before and after intervention have long been sought, but only now is it possible to achieve accurate, high-resolution foot pressure distributions with high sampling rates and easily interpreted graphic displays. The development and principles of these devices and their clinical applications were reviewed.

Assessment Techniques.—There have been several reports on the instrumented shoe technique of dynamic plantar assessment, using various transducers and load cells mounted in or on the soles of shoes. Padlike multifield pressure-sensitive transducers and in-shoe transducers applied to the sole of the foot also have been described. Floor-mounted devices have been in use for many years. Force plate analysis techniques now are used for dynamic analysis of foot-to-ground contact forces. Floor-mounted transducer matrices are used to measure forces under specified areas of the foot, and portable capacitance mats also have been described and marketed. Other techniques include the critical light reflection technique, polyurethane photoelastic plastic sheets, and shear-sensitive liquid crystals.

Clinical Applications.—The techniques described have been used in studies of normal walking, the effects of shoe wear and immobilization devices, running, neuropathic and diabetic foot problems, the rheumatoid foot, and situations (e.g., hallux valgus, first metatarsophalangeal silastic arthroplasty, heel pain, and talonavicular and triple arthrodesis). Sometimes the selection of technique depends on the problem to be examined. Floor-mounted transducer matrices and foil-covered translucent force platforms can help in planning pedorthic and surgical intervention, but they do not address the effectiveness of orthotics and shoe wear. Floor-mounted and in-shoe devices both have a place in research. Clinically, the Harris mat is useful and economical, but eventually the critical light reflection foil technique without transducers or the photoelastic sheet method will become reasonably affordable.

Conclusion.—Some devices can provide objective documentation for prospective studies of a variety of foot problems, which should ultimately improve patient care.

▶ Multiple devices have been used to assess foot-to-ground contact forces and plantar pressure distribution. This article outlines the development and explains the principles of operation of these devices. Clinical applications of these instruments are reviewed. Evidence from these prospective studies supporting or refuting the efficacy of currently used therapeutic techniques should improve the overall care of patients with foot and ankle problems. The quantitative accuracy in resolution of these tools will likely improve as research in the area keeps pace with advancing technology.—K.A. Johnson, M.D.

7 Musculoskeletal Neoplasia

Introduction

Although it seems that progress in the management of musculoskeletal tumors is slow, progress is being made. The number of patients with osteosarcoma or Ewing's sarcoma that have been cured during the past decade that would have died if they had presented in the preceding decade is remarkable. The number of amputations that would have been done in the 1970s that was not done in the 1980s for the patients with osteosarcoma is astounding. But more needs to be done.

The first 5 articles in this chapter concern the treatment of Ewing's sarcoma. Before 1970 almost every patient with a Ewing's sarcoma died of their disease. Then, during the 1970s, adjuvant chemotherapy was found to be of great benefit, and more than half of all patients with Ewing's sarcoma can now expect to be cured. Irradiation has been the treatment of choice for the primary Ewing's sarcoma, but it has been used mainly because the prognosis was so bad that surgery was felt to be unjustified. Now that the prognosis is improving, we need to decide if surgery should be done. There is an increasing amount of data that suggests that surgery is the treatment of choice for Ewing's sarcoma, but the answer is still not definite.

Limb salvage is here to stay, and we now know that it is oncologically safe for patients with malignant bone tumors. The methods of reconstruction have improved during the past decade, and options are greater. We still need to develop a reliable permanent reconstructive solution. A review of retrieved allografts and a long-term review of endoprosthetic reconstruction reported this past year help us to understand the current state of the art and show the problems we still face in providing a useful extremity for patients who must have a major bone resection.

One of the major deficits, if not the major deficit, in musculoskeletal oncology is our limited ability to predict the natural history of an individual patient's tumor. Many patients are receiving adjuvant chemotherapy who do not need it, and many are receiving chemotherapy that is not optimal. Numerous laboratories are working on finding better tools for predicting a tumor's behavior. So far, not much has been useful, but progress is being made. We are learning that the histologic tissue type is only 1 of several variables that are predictive. There are better ones somewhere, and they should be found soon.

Musculoskeletal pathology and musculoskeletal oncology are young disciplines and have a ways to go before they catch up with the other specialties, but ground is gained each year. In the future we should see novel approaches to classifying musculoskeletal tumors and novel treatments. It is possible that the classification of musculoskeletal tumors based on their histologic appearance will prove not to be the best method, and we will classify them from their genetic makeup or behavior in culture. The future is exciting.

Dempsey S. Springfield, M.D.

Ewing's Sarcoma

Long-Term Follow-Up of Ewing's Sarcoma of Bone Treated With Combined Modality Therapy
Kinsella TJ, Miser JS, Waller B, Venzon D, Glatstein E, Weaver-McClure L, Horowitz ME (Natl Cancer Inst; Univ of Wisconsin, Madison)
Int J Radiat Oncol Biol Phys 20:389–395, 1991   7–1

Background.—Initial trials of combined modality treatment for Ewing's sarcoma of bone showed significant improvements in 2– to 3–year disease-free survival compared with radiation treatment or surgery alone. The long-term follow-up data on 107 patients treated for Ewing's sarcoma in 3 sequential combined modality trials during a 12-year period were reviewed.

Methods.—Patients received 4 cycles of either a 2-drug regimen (cyclophosphamide and vincristine or a 3-drug regimen (cyclophosphamide, vincristine, and either actinomycin D or doxorubicin). They also received 50 Gy of local irradiation to the involved bone. Initially 80 patients had localized and 27 had metastatic disease; 11 had more than 1 site of metastasis.

Results.—With a median potential follow-up period of longer than 15 years 28 patients (27%) remained alive. Disease-free and overall survival decreased most rapidly in the first 5 years of follow-up, with a 5-year disease-free survival rate of 29% and a 5-year overall survival rate of 39%. Only 2 patients with metastases survived longer than 5 years. The disease-free survival rate was 52% at 2 years, 37% at 5 years, 35% at 10 years, and 33% at 15 years for patients with localized disease (table). The overall survival rate was 68% at 2 years, 51% at 5 years, 39% at 10 years, and 34% at 15 years. The first site of failure was local relapse in

Long-Term Follow-up Data for Patients With Localized Disease (N = 80)				
	2 yr	5 yr	10 yr	15 yr
Disease-free survial (%)	52	37	35	33
Overall survival (%)	68	41	39	34
Local control (%)	92	84	80	80

(Courtesy of Kinsella TJ, Miser JS, Waller B, et al: *Int J Radiat Oncol Biol Phys* 20:389–395, 1991.)

11 patients. The variable with the most significant effect on disease-free and overall survival was metastatic disease, followed by age older than 25 years, high lactate olehydrogenase level in localized disease, and central primary tumor in localized disease.

Conclusions.—Most patients with Ewing's sarcoma of bone receiving combined-modality treatment appear to relapse within 5 years, and relapse may occur as late as 15 years. Local failure is not uncommon but does not appear to affect overall survival.

▶ Multidrug adjuvant chemotherapy for Ewing's sarcoma began in 1968. Before that time patients with a Ewing's sarcoma usually were treated with local irradiation and observation. The success of this treatment was poor, with less than 15% of these patients surviving 5 years. This report by Kinsella and associates tells us about the outcome of those patients treated between 23 and 12 years ago. By today's standards the protocols used would be considered timid, but they do give us an indication of how much the chemotherapy has improved the prognosis of the patient with Ewing's sarcoma. Those patients with metastatic disease at the time of presentation continue to have a poor prognosis. On the other hand, the cure rate of those patients with localized disease is more than double the rate expected without adjuvant chemotherapy. This is evidence of a significant benefit of adjuvant chemotherapy. The long-term follow-up and flat survival curves after 5 years reveal that the increased early survival is not simply chemotherapy delaying relapse but a true increase in patients cured. The other piece of information reported is the 20% incidence of local failure when the patients were treated with irradiation and adjuvant chemotherapy. This is another report suggesting that irradiation and chemotherapy are not adequate to control the primary site of the Ewing's sarcoma. Current protocols are evaluating the role of irradiation of the primary Ewing's sarcoma, as there is retrospective evidence that surgical resection results not only in better local control but also in a higher rate of cure.—D.S. Springfield, M.D.

Ewing's Sarcoma: Local Tumor Control and Patterns of Failure Following Limited-Volume Radiation Therapy
Arai Y, Kun LE, Brooks MT, Fairclough DL, Fontanesi J, Meyer WH, Hayes FA, Thompson E, Rao BN (St Jude Children's Research Hosp, Memphis; Univ of Tennessee, Memphis)
Int J Radiat Oncol Biol Phys 21:1501–1508, 1991   7–2

Background.—In Ewing's sarcoma tumor parameters that affect treatment outcome seem to include primary tumor size, primary tumor site, and soft tissue tumor extension before chemotherapy. However, radiation dose and radiation volume do not seem to affect local tumor control significantly according to major clinical series. A prospective treatment protocol for localized osseous Ewing's sarcoma, included induction chemotherapy, a surgical option after initial tumor response, and radiation treatment with limited radiation volume and, in selected patients, reduced radiation dose. Sixty consecutive children were treated according to this protocol between 1978 and 1988.

Methods.—Induction chemotherapy began with cyclophosphamide doxorubicin hydrochloride (Adriamycin), after which irradiation or surgery, or both, were used. Then maintenance chemotherapy with cyclophosphamide, Adriamycin, dactinomycin, and vincristine was administered for 10 months. After induction chemotherapy, 43 patients received primary radiation treatment to limited radiation volumes, including 3-cm margins beyond the defined radiation tumor volume. Thirty-one patients with objective response to induction chemotherapy received 30–35 Gy; 12 patients with poor responses to induction chemotherapy or with tumors of at least 8 cm received 50–60 Gy. Fourteen patients who had total tumor resection received no irradiation. Patients undergoing surgical resection included 17 with negative or only microscopically positive margins.

Results.—The overall event-free survival at 5 years was 59%, and local tumor control was 68%. The initial relapse sites were local alone in 12 patients, distant alone in 6, and both local and distant in 7. Local tumor control was significantly better with tumors less than 8 cm in their greatest dimension. The presence of residual tumor had no effect on event-free survival or local tumor control. Among 17 patients undergoing surgical resection, the event-free survival rate was 75% at 5 years, significantly better than that of patients who received irradiation alone (53%). All patients who underwent surgical resection had maintained local tumor control compared to 58% of those who received radiation alone.

Conclusions.—Overall the event-free survival rate of 59% at 5 years was similar to previous series. A high proportion of local failures occurred. These findings suggest that tumor size is an important factor for both local tumor control and survival but leave unclear the impact of surgical resection. The relative roles of surgery and irradiation in Ewing's sarcoma are still controversial.

▶ The proper management of the primary site of a Ewing's sarcoma remains controversial. Irradiation has been the conventional treatment of the primary tumor, but this is based on the facts that the tumor clinically shrinks when treated and that, in the past, the survival was so poor that local control was not as important because almost all of the patients died of distant metastasis. The recent increase in survival has prompted a re-examination of the issue of treatment of the primary tumor. There have been numerous retrospective reports suggesting that surgical resection of the primary tumor results in an improved survival compared to irradiation. Arai and associates have reported on their experience with 60 patients with nonmetastatic Ewing's sarcoma treated with adjuvant chemotherapy and irradiation, irradiation and surgery, or surgery. The patient groups were not controlled, and the decision as to who was irradiated, who had irradiation and surgery, and who had surgery alone was made in a nonrandom manner. Despite the absence of a controlled study, we can learn some things. The 5-year disease-free rate was almost 60%—twice that reported in Kinsella's paper (Abstract 7–1)—suggesting continued improvement in systemic control. Irradiation alone was not an effective method of achieving local control of Ewing's sarcoma in this group. All of the patients who had a surgical resection had local control, and these patients had a better chance of surviving. The problem with deducing that patients with Ewing's should have a surgical resection of their primary tumor, although this may be correct, is that irradiation was used for the larger tumors and surgery for the smaller ones. Size is an important prognostic variable, and, before we decide that all Ewing's tumors should be surgically removed, we must show that surgery is better than irradiation in controlling the large tumors as well as the small tumors. Irradiation seems to be able to control the small tumors just as well as surgery. A controlled study needs to be done.—D.S. Springfield, M.D.

Radiation Therapy as Local Treatment in Ewing's Sarcoma: Results of the Cooperative Ewing's Sarcoma Studies CESS 81 and CESS 86
Dunst J, Sauer R, Burgers JMV, Hawliczek R, Kürten R, Winkelmann W, Salzer-Kuntschik M, Müschenich M, Jürgens H, Cooperative Ewing's Sarcoma Study Group (University of Erlangen, Germany; The Netherlands Cancer Inst, Amsterdam; University of Vienna; University of Düsseldorf, Germany; University of Münster, Germany)
Cancer 67:2818–2825, 1991   7–3

Background.—Ewing's sarcoma has become curable with the use of adequate systemic and local treatment in a substantial number of patients. Definitive local control of the primary tumor is a prerequisite of cure because local failure is associated with an extremely poor prognosis. Two treatment trials, the Cooperative Ewing's Sarcoma studies of 1981 and 1986 (CESS 81 and CESS 86), were conducted.

Methods.—From January 1981 to November 1989 a total of 590 patients were registered from 83 participating institutions, 230 of whom were eligible to be protocol patients. Ninety-three patients were enrolled in CESS 81, and 137 were enrolled in CESS 86. Local treatment consisted of radical surgery, resection plus postoperative irradiation, or definitive radiation treatment. The type of local treatment was selected individually for each patient, not randomized.

Results.—The overall relapse-free survival in CESS 81 was 55% after 3 years and 54% after 5 years. In CESS 81 the 5-year relapse-free survival was 43% after primary irradiation compared with 54% after surgery and 68% after surgery plus postoperative radiation treatment. However, the outcome in CESS 86 was different in that the prognosis for irradiated patients was as good as that for surgically treated patients. The 3-year relapse-free survival rate for CESS 86 was 67% after radiation treatment, 65% after surgery, and 62% after resection plus postoperative irradiation. Compared with CESS 81, the results after radiation treatment have improved, whereas the results after surgery have remained almost unchanged. The overall local failure rate was lowest after radical surgery in both trials (6% in CESS 81; 4% in CESS 86). The highest local failure rate occurred after radiation treatment in both trials, but the incidence of local relapse markedly decreased from 50% in CESS 81 to 13% in CESS 86. Surgically treated patients had higher local control rates for all tumor sites.

Conclusions.—The data from CESS 81 indicate that larger lesions, especially those in the pelvis, thorax, or femur, are at higher risk of local failure if irradiation is the sole local treatment. Optimal radiation treatment is not only a matter of available technical equipment; it also requires personal experience with the treatment of this disease, especially if radiation treatment is part of a combined modality regimen. Radiation treatment and surgery as sole local treatment in Ewing's sarcoma can yield good results, but careful selection of patients for each treatment modality is essential.

▶ The Europeans have been working together to study treatment protocols for a number of malignancies, including Ewing's sarcoma. The CESS data are important and should help us decide how best to treat patients with this sarcoma. As is the case with other studies, all the patients received adjuvant chemotherapy but had the primary sarcoma treated with irradiation, surgery, or a combination of the 2. The patients were not randomly assigned to these groups. A significant finding was that, with the later chemotherapy protocol, the benefit of a surgical resection that was seen with the earlier chemotherapy protocol was not observed. Surgical resection of the primary tumor was associated with better local control in both protocols, but local control with irradiation was almost equal to surgery in the later chemotherapy protocol. The improved local control in the later protocol probably reflects better selection of patients for irradiation alone compared to the earlier protocol. It seems clear that small lesions can be treated effectively with either irradiation or surgery but that larger tumors, especially those in the pelvis, probably should be resected, and if the margins are not free of tumor the patient should also receive irradiation.—D.S. Springfield, M.D.

Local Control and Function After Twice-A-Day Radiotherapy for Ewing's Sarcoma of Bone

Marcus RB Jr, Cantor A, Heare TC, Graham-Pole J, Mendenhall NP, Million RR (Univ of Florida, Gainesville)

Int J Radiat Oncol Biol Phys 21:1509–1515, 1991   7–4

Background.—Ewing's sarcoma of bone is commonly treated locally with radiation. Recently, the effectiveness of radiation treatment alone for local control of this disease has been questioned, as has the long-term functional result of such treatment. A twice-a-day radiation protocol was tested.

Methods.—Thirty-nine patients with Ewing's sarcoma who received twice-a-day radiation treatment included 4 patients who also received surgery. All patients received chemotherapy. Between 1982 and 1987 some received the standard risk regimen (SR-1); the HR-2 regimen was administered to patients at high-risk between 1982 and 1984, and a different HR-3 regimen was administered to patients at high-risk thereafter. All patients received 3,600 cGy (120 cGy twice a day to the volume of the original tumor at diagnosis), plus a 4-cm margin. Additional boost doses, ranging from 1,440 to 2,400 cGy depending on the result of induction chemotherapy, were administered at the residual lesion present at the start of radiation treatment plus a 2-cm margin. Boost doses were also administered at 120 cGy twice a day. Thirteen patients on the HR-3 regimen received an additional 800 cGy of total body radiation treatment. Patients were observed for local control, functional status, and survival.

Results.—The local control rates at 5 years were 88% for patients on the SR-1 protocol, 92% for those on the HR-2 protocol, and 80% for patients on the HR-3 protocol. Twice-a-day radiation treatment seemed to give superior local control for patients with large primary lesions (Fig 7–1). The radiation regimen was tolerated satisfactorily by all patients. Seventeen of 35 patients who received radiation treatment alone to the primary lesions are alive, and 12 were evaluated by formal functional analysis. Only 4 patients had fibrosis, mild or grade 2 at worse, and none of 4 patients with lower extremity lesions had measurable differences in extremity lengths. Range of motion deficits had the largest deficits of any observed parameter. Four patients had a 1 cm and 1 patient had a 1.5 cm difference in circumference between a treated and a nontreated extremity. Three of 4 patients with lower extremity primary tumors had a normal gait, and none had permanent edema. No pathologic fractures occurred in any of the 20 patients with extremity lesions.

Conclusions.—Twice-a-day radiation treatment resulted in good local

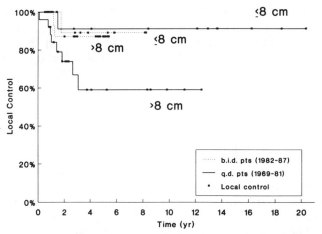

Fig 7–1.—Local control (product-limit method) for hyperfractionated radiation therapy versus conventional radiation therapy according to size of tumor. (Courtesy of Marcus RB Jr, Cantor A, Heare TC, et al: *Int J Radiat Oncol Biol Phys* 21:1509–1515, 1991.)

control and excellent functional results in these patients. The success of local control seemed to be related to that of systemic control.

▶ Irradiation for Ewing's sarcoma is still the standard treatment, and radiation oncologists have improved their treatment methods through the years. Treating a patient with an accelerated course is a method that may have advantages. The accelerated course of irradiation is supposed to be better than the standard course because the tumor has less time to recover between treatments and the concentrated dose schedule will theoretically kill more tumor cells. The 92% local control rate is the highest reported for irradiation alone, although in other studies surgery and surgery with irradiation usually achieves 100% local control. In some centers therapeutic doses of irradiation to the extremities of young patients has produced significant functional deficits. The twice-a-day irradiation protocol seems to be tolerated both acutely and in the long run better than the once-a-day regimen. These data suggest that, with intense chemotherapy and well planned and administered irradiation, it may be possible to treat patients with Ewing's sarcoma successfully without a surgical resection.— D.S. Springfield, M.D.

Multimodal Therapy for the Management of Localized Ewing's Sarcoma of Pelvic and Sacral Bones: A Report From the Second Intergroup Study
Evans RG, Nesbit ME, Gehan EA, Garnsey LA, Burgert O Jr, Vietti TJ, Cangir A, Tefft M, Thomas P, Askin FB, Kissane JM, Pritchard DJ, Neff J, Makley JT, Gilula L (Mayo Clinic and Found, Rochester, Minn; Univ of Minnesota, Minneapolis; Univ of Texas, Houston; Washington Univ, St Louis; Rhode Island Hosp, Providence, et al)
J Clin Oncol 9:1173–1180, 1991   7–5

Background.—Early results from the first Intergroup Ewing's Sarcoma Study (IESS-I) suggested that doxorubicin or pulmonary irradiation is helpful when added to treatment with vincristine, dactinomycin, and cyclophosphamide in patients with primary nonpelvic lesions but not in those with a pelvic primary lesion. This prompted development of a protocol for patients with Ewing's sarcoma localized to the pelvis and sacrum, which was evaluated in the second IESS (Fig 7–2).

Methods.—Data on 59 patients with disease in the pelvic and sacral bones were compared with those on 68 patients who were previously entered in IESS-I. Patients received high-dose intermittent treatment with vincristine, cyclophosphamide, doxorubicin, and dactinomycin for 6 weeks before and 70 weeks after local treatment. Those not having complete resection received a dose of 55 Gy to the tumor bed.

Results.—A significant advantage was apparent for the patients in IESS-II. Their survival at 5 years was 63% compared with 35% for those in IESS-I. The respective rates of complete remission were 68% and 13%. Local recurrences were more than twice as frequent in the IESS-I group. Intensified treatment appeared to control lung metastasis more effectively

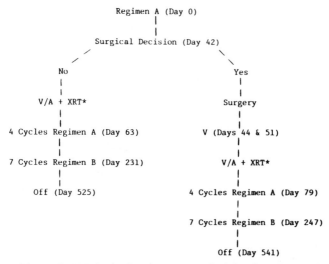

Fig 7–2.—Schema of IESS-II, localized Ewing's sarcoma of pelvic and sacral bones. Doses: vincristine *(V)*, 1.5 mg/m²; V/A: V, 1.5 mg/m² (day 1), Adriamycin *(A)*, 75 mg/m² (day 2). Regimen: A, 1.5 mg/m² (day 1); A, 75 mg/m² (day 2); V, 1.5 mg/m² (day 22; cyclophosphamide *(c)*, 1,400 mg/m² (day 23). *Asterisk* indicates omit if completely resected with no evidence of microscopic residual disease. Maximum single doses of V and D and 2 mg and .5 mg, respectively. (Courtesy of Evans RG, Nesbit ME, Gehan EA, et al: *J Clin Oncol* 9:1173–1180, 1991.)

than the IESS-I protocol, and bone metastases also were less frequent. More than 60% of patients had severe toxicity, and 1 died of congestive failure secondary to doxorubicin; 3 patients had life-threatening cardiotoxicity.

Conclusion.—High-dose chemotherapy and radiotherapy have improved the survival of patients with Ewing's sarcoma of the pelvic and sacral bones to the level reported for those having disease in nonpelvic sites.

▶ It is clear from numerous previous reports that patients with a Ewing's sarcoma arising in the pelvis or sacrum have a worse prognosis than patients with Ewing's sarcoma in other locations. This is probably a result of the larger size of these pelvic and sacral tumors. The Intergroup is composed of a large number of physicians from different institutions who agree to treat patients with similar sarcomas in a similar manner for the purpose of discovering the best treatment regimen. In this report they say that with increased intensity of the chemotherapy and more aggressive surgery and irradiation the local control and overall survival of patients with a pelvic and sacral lesion can equal those of the Ewing's tumors in other sites. This information does not tell us if surgery is necessary for these larger lesions, as has been suggested by other articles abstracted in this issue of the YEAR BOOK. The survival of patients at 5 years was higher for those that had a surgical resection than for those treated with irradiation, but we are told that the differences are not significant. The role of surgery remains controversial, although I think there is sufficient data to support surgical resection of all Ewing's sarcomas.—D.S. Springfield, M.D.

Osteosarcoma

Incidence and Survival Rates of Children and Young Adults With Osteogenic Sarcoma

Homa DM, Sowers MFR, Schwartz AG (Univ of Michigan, Ann Arbor; Michigan Cancer Found, Detroit)
Cancer 67:2219–2223, 1991   7–6

Background.—Few trials have assessed the incidence and survival rates of both children and young adults with osteogenic sarcoma, and no study has assessed gender- and race-specific survival differences in young persons with this disease. The incidence of osteogenic sarcoma and these survival trends were investigated in 350 microscopically confirmed cases.

Methods.—All patients, whites and blacks, aged 24 years or younger at diagnosis of primary osteogenic sarcoma who were identified from 1973 to 1986 at 8 surveillance, epidemiology, and end results registries were included. Follow-up extended through 1988.

Results.—The overall survival rates were 81% at 1 year, 49% at 3 years, and 44% at 5 years, with a median survival time of 36 months. Although there were no significant gender differences in age at diagnosis or in overall incidence, females had a median survival time of 74 months, significantly longer than the 29-month median survival time for males. There was no significant racial difference in age at diagnosis, nor were there significant racial differences in incidence rates after controlling for multiple comparisons. At 1, 3, and 5 years, white males had survival rates of 77%, 41%, and 36%; white females had survival rates of 82%, 58%, and 52%; black males had survival rates of 97%, 48%, and 43%; and black females had survival rates of 78%, 54%, and 49% (Fig 7–3). The median survival time was 94 months for white females, 41 months

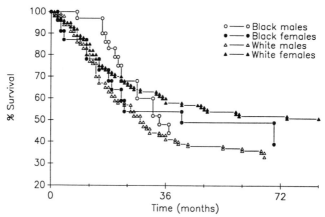

Fig 7–3.—Race-specific and gender-specific survival distributions of osteogenic sarcoma in whites and blacks, 0–24 years of age. Surveillance, Epidemiology, and End Results (SEER), 1973–1988. Events also observed in white females at 94 months (% survival, 49) and 123 months (% survival, 47). (Courtesy of Homa DM, Sowers MFR, Schwartz AG: *Cancer* 67:2219–2223, 1991.)

for black females, 34 months for black males, and 28 months for white males. Girls had higher rates of incidence than boys only in the 10- to 14-year-old age range.

Conclusions.—In children and young adults with osteogenic sarcoma, no significant difference in survival rates between blacks and whites was noted. However, females, especially whites females, have greater survival rates than males. Further studies of this observation are needed.

Osteosarcoma in Young Children
Kozakewich H, Perez-Atayde AR, Goorin AM, Wilkinson RH, Gebhardt MC, Vawter GF (Children's Hosp; Boston; Dana-Farber Cancer Inst; Boston)
Cancer 67:638–642, 1991   7–7

Background.—Osteosarcoma is a rare disease among young children. At 2 centers, only 12 children younger than 6 years of age were treated for this disease between 1918 and 1988. The clinicopathologic features of the disease were analyzed in these 12 children to investigate whether these features differ in young children from those in older children and adolescents.

Patients and Methods.—Patients included 8 girls and 4 boys ranging from 3.4 years to 5.8 years of age. Medical records and histologic slides for all patients were reviewed. Radiographs were available for 7 patients, and radiographic reports were available for the remaining 5.

Results.—No patient appeared to have metastases at the time of presentation. Six patients had tumors in the distal femur, 3 in the proximal humerus, 2 in the proximal tibia, and 1 in the distal tibia. All tumors involved at least one third of the bone shaft; there was no epiphyseal involvement according to radiographic evidence. Eight tumors were mainly osteolytic, and 3 were mainly osteoblastic. All were high-grade sarcomas with at least focal direct production of osteoid bone or immature bone or both. In 1972, treatments with high-dose methotrexate and leucovorin rescue were instituted. Only 1 of 6 children treated before 1972 experienced long-term survival, compared with 4 to 6 children treated after 1972, who were disease-free after an average follow-up of 8.8 years. Those survival times were similar to those of older children and adolescents treated at these institutions.

Conclusions.—Osteosarcoma in young children appears to have clinicopathologic features similar to those of older children and adolescents. This highly malignant tumor should be treated with a combination of complete (wide) surgical resection or amputation and aggressive chemotherapy.

▶ There continues to be the need for better predictors and indicators of metastasis in patients with osteosarcoma. From data obtained in the past, before the use of routine adjuvant chemotherapy, it is known that at least 80% of patients with a high-grade classic osteosarcoma have pulmonary metastasis at the time they first present to a physician. It has not been possible to predict which patients have the metastasis and which do not. Through experience and analysis of variables, a few predictive risk factors indicating increased risk of metastasis have been identified, such as a tumor larger than 10 cm, a very high serum alkaline phosphatase level, an elevated lactic dehydrogenase level, and microscopic vascular invasion. Females are said to have a better survival rate than males, and age has been suggested to be predictive, although the data are not strong. Kazakewich and associates (abstract 7-7) tell us that even the very young patients with osteosarcoma must be treated with the high-dose multidrug chemotherapy regimens, as are the older patients. Homa and associates (abstract 7-6) found that white females had a significantly higher survival rate than black males. The differences are minimal and do not help select patients that should be treated differently. The presence of greater than 90% necrosis in the primary tumor after preoperative chemotherapy is still the only significant predictive variable we have. The patients who have tumors with greater than 90% necrosis after preoperative chemotherapy have a significantly better survival rate compared to the patients with less necrosis after the chemotherapy. We need to find better indicators of each patient's prognosis. With our current knowledge, we must treat all patients with an osteosarcoma with 3 or 4 chemotherapeutic drugs, even though we know that 20 out of each 100 would be cured with surgery alone and that, almost certainly, many of the other 80 would be treated successfully with less aggressive adjuvant chemotherapy.—D.S. Springfield, M.D.

Soft Tissue Sarcomas

Pediatric Nonrhabdomyosarcomas of the Extremities: Influence of Size, Invasiveness, and Grade on Outcome

Rao BN, Santana VM, Parham D, Pratt CB, Fleming ID, Hudson M, Fontanesi J, Philippe P, Schell MJ (St Jude Children's Research Hosp, Memphis; Univ of Tennessee, Memphis)

Arch Surg 125:1490–1495, 1991   7-8

Background.—No standard treatment has been generally accepted for children with nonrhabdo soft tissue sarcoma (NRSIS). Surgery is generally the primary treatment when possible, after which radiation treatment is administered if margins are considered inadequate. However, this protocol has been estimated to result in a disease-free survival rate of only 50%. A retrospective review was designed to identify subsets of patients who might benefit from additional treatment.

Methods.—Data were examined on 64 children and adolescents with NRSTS treated between 1965 and 1990. Survival rates were analyzed based on the size of the lesion, grade according to the American Joint Committee on Cancer staging system, and invasiveness according to this system.

Results.—Five patients had metastases at the time of diagnosis. Only 2 of 32 patients who underwent regional lymph node dissection had evidence of nodal involvement. In 11 of 31 patients who underwent reexcision suspected residual disease was found. Survival was associated with

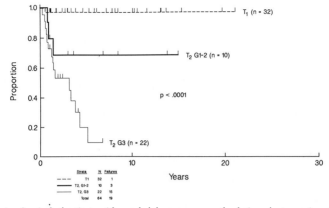

Fig 7–4.—Survival of patients with nonrhabdomyosarcoma of soft tissue by tumor invasiveness and grade. Tick marks indicate censored observations. There is considerable difference in survival of patients with T1 lesions versus those with T2 lesions; survival of patients with G1-2 lesions versus those with T2/G3 lesions is highly significant. Number of patients experiencing failure was T1, 1 patient; T2/G1-2, 3 patients; and T2/G3, 18 patients. (Courtesy of Rao BN, Santana VM, Parham D, et al: *Arch Surg* 125:1490–1495, 1991.)

tumor invasiveness, grade, and size (Fig 7–4). Seventeen patients had relapses at a median of 11 months, and 14 survived a median of 4 months after relapse. Forty-six patients did not require amputation initially but were treated with wide local excision or en bloc resection; 2 of these subsequently required amputation for local control. Sixteen patients received 36–60 Gy of radiation, and all of them achieved local control. Twenty-eight patients received adjuvant chemotherapy, which was not associated with invasiveness, size, or grade.

Conclusions.—A wide local excision, including a 2-cm rim of normal tissue, is the initial treatment of choice for patients with NRSTS. Tumor invasiveness and grade significantly influence survival. The role of adjuvant chemotherapy is still unclear.

▶ Rhabdomyosarcoma is the most common soft tissue tumor in children. It occurs in all anatomical sites. It responds to systemic chemotherapy and limited surgical resection or irradiation. Rhabdomyosarcoma, although once diagnosed in adults with regularity, is now thought to be uncommon in adults. Most of the adult soft tissue tumors thought to be rhabdomyosarcoma in the past are now called malignant fibrohistiocytoma. Nonrhabdomyosarcoma soft tissue sarcomas in children are unusual. Rao and associates have reviewed 64 patients with a NRSTS in an attempt to reveal important prognostic information that might indicate how they should be treated. In brief, it can be said that soft tissue sarcomas in the pediatric-aged patient have the same behavior as those that occur in adults. In adults the benefits of adjuvant chemotherapy have not been realized, but in children larger doses and a more aggressive protocol is tolerated; therefore, adjuvant chemotherapy probably should be used in the young patient with a high-grade nonrhabdomyosarcoma.—D.S. Springfield, M.D.

DNA Content Prognostic in Soft Tissue Sarcoma: 102 Patients Followed for 1–10 Years

Bauer HCF, Kreicbergs A, Tribukait B (Karolinska Instit and Hospital, Stockholm)
Acta Orthop Scand 62:187–194, 1991   7–9

Introduction.—Histogenetic classification has become more accurate with the aid of immunohistochemical markers and electron microscopy, but it remains of limited prognostic value. Although malignancy grading appears to be of greater relevance, there is still a need for improved characterization of soft tissue sarcomas for both prognostic and therapeutic purposes. Previous reports have shown that cellular DNA content in soft tissue sarcoma is related to histologic grade. A prospective trial was designed to relate the DNA content of soft tissue sarcoma to the clinical course of the disease.

Patients.—The population consisted of 102 patients with soft tissue sarcoma. All patients were treated surgically without previous chemotherapy or radiation treatment.

Results.—Based on DNA flow cytometry, 37 lesions were diploid and 65 were nondiploid. The incidence of nondiploidy increased with increasing histologic grade. The 5-year metastasis-free survival rate for the entire series of 102 patients was .59. Bivariate analysis demonstrated that survival was related to both tumor grade and level of ploidy. Cox regression analysis identified 3 independent risk factors for metastasis: tumor size with a relative risk of 1.2 for each cm increase, nondiploidy with a relative risk of 4.5, and male sex with relative risk of 2. The risk of metastasis was strongly related to the number of risk factors present. The 5-year

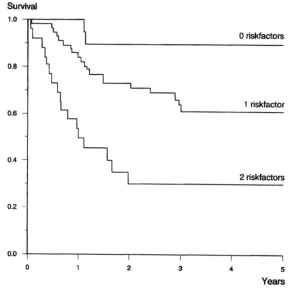

Fig 7–5.—Life-table curve of metastasis-free survival in relation to risk factors. (Courtesy of Bauer HCF, Kreicbergs A, Tribukait B: *Acta Orthop Scand* 62:187–194, 1991.)

survival rate was .9 for patients with no risk factors, .6 for those with 1 risk factor, and .3 for those with 2 risk factors (Fig 7–5). Contrary to most investigations of soft tissue sarcoma, histologic malignancy grading yielded no independent prognostic information.

Conclusions.—Identification of patients who are at high risk for metastasis may be valuable in trials with adjuvant chemotherapy, whereas those at low risk should be excluded from adjuvant chemotherapy. The risk of metastasis in soft tissue sarcoma is related to DNA content and tumor size. Both parameters can be assessed by objective means.

▶ As is the case with osteosarcoma, better indicators of the risk of metastasis are needed for patients with soft tissue sarcomas. Currently, histologic grade and tumor size are the only significant prognostic variables recognized. The DNA content has been found to be a predictor in some carcinomas and seems to be an indicator in osteosarcoma, although its significance in osteosarcoma is not yet clearly established. Bauer and associates have determined the DNA content for 102 soft tissue tumors to determine if it was predictive. A close look at their data reveals that there were 17 patients who had a high grade (3 or 4) malignant tumor but a diploid DNA pattern; 9 of these patients are alive and free of disease, and 8 are dead. There were only 3 patients with a grade 1 tumor, and all 3 were diploid, but 5 of the grade 2 tumors were nondiploid. Two of these patients are dead, but 3 are alive without disease. Thus, for the patients with a discrepancy between their tumor's histologic grade and DNA content, it was impossible to tell who would have a metastasis develop and who would not. The DNA content will not yet give us a sufficiently accurate prediction of metastatic risk.—D.S. Springfield, M.D.

Treatments

Chemotherapy for Children With Aggressive Fibromatosis and Langerhans' Cell Histiocytosis

Raney RB Jr (Univ of Texas, Houston)
Clin Orthop 262:58–63, 1991   7–10

Introduction.—Many of the drugs that now cure childhood cancers produce some acute side effects and may cause long-term damage. Such drugs have also been used to treat nonmalignant proliferations of fibrous tissue or histiocytes in children. Because the use of chemotherapy for nonmalignant masses is problematic, guidelines were created for the initiation of multiple-agent chemotherapy in aggressive fibromatosis and Langerhans' cell histiocytosis (LCH).

Aggressive Fibromatosis.—Surgical removal is the mainstay of treatment in children with aggressive fibromatosis or an extra-abdominal-wall desmoid tumor of soft tissue. However, local recurrence is frequent, even after wide excision. Radiation treatment, with or without chemotherapy, is used when some of the mass is recurrent or inoperable. Because radiation can affect bone growth and cause cancer, multiple-agent chemotherapy may be more attractive. A combination of vincristine, actinomycin

D, and cyclophosphamide was successful in several young patients with aggressive fibromatosis. A minimum of 12 weeks of this combination should be considered, using Regimen 25 of the Intergroup Rhabdomyosarcoma Study. If no response is seen by 16–20 weeks, doxorubicin (Adriamycin) or dacarbazine may be helpful. Myelosuppression may be an immediate consequence of vincristine-actinomycin D-cyclosphosphamide and of Adriamycin plus dacarbazine. Long-term, dose-related complications include bladder fibrosis and decreased fertility. Children treated with these agents should be observed by the pediatric oncologist and surgeon.

Histiocytosis.—Children are more frequently affected by LCH, a heterogeneous disorder of unknown origin, than are adults. Biopsy is always indicated for diagnosis. Because LCH is commonly disseminated at the time of diagnosis, chemotherapeutic agents were used in treating the disorder as soon as they became available. Now, chemotherapy is used more conservatively unless the lesions result in systemic symptoms or dysfunction of the liver, spleen, or lungs. Patients with a surgically inaccesible mass threatening an important structure may benefit from low-dose radiation treatment, 450–600 cGy in 3 or 4 treatments. Equally effective may be the rapid administration of high-dose steroids and an antimetabolite or vinca alkaloid.

Radiation Therapy for Aggressive Fibromatosis: The Experience at the University of Florida

McCollough WM, Parsons JT, Van Der Griend R, Enneking WF, Heare T (Univ of Florida, Gainesville)
J Bone Joint Surg 73-A:717–725, 1991   7–11

Background.—It has been suggested that radiation treatment may control unresectable aggressive fibromatosis and decrease the risk of local recurrence when the resection margin is close to the tumor.

Methods.—Radical courses of radiation were administered to 30 sites in 29 patients with histologically confirmed aggressive fibromatosis. Follow-up for all patients was at least 2 years, and 76% had follow-up for more than 5 years. A minimum of 5,000 cGy was administered to 27 sites, and 12 patients received twice-a-day treatments. Postoperative radiation was administered for 14 sites with known or presumed microscopic residual aggressive fibromatosis; local control was achieved in 11 of these. Postoperative treatment was administered for 16 sites with grossly apparent residual disease; local control was achieved in 14 of these.

Results.—Control of disease was achieved in 83% of sites, and the 6-year actuarial rate of local control was 79%. There were 5 local recurrences at 4, 11, 34, 61, and 68 months after the start of treatment, 2 of them occurring in the high-dose radiation field in patients treated for grossly apparent disease. The other 3 occurred at the margin of the irradiated field in patients treated for microscopic residual disease. Rate of local control appeared to be no different in patients treated for primary aggressive fibromatosis compared with those treated for recurrence.

Conclusions.—Local control of aggressive fibromatosis appears to improve substantially with postoperative radiation treatment when operative margins are less than wide. On its own, radiation treatment appears to be an effective alternative to radical surgery or for patients with unresectable lesions.

▶ Fibromatosis or extra-abdominal desmoid is often a difficult disorder to manage. The local disease is infiltrative of soft tissues and can infiltrate bone. Even with an apparently wide surgical margin, it often recurs. Surgical resection will control approximately half of the lesions, but the other half are very difficult to treat successfully, and, even after an amputation, fibromatosis can recur. It does not metastasize and does not have a significant incidence of malignant degeneration. Numerous nonsurgical treatment methods have been tried, and these 2 reports give us some hope. Raney and associates (Abstract 7–10) suggest using a combination of 3 antimetabolites to control those patients with recurrent disease who are not good surgical candidates. McCollough and associates (Abstract 7–11) recommend using irradiation and report their experience. These 2 reports support the use of nonsurgical means of managing recurrent fibromatosis, but both treatment protocols have short- and long-term risk and should be used cautiously.—D.S. Springfield, M.D.

Cryosurgery and Acrylic Cementation as Surgical Adjuncts in the Treatment of Aggressive (Benign) Bone Tumors: Analysis of 25 Patients Below the Age of 21

Malawer MM, Dunham W (Children's Hosp, Bethesda, Md; Univ of Alabama, Birmingham)

Clin Orthop 262:42–57, 1991   7–12

Background.—Curettage and bone grafting is the classic treatment of most benign, aggressive bone tumors. Cryosurgery and acrylic cementation (polymethylmethacrylate [PMMA]), developed during the past 2 decades, are used to decrease the high rate of local recurrence. The clinical and biologic basis of these adjuvant modalities were evaluated in the treatment of aggressive, benign bone sarcomas.

Cementation.—Use of cementation was based on the hypothesis that PMMA might kill the residual tumor cells after curettage. Analysis of 20 patients so treated between 1972 and 1985 revealed only 3 local recurrences; similarly, the overall recurrence rate in a group of 240 patients was 10%. With curettage and cementation, the joint is preserved, functional result is improved, local recurrence is easier to detect, and other therapeutic options still exist. Used with the mechanical burr, PMMA immediately stabilizes a large defect and decreases the risk of fracture during healing. The tumorcidal effect of PMMA may be attributed to hyperthermia from the heat of polymerization or a possible direct toxic effect of the monomer. The need for PMMA removal has little support in clinical or scientific data.

Cryosurgery.—The use of extreme cold ($-21°$ to $-60°$) results in cellular necrosis. The extent of necrosis is increased by repeated freeze–thaw cycles. There was only 1 tumor recurrence in 25 patients younger than age 21 years treated by cryosurgery. Nineteen lesions involved the lower extremity, and 6 involved the upper extremity. Tumor types were giant-cell tumor, chondroblastoma, aneurysmal bone cyst, and malignant giant-cell tumor. No infections occurred, but 5 patients required an additional procedure. Of 24 patients evaluated for function, 20 had an excellent result.

Conclusions.—Computed tomography and MRI are recommended before surgery to evaluate carefully the extent of the tumor. A pathologic fracture is a contraindication to cryosurgery. However, in most patients cryosurgery and PMMA reduce the incidence of recurrence and the need for reconstructive procedure.

▶ Giant cell tumor of bone and, to a lesser extent, chondroblastoma and aneurysmal bone cyst are benign tumors that can be difficult to control with only a curettage. Local recurrence is more common than one wants, with only a curettage, especially for giant-cell tumor of bone, and recurrent disease has prompted surgeons on occasion to do a major resection. In an attempt to reduce the incidence of recurrence and to save more joints, a number of surgeons have used local adjuvants with a curettage. Freeze-thawing of tumors has been one of the adjuvants used, but there have been a significant number of complications, including late fractures. Malawer and Dunham report on the use of the freeze–thaw technique, but with PMMA used to support the injured bone so that it will not fracture. This is a difficult surgical technique but one that does work. It probably should be done only by those surgeons who are taught the technique and who use it regularly.—D.S. Springfield, M.D.

Autograft Versus Allograft for Benign Lesions in Children
Glancy GL, Brugioni DJ, Eilert RE, Chang FM (Children's Hosp, Univ of Colorado, Denver)
Clin Orthop 262:28–33, 1991   7–13

Background.—Surgical curettage with bone grafting is the standard method of treating benign bone lesions in children. In some children, the lesion is so large that an autograft cannot restore bone integrity. Autografts and allografts were compared to determine if there were any significant differences in outcome between the 2 types of grafts.

Methods.—Data were obtained from the medical records and roentgenograms of children who had curettage and bone grafting of benign lesions between 1976 and 1988. Fifty-four patients with 61 lesions were included. The children's mean age at surgery was 8.9 years; the mean follow-up period was 29 months. Lesions were classified as small (<60 mL) or large (>60 mL) volume and separated into 4 groups: small-volume autograft, large-volume autograft, small-volume allograft, and large-volume allograft.

Results.—Outcome appeared comparable for the 2 types of grafts when small-volume lesions were treated. Allografts required a slightly longer average healing time (27 months) than autografts (21 months). The allograft large-volume group had the highest incidence of complications. Cases of no healing ranged from 10% in the small-volume allograft group to 33% in the large-volume allograft group. Lesions healed completely in 91% or partially in 9% of the small-volume autograft group, and lesions healed completely in 69% or partially in 31% of large-volume autograft group.

Conclusion.—In small, solitary lesions in children, allografts offer results nearly comparable to those of autografts. However, the larger lesions (>60 mL) remain an orthopedic challenge. Autografts will give a higher success rate in older children with large lesions, but a young child with multicentric or polyostotic lesions can achieve successful incorporation with allografts.

▶ Benign bone lesions often must be curetted, and most of them are in children. The defect created by the curettage is filled with bone in an attempt to speed the healing and to be sure that the entire cavity fills with bone. Not uncommonly, the defect is so large that either the patient does not have sufficient bone or filling the defect would require harvesting most of the patient's iliac crest. Allograft has been used to fill these large defects with clinical success. Because of the clinical success with allograft in large defects, it has been used more frequently to fill small defects as well as that patients will not have to have their own bone harvested. What Glancy and associates showed was not unexpected. The small lesions healed well with either type of graft, but the larger defects did better with autograft. This still does not indicate that autograft should be used for the larger lesions. The surgeon must weigh the risk of harvesting enough bone from the patient to fill a large lesion, and often it is better to accept slower filling than to harvest the patient's own bone. One issue not discussed was whether any of the defects require bone grafting. In all likelihood the small cavities would fill in without bone graft, and many of the larger cavities may do so as well. A study of bone graft vs. no bone graft should be done.—D.S. Springfield, M.D.

Prosthetic Replacement of the Distal Femur for Primary Bone Tumours
Roberts P, Chan D, Grimer RJ, Sneath RS, Scales JT (Royal Orthopaedic Hospital, Birmingham, England)
J Bone Joint Surg 73-B:762–769, 1991   7–14

Background.—Chemotherapeutic advances in tumor control have made limb salvage surgery common in patients with malignant bone tumors. A 16-year experience in prosthetic replacement of the distal femur in such patients is described.

Methods.—One hundred thirty-five patients were treated. All were skeletally mature and had malignant or aggressive benign primary tumors of bone requiring prosthetic replacement of the distal femur. Osteosarcoma was the most common diagnosis; the patients' median age was 22 years. The prostheses were custom-made, based on the fully constrained Stanmore-type knee replacement (Fig 7–6). The stems were grouted into the intramedullary cavity using bone cement. Survivorship analysis and functional assessment were done, and rates of revision surgery and infection were reviewed.

Results.—Follow-up ranged up to 156 months (median, 34 months). Of 133 patients available for follow-up, 13 required amputation. Another 13 patients required revision surgery for infection, loosening, or stem fracture. At 5 years there was an 88% likelihood of avoiding amputation, a 75% chance that the original prosthesis would be in place, and a 72% chance that the prosthesis would be asymptomatic. Functional assessment was good or excellent in 91% of patients. Infection rate was 6.8%; this was the major complication.

Conclusions.—In prosthetic replacement of the distal femur for patients with primary bone tumors, success rates similar to those of conventional Stanmore prostheses can be obtained. Functional recovery is impressive, and there is no greater survival risk than there is for amputation.

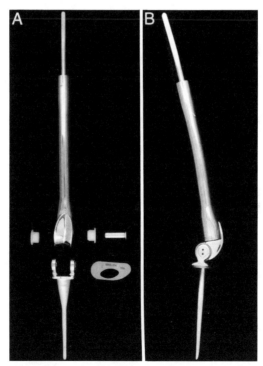

Fig 7–6.—An example of a custom-made distal femur and knee prosthesis. (Courtesy of Roberts P, Chan D, Grimer RJ, et al: *J Bone Joint Surg* 73-B:762–769, 1991.)

▶ During the past decade the number of limb salvage resections done for malignant bone tumors has increased dramatically. Currently, somewhere around 80% of patients with osteosarcoma will have a limb-sparing resection. Usually the resection includes an articular surface, and most early reconstructions were arthrodeses. With the development of improved endoprostheses, an increasing number of reconstructions were done with articulating custom endoprosthetic replacements. Roberts and associates report from one of the major centers involved in the development and use of these custom endoprostheses. The other alternatives include an arthrodesis or an osteoarticular allograft replacement. The advantages of the endoprosthesis are that it works almost immediately and that the patient is back walking within a few weeks of surgery with an almost normal extremity. The disadvantage is that if the patient survives, the endoprosthesis will eventually fail. It was originally thought that the endoprosthesis would fail quickly. As is reported by these authors, the endoprostheses have survived extremely well, and the 10% revision is certainly acceptable. During the next decade more of these reconstructions will require revision, but it is hoped that with the new designs even longer survival of the endoprosthesis can be expected.—D.S. Springfield, M.D.

Observations on Massive Retrieved Human Allografts

Enneking WF, Mindell ER (Univ of Florida, Gainesville, Fla; State Univ of New York, Buffalo)

J Bone Joint Surg 73-A:1123–1142, 1991   7–15

Methods.—Radiographic and histologic findings in 16 massive human allografts were used to reconstruct defects created by extremity-salvaging resection in the treatment of musculoskeletal tumors. The allografts had been in situ for 4–65 months, but most were retrieved less than 2 years after implantation. Eight specimens were osteoarticular grafts, 3 were intercalary grafts, and 5 had been used as composites with prosthestic joints. Allograft recipients ranged in age from 13 to 66 years.

Results.—Union between allograft and host at cortical junctions occurred slowly by the gradual formation of an external callus derived from the cortex of the host. The callus extended from the host bone onto the external surface of the allograft. Union was usually evident externally before the radiolucent gap was obliterated. Union at the cancellous junctions occurred more rapidly by internal callus advancing from the host into the allograft without formation of external callus. The pattern of revascularization and internal repair appeared consistent. On the external surface of the graft a thin 1- to 2-mm layer of bone was laid down by mesenchymal proliferation derived from adjacent host cells. Resorption often did not reach the peripheral cement line about the canal, and this in turn led to partial repair of osteons with a near-complete absence of cutting cones crossing the peripheral cement line and extending into the interstitial lamellae. On most surfaces adjacent soft tissue was firmly adherent to the underlying allograft. There was solid healing in all specimens except in those obtained after rejection. If suture material had not marked the sites of repair, it would have been hard to identify the junction sites grossly because the tissues were so well integrated. However, the junction sites were identified easily on histologic study. A few millimeters from the allograft junction, tissue consisted of acellular mature bundles of collagen arranged in an orderly pattern. The interface between allograft and cement was secure as seen on gross inspection and on microscopy. Histologic examination revealed no evidence of revascularization of the allograft adjacent to cement and no evidence of tissue ingrowth between cement and adjacent allograft. The remaining cartilage in all osteoarticular specimens was acellular, and there was no evidence of metabolic activity in the matrices. Despite the lack of chondrocyte survival, the architecture of the matrix was well preserved in specimens retrieved at 6–25 months. Only 1 distal femoral specimen retrieved at 25 months had moderately severe degenerative changes.

Conclusion.—These findings of this study suggest that large frozen allografts in human beings are osteoconductive rather than osteoinductive.

▶ Large fresh-frozen allografts have been increasingly used as a means of reconstructing the skeleton after tumor resections and for the revision of a failed total joint. Although animals studies have been done and the clinical course of humans with allograft bone implants have been observed, little is known about what happens to a large allograft bone in a human. Enneking and Mindell have studied 16 retrieved human allografts. The 3 most important findings include incorporation of the allograft without signs of an immunologic reaction, no resorption of bone adjacent to the polymethylmethacrylate, and healing of the patient's ligaments to the allograft bone and ligaments. One of the objections to the large metallic endoprostheses is that muscle attachments do not heal to them so that for the proximal femur with its abductors and the proximal tibia with the patellar tendon the lack of a satisfactory attachment for these muscles means the patient has weak hip abduction or knee extension, respectively. The ability of these tendons to heal is an advantage for the allograft, as shown by this report. The other finding, which is not surprising although it is disappointing, was the lack of articular cartilage survival. Degenerative arthritis is the fate of the osteoarticular allografts, although clinically it is not as big a problem as would be predicted by the finding in this report. The major challenge for the future is learning how to transplant living cartilage with the bone successfully. This analysis makes one wounder whether the use of a conventional endoprosthesis with an allograft may offer the best method of reconstruction for the proximal femur, distal femur, and proximal tibia.—D.S. Springfield, M.D.

Metastatic Disease

Prognostic Indicators of Metastatic Bone Disease in Human Breast Cancer
Kamby C, Rasmussen BB, Kristensen B (Copenhagen Univ Hosp)
Cancer 68:2045–2050, 1991   7–16

Background.—The most common site of metastasis in breast cancer is bone. Detection of metastatic bone disease (MBD) in patients with first recurrence of breast cancer is important because survival after recurrence can be several years. Prognostic indicators in the development of MBD were sought.

Methods.—Included were 221 consecutively seen patients with recurrent breast cancer without MBD at the time of initial recurrence. Mean age at recurrence was 53 years, with recurrence detected at a median of 27 months. All patients had mastectomies, and none had bone metastases on radiographic survey or bone marrow carcinosis demonstrated on iliac crest biopsy examination. Follow-up after first recurrence was for a median of 46 months.

Results.—At follow-up, 60% of the patients had died. Eighty-nine patients died without MBD. Twenty-five percent of all patients had MBD demonstrated by radiography, with 14% showing recurrence in bone after 1 year and 27% after 2 years. Univariate survival analysis showed that node-positive patients were more likely to have MBD than node-negative patients. Eighty-five percent of patients had metastases in only a single site. Patients with visceral metastases had shorter times to bone metastasis than patients with soft-tissue recurrences. Nineteen percent of patients with abnormal results of bone scintigraphy at the time of recurrence had MBD at 1 year, significantly more than the 9% of those with normal bone scans. Elevated levels of serum alkaline phosphatase and lactate dehydrogenase were both associated with significantly shorter times to bone metastasis. The presence of micrometastases in bone marrow, as detected by monoclonal antibodies, was not associated with development of MBD.

Conclusions.—In the patients reviewed, the 2 most important independent predictors of the time to bone metastasis were the presence of visceral metastases and positive bone scintigraphic scans. These findings provide further evidence that radiographic examinations often yield false negative results and that bone scintigraphy is more sensitive than radiography.

Breast Cancer With Bone-Only Metastases: Visceral Metastases-Free Rate in Relation to Anatomic Distribution of Bone Metastases
Yamashita K, Ueda T, Komatsubara Y, Koyama H, Inaji H, Yonenobu K, Ono K (Osaka University, Japan)
Cancer 68:634–637, 1991   7–17

Background.—Metastases from breast cancer confined to bone often remain localized for a long time. Most patients however, eventually die of visceral metastases. Retrograde venous seeding, rather than dissemination through the lungs, appears to be the pathway for bone-only metastases from breast cancer. Although bone-only metastases cannot be identified clinically, their distribution may provide a clue to the seeding pathway from breast cancer. The distribution of bone-only metastases in relation to the visceral metastases-free rate was examined by retrospective review of records.

Patients.—The patient population included 82 women aged 31–80 years who had relapse with bone-only metastases from breast cancer. Because tumors may spread to bones near the primary site directly by retrograde venous seeding, the boundary for the area to which breast cancer can spread directly via this pathway was arbitrarily defined as the lumbosacral junction. On the basis of the distribution of bone metastases on the bone scans, patients were divided into 3 groups. Forty-six patients (56%) had bone metastases exclusively cranial to the lumbosacral junction, 6 (7%) had metastases exclusively caudal to the junction, and 30 (37%) had metastases both cranial and caudal to the junction.

Results.—Patients with bone metastases exclusively cranial to the lumbosacral junction had a significantly higher visceral metastases-free rate than did those in either of the other 2 groups (Fig 7–7). Serial bone scans and radiographs in those patients revealed that bone lesions cranial to the lumbosacral junction rarely developed into visceral metastases, whereas bone lesions caudal to the junction often developed into visceral metastases.

Conclusion.—The presence of bone metastases caudal to the lumbosacral junction in patients with bone-only metastases from breast cancer is predictive of visceral metastases. This finding may be helpful in selecting the most appropriate treatment for individual patients with bone-only metastases from breast cancer.

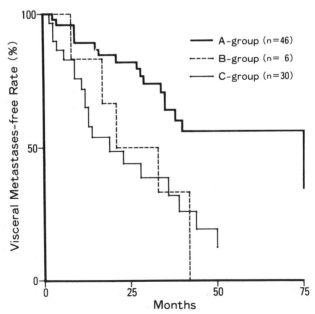

Fig 7–7.—Visceral metastases-free rate from the diagnosis of bone metastases according to the distribution of bone metastases: group A (n = 46), group B (n = 6), and group C (n = 30). The differences between groups A and B and between groups A and C were significant at $P < .05$ and $P < .005$ levels, respectively. The difference between groups B and C was not significant. (Courtesy of Yamashita K, Ueda T, Komatsubara Y, et al: *Cancer* 68:634–637, 1991.)

▶ Bone metastasis from breast cancer is a common clinical problem. If we could predict which patients are going to have bone metastases and what the natural history for those patients will be, it would be easier to manage their disease. Abstract 7–16 gives the reader a few indicators of who is at greatest risk of having bone metastasis develop. Those patients with an increased risk should be followed more closely than those without these risks. Bone scans should be done as a routine, and we should not rely on plain radiographs to identify bone metastasis. Abstract 7–17 suggests that some (and maybe a majority of) patients with breast cancer that has metastasized to bone have direct extension from the breast to bone. The authors are suggesting a new pathway for the spread of tumor cells from the breast to bone. This is an interesting concept that may prove to be true, but additional evidence is required. If true, it suggests that patients with metastasis above the lumbosacral junction will survive longer than those with metastases below this level.—D.S. Springfield, M.D.

Scoring System for the Preoperative Evaluation of Metastatic Spine Tumor Prognosis
Tokuhashi Y, Matsuzaki H, Toriyama S, Kawano H, Ohsaka S (Nihon University, Tokyo)
Spine 15:1110–1113, 1990   7–18

Purpose.—A simple scoring system was designed for the preoperative evaluation of the prognosis of metastatic spinal tumors or of cancer with spinal cord palsy and progressive pain. The scoring system is based on experience with patients who had been treated surgically.

Methods.—A group of 64 patients who were operated on between 1978 and 1988 were included. Six parameters were used to assess the severity of vertebral collapse resulting from metastatic spine tumors: general condition, number of extraspinal bone metastases, number of metastases in the vertebral body, metastases to the major internal organs, primary cancer site, and severity of spinal cord palsy. Each parameter was scored for a range of 0 to 2 points (table). Each score and the grand total were examined in relation to the prognosis and for their potential usefulness as criteria for surgical treatment.

Results.—The mean postoperative survival was less than 3 months for patients with the primary lesion in the lung or stomach, but it was more than 1 year for those with the primary lesion in the thyroid, breast, prostate, or rectum. The prognosis could not be predicted from a single parameter, but total scores were useful in selecting the type of surgical treatment. Patients with a total score of 5 or less survived 3 months or less on average, whereas those with a total score of 9 or more survived an average of 12 months or more. Thus, excisional operation is indicated in patients with total scores of 9 or more, whereas palliative treatment is indicated for patients with total scores of 5 or less.

Conclusions.—Progressive pain from radioresistant tumors, spinal cord palsy, and an unstable spine caused by vertebral dysfunction are

Evaluation System for Prognosis of Metastatic Spine Tumors

		Score
1. General condition (performance status)		
Poor	(PS 10-40%)	0
Moderate	(PS 50-70%)	1
Good	(PS 80-100%)	2
2. Number of extraspinal bone metastases foci		
≧ 3		0
1-2		1
0		2
3. Number of metastases in the vertebral body		
≧ 3		0
2		1
1		2
4. Metastases to the major internal organs		
Unremovable		0
Removable		1
No metastases		2
5. Primary site of the cancer		
Lung, stomach		0
Kidney, liver, uterus		1
Others, unidentified		
Thyroid, prostate, breast		2
Rectum		
6. Spinal cord palsy		
Complete		0
Incomplete		1
None		2
		Total = 12

(Courtesy of Tokuhashi Y, Matsuzaki H, Toriyama S, et al: *Spine* 15:1110–1113, 1990.)

generally considered to be indications for surgical treatment. However, when there is a delay of less than 24 hours between the onset of symptoms and the appearance of a full-blown neurologic syndrome, the prognosis for recovery is poor, regardless of which treatment is offered. In quite a few patients an excision performed in the hope of prolonging the patient's life resulted in the patient's death within 3 months or in a postoperative infection that led to additional hospitalization for most of the already short period of life remaining.

Spinal Instability Secondary to Metastatic Cancer

Galasko CSB (University of Manchester, England)
J Bone Joint Surg 73-B:104–108, 1991   7–19

Background.—In about 10% of patients with disseminated carcinoma, the back pain is attributable to spinal instability. The management and outcome in 55 patients with severe pain from thoracic or lumbar instability secondary to spinal metastatic cancer were reviewed.

Patients.—All patients had been referred for surgical stabilization of

Results and Complications in 54 Patients Who Had
Operations for Spinal Instability Caused by Metastases

	Number
Relief of pain	
complete	49
partial	2
Loosening of implant	2
Infection resulting in removal of implant	1
Complications*	
infection treated successfully	1
wound breakdown, successful secondary suture	1
fracture of a Luque L rod requiring additional anterior stabilisation	1
fracture of a Hartshill rectangle (at five years)	1

*In 51 patients with relief of pain.
(Courtesy of Galasko CSB: *J Bone Joint Surg* 73-B:104–108, 1991.)

the spine after chemotherapy and irradiation had failed to control their pain. None of the patients were deemed in terminal condition, and none had malignant hypercalcemia. All patients but the first underwent routine preoperative myelography with decompression if there was any evidence of extradural tumor. All patients were referred for consideration of postoperative irradiation.

Results.—Surgical stabilization was not feasible in 1 patient. The remaining 54 underwent 55 spinal stabilizations. One patient was operated on for lumbar instability 22 months after successful dorsal stabilization. Forty-nine patients (89%) had complete relief of pain, and 2 had partial relief of pain (table). Twenty-eight patients had some clinical evidence of spinal cord compression or cauda equina, usually weakness of the lower extremities severe enough to affect walking or standing. Twenty of these 28 patients (71%) obtained major recovery of neurologic function, which was sufficient to allow them to walk without aids and to restore bladder function in cases where it had been compromised.

Conclusions.—Instability of the dorsal or lumbar spine secondary to metastatic cancer can be treated adequately in most patients by posterior stabilization alone. The implant should be fixed to at least 2 and preferably 3 vertebrae above and 3 vertebrae below the area of instability. All patients in this series had pain secondary to spinal instability, and none had cord or cauda equina compression initially. Whenever possible, the lesion should be irradiated after stabilization, and the patient should receive chemotherapy or endocrine therapy to prevent further tumor growth.

▶ In autopsy studies, the vertebral bodies are the most common site for metastatic deposits of carcinoma, but, fortunately, most of these deposits are not symptomatic, and most of those that produce systems can be managed with irradiation. Surgical management of metastatic disease to the spine is complicated and not well addressed in texts or the literature. Abstract 7–18 describes a scoring system to decide who should undergo operation. The system offers an objective means of weighing the clinical information before deciding whether to do an operation on a patient with a spine metastasis. This scoring system should make the decision process better. Abstract 7–19 concerns the rare problem of spinal instability caused by metastatic disease. These patients often are not operated on because of their metastatic disease and lack of significant neurologic findings. Galasko suggests that spinal stabilization is indicated in patients who had pain, instability, and more than a few weeks to live. His results are impressive with respect to relief of pain and lack of complications in a group of patients who are most difficult to treat. The method of fixation is not the important variable—they are the surgeon's ability to select the patient to operate on and the surgeon's technical skills. Operative stabilization is indicated for the patient with metastatic disease who has an unstable spinal condition.—D.S. Springfield, M.D.

8 Hand

Introduction

This chapter is dedicated to the hand and wrist. The goal has been to select a spectrum of articles addressing both acute and chronic disorders as well as relevant research. The first series of articles addresses fractures and the resulting problems from failing to gain or being unable to gain a good reduction in intra-articular injuries. Functional treatment of fractures, a principle well established for the larger bones, is possible for metacarpal injuries as well.

Occupational disorders, especially carpal tunnel syndrome, are almost epidemic in the workplace. This may well be the next significant problem of major interest for surgeons interested specifically in care of problems of the hand and upper extremity. Occupational carpal tunnel syndrome differs from the familiar idiopathic carpal tunnel. Its occurrence can be well correlated with jobs that require multiple repetitive motions, especially when high frequency and high force is required, and it is seen in a different sex and age distribution. Addressing the job requirements will be far more essential for the treating physician than surgical procedures. Dupuytren's disease in the workplace is also problematic when defining causality, and some basic guidelines are suggested.

Continued interest in problems of the wrist and distal radioulnar joint are reflected in the large series of articles addressing this problem. Reconstructive procedures to date have been secondary rather than repairing the original lesion. The surgeon has to choose among an increasingly large menu of alternatives. Now, with further definition of the vascularity of the triangular fibrocartilage, repairs, as is desirable in certain meniscal lesions of the knee, should be encouraged. Selective intercarpal arthrodeses may also be useful, especially in the rheumatoid wrist, in both correcting deformity and delaying further progression.

Imaging techniques are increasingly helpful, especially in scaphoid fractures. Defining both the alignment of the fractures as well as vascularity of the proximal pole hopefully will sharpen one's indications for surgery as well as predicting results. Perhaps we should all be more aggressive surgically in the acutely fractured scaphoid, at least when displacement is present.

The last series of articles covers a spectrum from compression neuropathies in reflex sympathetic dystrophy to correction of deformities of the spastic thumb. Among them is an important article defining the injury beneath a tourniquet rather than distal to it as has been studied previously. It graphically demonstrates what we all suspect (i.e., the lowest pressure for the shortest period of time is preferable).

Barry P. Simmons, M.D.

Augmented External Fixation of Unstable Distal Radius Fractures

Seitz WH Jr, Froimson AI, Leb R, Shapiro JD (Mt Sinai Med Ctr, Cleveland)
J Hand Surg 16-A:1010–1016, 1991   8–1

Background.—New techniques and fixation devices have improved the management of unstable distal radius fractures using ligamentotaxis through external fixation. However, reduced fractures sometimes suffer late displacement or collapse with loss of articular congruity. Thus augmentation of fixation with percutaneous Kirschner wires and, when necessary, supportive bone grafting have come into use. The outcome in a series of fractures treated in this way was evaluated.

Methods.—The 51 patients were all adults (average age, 50 years); follow-up averaged 2.5 years. All had unstable intra-articular distal radius

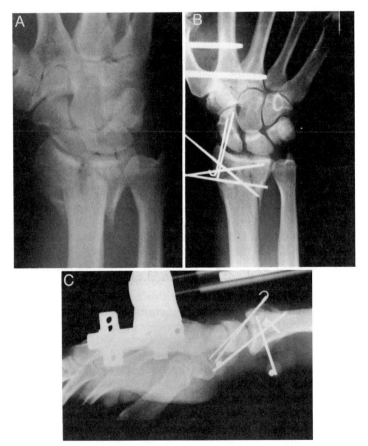

Fig 8–1.—A, unstable intra-articular distal radius fracture in a 60-year-old man. **B-C,** external fixation has been augmented using radial styloid and subarticular lunate fossa pins with subarticular supportive bone graft. Kirschner wires have secured a concomitant scaphoid fracture. (Courtesy of Seitz WH Jr, Froimson AL, Leb R, et al: *J Hand Surg* 16-A:1010–1016, 1991.)

fractures with a major radial styloid fragment, a lunate fossa fragment, and substantial dorsal or volar comminution. Bone grafting was done in 9 patients.

Technique.—Pins are inserted by a limited open surgical approach. The radius is visualized directly to allow predrilling and central insertion. The distal pin insertion is also made under direct vision with image intensification. The proximal pin is passed through the metaphyseal bases of the index and middle metacarpals, and the distal pin is passed through the index metacarpal shaft. The external fixation device is applied followed by fracture reduction. After overall length and radial tilt are restored, 2 mm more of traction is applied to increase the joint space of the radioscapholunate articulation by 2 mm. This keeps the ligaments taut during immobilization. The radial styloid is aligned to the shaft and a smooth .062 Kirschner wire placed from the tip of the styloid and secured in the ulnar cortex of the shaft. A second wire is placed dorsally to elevate the lunate fossa fragment and a third from the radial aspect of the styloid fragment directly underneath the subchondral bone of the elevated die-punch fragment. Additional wires are placed according to the degree of comminution. Bone grafts are placed if radiographs show significant lucency of the supportive bone stock.

Outcome.—There were 47 acceptable and 4 unacceptable results (Fig 8–1). One patient had reflex sympathetic dystrophy and articular collapse resulting from inadequate reduction and fixation.

Conclusions.—In unstable distal radius fractures, augmentation may be done to prevent late settling of initially well-reduced fractures. The major radial styloid fragment is fixed with a Kirschner wire and buttresses the lunate fossa and comminuted fragments. If the lunate fossa needs to be elevated 5 mm or more after styloid fixation, a supportive bone graft should be used. Immediate rehabilitation and patient education in activities of daily living and pin-site care are essential.

▶ The good results in this paper re-emphasize the need to obtain as near an anatomical reduction of distal radius fracture as possible. The combination of external fixation, augmentation with pins or a graft, or both, allows maintenance of reduction in a large percentage of the cases. In addition, the absence of complications from the external fixator, up to 40% in some series, emphasizes the necessity for direct visualization of the skeleton for pin placement.—B.P. Simmons, M.D.

Pilon Fractures of the Proximal Interphalangeal Joint

Stern PJ, Roman RJ, Kiefhaber TR, McDonough JJ (Univ of Cincinnati)
J Hand Surg 16-A:844–850, 1991   8–2

Background.—An axial loading injury of the proximal interphalangeal (PIP) joint resulting in comminution, central depression, and sagittal and coronal splay of the articular surface of the base of the middle phalanx is known as a pilon fracture. These injuries may result in pain, subluxation, stiffness, and flexion contracture of the PIP joint. The long-term results of 3 treatment methods—splinting, skeletal traction, and open reduction—were evaluated.

Methods.—Closed pilon fractures of the PIP joint were treated in 20 patients, 16 men and 4 women (average age, 31 years). The most common cause was being struck by a ball. Splinting, consisting of dorsal splint immobilization of the PIP joint in 30 degrees to 45 degrees of flexion, was done in 4 patients. Skeletal traction, consisting of a pin placed through the diaphysis of the middle phalanx and axial traction, was applied in 7 patients. Open reduction and stabilization were done in 9 patients. Results were assessed by range of motion, grip strength, pain, swelling, and radiographic appearance.

Results.—Splints were applied for an average of 5 weeks. Active range of motion was 20/85 for the PIP joint and 5/55 for the distal interphalangeal (DIP) joint. Arthrodesis had to be done for symptomatic PIP arthritis in 2 patients. The other 2 patients had pain at least with heavy activity, symptomatic PIP swelling, and limitation of motion. Radiographic findings included articular remodeling, central depression, and splaying. Traction was applied for an average of 4 weeks with active motion begun at 2.5 days. Range of motion was 10/90 for the PIP joint and 0/50 for the DIP joint. No surgery was needed. All patients had some fusiform PIP swelling, and radiographs revealed remodeling of the middle phalangeal base and varying degrees of splay. Pain was absent in 4 patients, present with axial loading in 2, and present with heavy activity in 1. In patients treated with open reduction, Kirschner pin immobilization lasted an average of 4 weeks. Results were satisfactory in 7 of 9 patients, with an average range of motion of 10/80 at the PIP joint and 5/55 at the DIP joint. One patient had PIP pyarthrosis at 3 weeks and another fell and sheared off the pin at 1.5 weeks. All patients had symmetric grip strength with mild swelling; 2 were free of pain, 4 had pain with axial loading, 1 had pain with heavy activity, and 2 had continuous pain. Radiographs showed lack of articular restoration and remodeling of the articular surface of the base of the middle phalanx.

Conclusions.—For pilon fractures of the PIP joint, skeletal traction is a safe treatment that gives results comparable to those of open reduction but without the risks. With motion, skeletal traction offers the advantage of cartilage and soft tissue nutrition. Splinting is not recommended.

▶ Comminuted, intra-articular fractures of the articular surface of the middle phalanx at the PIP joint defy good results, regardless of treatment. Early motion is to be encouraged. Although open reduction did not improve the results, the authors did not use bone graft; better reduction and maintenance of position might improve the results, especially in die-punch injuries.—B.P. Simmons, M.D.

Functional Treatment of Metacarpal Fractures: 100 Randomized Cases With or Without Fixation

Konradesen L, Nielsen PT, Albrecht-Beste E (County Hospital, Hillerød, Denmark)

Acta Orthop Scand 61:531–534, 1990

8–3

Background.—Consensus is lacking regarding the correct method of maintaining reduction and the acceptable angulation after metacarpal shaft and neck fractures. Results of treatment produced by immobilization of the wrist joints in an ulnar or dorsal plaster cast were compared with those produced while maintaining a full range of motion in a functional cast.

Methods.—One hundred patients with subcapital or diaphyseal fractures of the second through fifth metacarpal were randomized to be treated with a plaster or functional cast (Table 1). All fractures were reduced under local anesthesia using the method of Jahss. In the plaster cast group, the metacarpophalangeal (MCP) and the proximal interphalangeal joints of the involved and adjacent digits were immobilized, and the wrist was held in 20 degrees to 30 degrees of extension. The functional cast allowed free range of motion (Fig 8–2), with reduction performed after application. Both casts were removed at 3 weeks.

Results.—The functional group maintained a more anatomic reduction than the plaster cast group (Table 2). In the plaster cast group, 28 patients had a 25-degree restriction of joint movement and 24 had a 20-degree restriction in the MCP joints. In comparison, in the functional group, 4 patients had a 10-degree restriction of joint movement and 14 had a 20-degree restriction in the MCP joints. A restriction of 10 degrees in the PIP joints was seen in 16 patients in the plaster cast group compared to

TABLE 1.—Data on 100 Patients With Subcapital or Diaphyseal Metacarpal Fractures Randomized to 2 Different Treatments

Site	n	Age	Metacarpals				Hand [*]		Work cat. [†]			
		median	2.	3.	4.	5.	D	non-D	1	2	3	4
		(range)										
Subcapital												
plaster	30	20 (12-62)	4	3	4	22	22	8	9	4	11	6
functional	28	23 (16-56)	0	2	4	26	19	9	8	6	9	5
Diaphyseal												
plaster	20	24 (14-60)	2	1	6	8	11	9	6	8	2	4
functional	22	22 (14-63)	2	4	8	4	9	13	9	4	2	7

[*]D indicates dominant hand; *non-D,* nondominant hand.
[†]1 indicates students; 2, white-collar workers; 3, light-equipment operators; 4, road-construction workers.
(Courtesy of Konradesen L, Nielsen PT, Albrecht-Beste E: *Acta Orthop Scand* 61:531–534, 1990.)

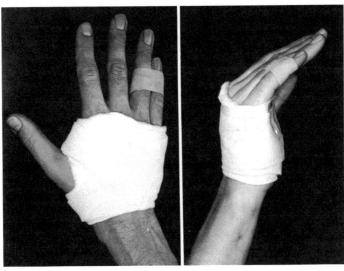

Fig 8–2.—Functional splintage of a metacarpal fracture allowing the wrist and digits a free range of motion. (Courtesy of Konradesen L, Nielsen PT, Albrecht-Beste E: *Acta Orthop Scand* 61:531–534, 1990.)

2 patients in the functional group. Grip strength was superior in the functional group at the time of cast removal, but at 3 months both groups had full grip strength. The functional cast group was able to return to work in one third of the time required for the plaster cast group (Table 3).

Conclusion.—In patients with metacarpal fractures, functional splintage appears to reduce fracture angulation and to shorten the impairment time compared to immobilization.

TABLE 2.—Comparison of Subcapital and Diaphyseal Metacarpal Fracture Angulation Before and After Reduction and Splintage and After Cast Removal

Site	Before reduction	After reduction	Cast removal
Subcapital			
plaster	27 (0-36)	27 (0-30)*	25 (0-37)*
functional	25 (0-30)	18 (0-34)	16 (0-30)
Diaphyseal			
plaster	15 (0-30)	12 (0-20)*	14 (0-25)[†]
functional	16 (0-24)	5 (0-10)	5 (0-10)

Note: Degrees are median and range.
*Plaster cast vs. functional cast, $P < .05$.
[†]Plaster cast vs. functional cast, $P < .01$.
(Courtesy of Konradesen L, Nielsen PT, Albrecht-Beste E: *Acta Orthop Scand* 61:531–534, 1990.)

TABLE 3.—Time in Days (Median and Range) Before Patients Returned to Work Divided Into Groups According to Treatment and Work

Work categories	1	2	3	4
Plaster slab	7 (1-21)*	21 (14-27)*	24 (21-30)	21 (10-27)
Functional cast	1 (1-3)	7 (1-10)	10 (1-28)	8 (7-21)

Note: For work categories, see footnote in Table 1.
*Plaster cast vs. functional cast, $P < .05$.
(Courtesy of Konradesen L, Nielsen PT, Albrecht-Beste E: *Acta Orthop Scand* 61:531–534, 1990.)

▶ Stress across fractures decreases what has been called the "fracture disease." This randomized study confirms that the functional treatment of metacarpal fractures allows alignment to be maintained while decreasing stiffness and other soft tissue sequelae. After an initial period of healing, we have allowed athletes to compete in noncontact sports using this orthosis.—B.P. Simmons, M.D.

Occupational Carpal Tunnel Syndrome in Washington State, 1984–1988

Franklin GM, Haug J, Heyer N, Checkoway H, Peck N (Univ of Washington, Seattle; Dept of Labor and Industries, Olympia, Wash)
Am J Public Health 81:741–746, 1991   8–4

Background.—A large number of lost work days and high workers' compensation costs result from occupational carpal tunnel syndrome (OCTS). A recent report from the Centers for Disease Control on carpal tunnel syndrome (CTS) noted that about half of these cases are occupational in nature, and in specific industries prevalences up to 15% have been reported. The population-based incidence of OCTS was determined for a 4-year period in Washington State.

Methods.—Cases were identified from the Washington State Workers' Compensation database, using the codes of the International Classification of Disease for CTS or median nerve neuritis. A subset of medical records was reviewed to estimate the proportion of claims with a documented physician diagnosis and the proportion meeting the criteria of the National Institute for Occupational Safety and Health for OCTS (Table 1).

Results.—In 1984–1988, 7,926 incident OCTS claims were filed. The industry-wide incidence rate was 1.74 claims/1,000 full-time equivalent workers. A significant increase in OCTS claims occurred between 1984 and 1988. Mean age in this population was 37.4 years. The female/male ratio was 1.2:1; this reflected a younger age and lower incidence in women than in previous studies of nonoccupational CTS. The female-specific incidence rate rose significantly during the period. Food processing, carpentry, egg production, wood products, and logging industries had the highest incidence of OCTS (Table 2).

TABLE 1.—NIOSH Case Definition for Occupational Carpal Tunnel Syndrome (CTS)

A. One or more of the following *symptoms* affecting at least part of the median nerve distribution: paresthesias, hypoesthesia, pain or numbness; and
B. *Objective findings consistent with CTS:*
   Either
   1) *Positive physical examination findings* – (+) Tinel's or Phalen's or decreased or absent sensation to pin prick in median nerve distribution of the hand; or
   2) *Nerve conduction findings* indicative of median nerve dysfunction across the carpal tunnel; and
C. Evidence of work-relatedness—a history of a job involving one or more of the following activities prior to development of CTS symptoms:
   1) *Frequent, repetitive use of the hand or wrist,*
   2) *Regular tasks requiring the generation of high force by the hand,*
   3) *Regular or sustained tasks requiring awkward hand positions,*
   4) *Regular use of vibrating hand tools,*
   5) *Frequent or prolonged pressure over the wrist or base of the palm.*

(From Franklin GM, Haug J, Heyer N, et al: *Am J Public Health* 81:741–746, 1991. Adapted from Cummings K, Maizlish N, Rudolph L, et al: *MMWR* 38:485–489, 1989.)

Conclusions.—Work exposure may account for a considerable proportion of physician-reported CTS; and OCTS appears to be a distinct entity. Regional industry-specific rates will vary, but some industries, such as meat and poultry processing, carpentry, and fruit and vegetable canning, will be seen in many regions. Workers' compensation data can be useful for investigating occupational conditions for which there are no other good surveillance systems.

▶ Carpal tunnel syndrome is almost epidemic in certain occupations, especially those where forceful, highly repetitive activities are required. Of note is the younger age group and the more equal sex distribution in which OCTS is seen.—B.P. Simmons, M.D.

TABLE 2.—Rates and Cases of Carpal Tunnel Syndrome by Washington Industrial Classification (WIC), 1984–1988 (Sorted by Rate)

Industrial Class Description	Cases N	Rate/FTE 1000	Rate Ratio	95% Confidence Interval
Oyster, crab, clam packing	50	25.7	14.8	(11.2, 19.5)
Meat, poultry dealers	132	23.9	13.8	(11.6, 16.4)
Packing house	55	18.5	10.6	(8.1, 13.8)
Fish canneries processing	124	18.2	10.5	(8.8, 12.5)
Carpentry	37	11.3	6.5	(4.7, 9.0)
Fruit & vegetable canning	55	10.2	5.8	(4.5, 7.6)
Egg production	30	9.8	5.6	(3.9, 8.1)
Box, shook, pallet bin manufacturing	25	9.3	5.4	(3.6, 8.0)
Sawmills, operation & maintenance	139	9.3	5.3	(4.5, 6.3)
Foundries, steel casting	37	9.0	5.2	(3.8, 7.2)
Logging operations	143	8.9	5.1	(4.4, 6.1)
Wallboard installation	43	8.4	4.8	(3.6, 6.5)
Roofwork, all types	48	8.0	4.6	(3.4, 6.1)
Boat building repair	36	7.7	4.4	(3.2, 6.1)
Plywood manufacturing	54	6.8	3.9	(3.0, 5.1)
Plastic goods manufacturing	121	6.5	3.7	(3.1, 4.5)
Food sundries manufacturing/processing	30	6.4	3.7	(2.6, 5.3)
Wood products manufacturing & assembly	53	6.4	3.7	(2.8, 4.8)
Lumber remanufacturing	26	6.4	3.7	(2.5, 5.4)
Building construction iron/steel/concrete	102	6.3	3.5	(2.9, 4.2)

(Courtesy of Franklin GM, Haug J, Heyer N, et al: *Am J Public Health* 81:741–746, 1991.)

Recovery From Symptoms After Carpal Tunnel Syndrome Surgery in Males in Relation to Vibration Exposure

Hagberg M, Nyström Å, Zetterlund B (National Institute of Occupational Health, Solna, Sweden; University Hospital, Umeå, Sweden)
J Hand Surg 16-A:66–71, 1991

8–5

Background.—Atrophy and length of history of carpal tunnel syndrome (CTS) have been identified as predictors of improvement after sur-

Patients rating of symptoms

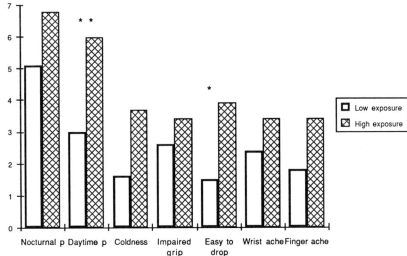

Fig 8–3.—Mean values for the patients' rating of symptoms according to Borg's new rating scale by exposure group before CTS surgery. *Low exposure* indicates the 13 operated hands with low exposure to hand-arm vibrations; *high exposure,* the 42 operated hands with high exposure to hand-arm vibrations; *nocturnal p,* nocturnal paresthesiae; *daytime p,* daytime paresthesiae; *impaired grip,* impaired grip strength; *double asterisk, P < .01; asterisk, P < .05.* (Courtesy of Hagberg M, Nyström Å, Zetterlund B: *J Hand Surg* 16-A:66–71, 1991.)

gery. The finding of persistent numbness in the hands of 10 patients with vibration syndrome after surgery for CTS prompted a follow-up investigation to determine if previous vibration exposure was a negative factor in recovery from CTS surgery.

Methods.—A total of 55 hands in 41 men undergoing surgery during a 10-year period were examined. Patients' mean age was 48 years. All had severe paresthesia and hand numbness at night, along with a positive Phalen test or distal motor latency of 4.5 ms or more in the median nerve. Mean follow-up was 5.8 years. Preoperative history of exposure to vibration was recorded in detail, including the number of hours of exposure, which hand was used, and what tool was used. Tools were then categorized according to vibration level, and an index was created by which patients were divided into high and low exposure groups.

Results.—The 13 patients in the low exposure group and the 42 in the high exposure group were similar as to age at surgery, mean values for distal latency in the median nerve, and duration between symptom onset and surgery. Mean duration of vibration for all hands was 9,816 hours, with the most common occupations being welder, concrete workers, truck and tractor driver, and chain saw operator. Both before and after surgery the high exposure group rated their symptoms of nocturnal and daytime paresthesia higher than did the low exposure group. Only 1 patient in the low-exposure group had nocturnal paresthesia at follow-up compared to 12 patients in the high exposure group (Figs 8–3 and 8–4).

Patients rating of symptoms

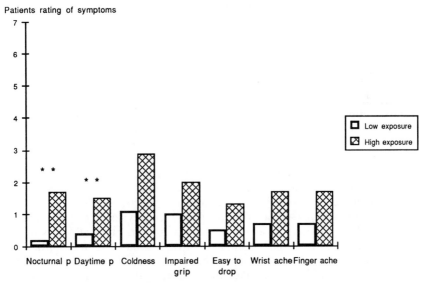

Fig 8–4.—Mean values for the patients' rating of symptoms according to Borg's new rating scale by exposure group at follow-up after CTS surgery. *Low exposure* indicates the 13 operated hands with low exposure to hand-arm vibrations; *high exposure*, the 42 operated hands with high exposure to hand-arm vibrations; *nocturnal p*, nocturnal paresthesiae; *daytime p*, daytime paresthesiae; *impaired grip*, impaired grip strength; *double asterisk*, P < .01; *asterisk*, P < .05. (Courtesy of Hagberg M, Nyström Å, Zetterlund B: *J Hand Surg* 16-A:66–71, 1991.)

Compared to the low exposure group, the high exposure group had a relative risk of 18 for nocturnal paresthesia after surgery.

Conclusions.—Recovery after carpal tunnel surgery may be affected by the patient's previous exposure to vibration. Ergonomic factors such as extreme wrist positions and repetitive power grips also may play important roles in the disorder. Workers exposed to vibration commonly report symptoms such as paresthesia.

▶ The second of 2 papers addressing CTS in the workplace, Hagberg and associates have shown that one can expect that results will not be as good when exposure has been prolonged. Early attention to symptoms and changes in the workplace are essential.—B.P. Simmons, M.D.

Dupuytren's Disease: Relation to Work and Injury
McFarlane RM (Victoria Hospital, London, Canada)
J Hand Surg 16-A:775–779, 1991   8–6

Introduction.—Current adjudication practices for workers' compensation cases involving Dupuytren's disease are inconsistent and unfair. A review of the characteristics of Dupuytren's disease relevant to manual-work and hand injury provided a basis for recommendations for consistency in the adjudication process.

Review.—Northern European peoples are most frequently affected by Dupuytren's disease. It is probably present in all races although it is rare in some. In addition, it is more common, occurs earlier, and is more aggressive in men than in women. Appearance is variable, but the typical patient is a man about 50 years of age with thickening of the palm in line with the ring or little finger that has become more pronounced. Many diseases such as diabetes mellitus, epilepsy, alcoholism, and AIDS may have a causal relationship with Dupuytren's disease; their presence decreases the probability of a work-related cause. There is no causal relationship between Dupuytren's disease and carpal tunnel syndrome, trigger finger or thumb, tenosynovitis, or degenerative arthritis. Increased diathesis to Dupuytren's disease is noted in patients with a family history of the disease, early onset, knuckle pads, or plantar nodules. There is no relationship between the occurrence of Dupuytren's disease and any specific work pattern.

Recommendations.—The occurrence of Dupuytren's disease in men younger than 40 years of age and women younger than 50 years of age suggests a causal relationship, unless the person has a strong diathesis to the disease. To exclude a strong diathesis in bilateral cases, the disease in the uninjured hand should have appeared after those ages. There should be objective evidence of injury to the hand, and Dupuytren's disease should be in the area of the injury. The disease should occur within 2 years of injury, and, if there is scar contracture, histologic proof of Dupuytren's disease should be obtained.

Conclusions.—Epidemiologic studies do not suggest that manual work hastens the onset or progression of Dupuytren's disease. In some individuals, a single injury can precipitate the onset of the disease.

▶ In the present climate of expanding worker's compensation claims and liability, this paper gives the reader some important guidelines. Although it would be more comforting to have data on the true cause of Dupuytren's disease, this approach guides one in determining whether there is or is not a causal relationship between Dupuytren's and the workplace.—B.P. Simmons, M.D.

The Sauvé-Kapandji Procedure: A Salvage Operation for the Distal Radioulnar Joint
Sanders RA, Frederick HA, Hontas RB (Hughston Orthopaedic Clinic, Columbus, Ga; Tulane Univ, New Orleans)
J Hand Surg 16-A:1125–1129, 1991   8–7

Background.—Injuries of the distal radioulnar joint and triangular fibrocartilage complex can pose difficult problems and sometimes have disabling effects. One method of treatment is arthrodesis with creation of a surgical pseudoarthrosis of the distal ulna, sometimes called the Lauenstein procedure but first described by Sauvé and Kapandji (Fig 8–5).

Methods.—Ten of 11 patients treated with the Sauvé-Kapandji procedure during a 3-year period were available for follow-up, which averaged 33 months. Posttraumatic arthritis was present in 9 patients and rheuma-

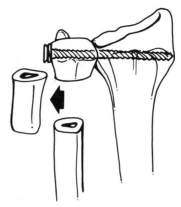

Fig 8–5.—The Sauvé-Kapandji procedure involves a distal radioulnar arthrodesis and creation of a pseudarthrosis in the distal ulna. (Courtesy of Sanders RA, Frederick HA, Hontas RB: *J Hand Surg* 16-A:1125–1129, 1991.)

toid arthritis was present in 1. Six were men and 4 women, (mean age, 36 years); they had previously had an average of 2.4 procedures on the involved wrist. Ulnar variance was determined preoperatively to determine the amount of ulna to be excised, and a 3.5-mm AO lag screw was used for permanent fixation.

Results.—There was clinical and radiographic evidence of healing at the arthrodesis site by 3 months in all patients. Results were excellent in 6 of 9 patients with posttraumatic arthritis, with an average 82 degrees of pronation and 83 degrees of supination. The other 3 patients had good results, with mild pain, average pronation of 83 degrees, and average supination of 82 degrees. In the patient with rheumatoid arthritis, results were considered excellent for 3 years, but the patient eventually required radiocarpal wrist fusion for radiocarpal arthritis. No major complications were noted; mild instability of the pseudoarthrosis site caused no functional problems. Eight patients were able to return to work at their previous level of activity.

Conclusions.—The Sauvé-Kapandji procedure is a reliable alternative for intractable disorders of the distal radioulnar joint. Recent reports discourage use of the Darrach procedure in younger patients. The Sauvé-Kapandji procedure gives good functional and cosmetic results despite mild, although sometimes painful, instability of the pseudoarthrosis.

The Darrach Procedure Defended: Technique Redefined and Long-Term Follow-Up
Tulipan DJ, Eaton RG, Eberhart RE (Hand Ctr at Roosevelt Hosp, New York)
J Hand Surg 16-A:438–444, 1991   8–8

Background.—Recently, the efficacy of the Darrach resection has been questioned, with regard to instability of the distal ulna, ulnar carpal

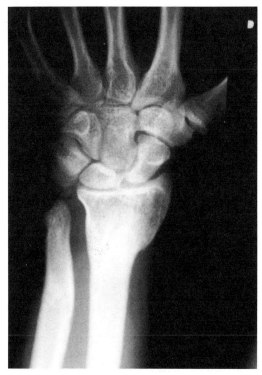

Fig 8–6.—Radiograph 26 months after operation of a student who had a severely displaced radius and ulnar fracture with residual radial shortening. The patient is free of pain, has extension, 45 degrees; flexion, 85 degrees; pronation, 80 degrees; supination, 80 degrees. As with most Darrach resections, 2–3 mm of new bone regeneration can be expected. (Courtesy of Tulipan DJ, Eaton RG, Eberhart RE: *J Hand Surg* 16-A:438–444, 1991.)

translocation, decreased grip strength, and pain. A modified Darrach procedure is described for the treatment of posttraumatic derangement of distal ulnar articulations.

Technique.—With the forearm in pronation, a dorsal hockey-stick incision is made over the distal ulna. The dorso-ulnar retinaculum is divided obliquely parallel to its fibers, creating distal, dorsal-based, and proximal, ulnar-based flaps. After subperiosteal exposure of the distal ulna, resection of the ulna begins at a level just proximal to the sigmoid notch of the radius. The osteotomy slants proximally to avoid a sharp dorsal subcutaneous prominence. Usually, less than 1 cm is resected. The periosteum is plicated in closure, and the palmar-based extensor retinaculum flap is advanced across the periosteal closure as an additional reinforcing layer. The extensor carpi ulnaris is mobilized proximally to create a straight line in its dorsal rerouting over the distal ulna. The distal extensor retinaculum flap is passed beneath the extensor carpi ulnaris tendon and sutured to itself and the dorsal retinaculum. This acts as a sling to maintain the tendon dorsally over the periosteal defect. The wrist is immobilized in slight extension to reduce tension on this sling.

Patients.—The modified Darrach distal ulnar resection was performed in 158 patients with pain and decreased range of motion after traumatic derangement of the distal radioulnar and ulnar–carpal joint; 33 were available for follow-up. Of the 33, 27 patients had Colle's or other distal radius fracture, and 7 had ulnar resection for ulnar–carpal derangement. Average follow-up was 54.4 months.

Results.—Postoperatively, extension increased by 58%, flexion by 40%, pronation by 40 degrees, and supination by 60 degrees (Fig 8–6); grip strength increased by 38%. All but 1 patient had a stable distal ulna. In 7 patients, CT scans showed no increased volar or dorsal displacement of the distal radioulnar joints when compared with the nonoperative side. Most patients had 2–3 mm of regeneration of the distal ulna. Ninety-one percent of patients had good or excellent results, and none complained of pain.

Conclusions.—The Darrach procedure is simple and can predictably provide pain relief in addition to improving strength and motion. Optimum results can be achieved with careful subperiosteal dissection of the distal ulna, minimal bony resection, and multiple layered dorsal reconstruction that includes plication of the periosteum.

▶ As Sandero et al. (Abstract 8–7) point out, results of a modified Darrach procedure in younger patients have been less than satisfactory. The Sauvé-Kapandji procedure is an attempt to solve the problem differently but makes the surgeon wary because of instability of the proximal ulna and insufficient reports of its use in traumatic cases. This article attempts to answer the question. However, the reader should take note that this is a small series. Furthermore, the inclusion of 1 patient with rheumatoid arthritis is inappropriate. In rheumatoid arthritis, despite initial good results, ongoing synovitis is likely to create degenerative joint disease between the ulna head and carpus with time. Abstract 8–8 again emphasizes that the modified Darrach procedure yields excellent results. However, it properly emphasizes that technique is important and that reconstruction rather than simple excision is mandatory. The reader should note that the average age of patients in Abstract 8–7 is 36 years and that in Abstract 8–8 is 50 years.—B.P. Simmons, M.D.

Management of Chronic Peripheral Tears of the Triangular Fibrocartilage Complex
Hermansdorfer JD, Kleinman WB (Indiana Ctr for Surgery and Rehabilitation of the Hand and Upper Extremity)
J Hand Surg 16-A:340–346, 1991   8–9

Background.—Triangular fibrocartilage injury is being more commonly recognized as a major cause of pain on the ulnar side of the wrist. Attritional perforation of the central hypovascular articular disk is more common than traumatic separation of the well-vascularized medial insertion of the triangular fibrocartilage complex (TFCC) at the fovea of the ulnar styloid. An experience with patients with chronic traumatic peripheral separation of the TFCC is described.

Methods.—Thirteen patients were treated, including 11 available for follow-up after more than 1 year. Avulsion–separation of the TFCC from the distal ulna was confirmed at surgery in all patients. The patients had severe, incapacitating ulnocarpal pain that interfered with their employment or activities of daily living and had tenderness on direct palpation that was well localized to the ulnar styloid, both dorsal and palmar. Standard hand and wrist radiographs were taken, including measurement of ulnar variance by zero rotation view. Eleven patients had a documented single episode of trauma. At arthroscopy, probing the TFCC disclosed an absence of usual resistance, or "trampoline effect"; open surgical reattachment of the avulsed portion of the TFCC to the ulna was then performed (Fig 8–7). Average follow-up was 23 months.

Results.—Eight of the 11 patients available for follow-up after more than 1 year achieved return to essentially normal activities without pain. Compared to the opposite side, grip strength averaged 87%; extension/flexion range of motion averaged 96%; radial/ulnar deviation averaged 97%; and pronosupination averaged 99%. Of the 3 patients who continued to have pain, 2 responded to subsequent distal ulna resection or ulnar shortening osteotomy. One patient, who sought no further treatment, was unable to return to competitive gymnastics.

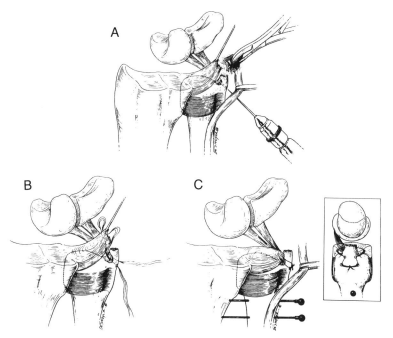

Fig 8–7.—**A,** débridement of chronic exuberant granulation and fibrous connective tissue from the injured periphery of the TFCC facilitates creation of a cancellous trough at the fovea; **B,** 3 3–0 nonabsorbable sutures are then placed through the retracted medial TFCC, and passed through drill holes at the medial base of the ulnar styloid; **C,** sutures are then tied securely to reconstitute normal resilience and tension after stabilizing the distal ulna to the radius with temporary extraarticular K-wires. (Courtesy of Hermansdorfer JD, Kleinman WB: *J Hand Surg* 16-A:340–346, 1991.)

Conclusions.—For patients with traumatic avulsion of the TFCC, surgical reattachment to the fovea at the base of the distal ulna reestablishes normal mechanics and the integral support system for the ulnar aspect of the wrist. Diagnosis requires a high index of suspicion, careful examination, and judicious use of diagnostic techniques including arthroscopy.

The Microvasculature of the Triangular Fibrocartilage Complex: Its Clinical Significance

Bednar MS, Arnoczky SP, Weiland AJ (Hosp for Special Surgery, New York)
J Hand Surg 16-A:1101–1105, 1991   8–10

Objective.—Tears of the triangular fibrocartilage complex (TFCC) may result in chronic ulnar wrist pain. Treatment choices include ulnar shortening, removal of some or all of the TFCC, or repair of the tear. Repair seems to be effective, but there are few data on the ability of the TFCC to respond in a reparative fashion. The microvasculature of the TFCC was examined to determine which patterns of tearing might respond to repair.

Methods.—Ten fresh or frozen cadaver wrists were used. The brachial or radial artery of 6 wrists was cannulated and then injected with India ink and sectioned. In the other 4 wrists, the TFCC was stained with hematoxylin and eosin fixed, sectioned, and examined by light and polarized microscopy.

Findings.—The original blood source for the TFCC was the soft tissue surrounding the ulnocarpal joint, with vessels from the peripheral capsular and synovial tissue penetrating the TFCC in a radial fashion and directed toward the center. Vascular penetration into the periphery of the TFCC varied from 10% to 40% of its width; the inner portion was always avascular. No vessels entered the complex from its radial attachment, and the fibrocartilage blended with the articular cartilage of the radius. The radial articular cartilage seemed to act as a barrier, preventing vessels from the subchondral bone from entering the TFCC.

Conclusions.—The blood supply of the TFCC is limited to the periphery; thus, tears in this area should have the potential for repair. Such tears, excluding those at the radial insertion, should be classified as type I. Those in the avascular center and at the radial insertion will not heal and should be classified as type II.

▶ For chronic ulnar-sided wrist pain attributable to an injury to the triangular fibrocartilage complex, repair is preferable to secondary procedures. Unfortunately, although surgically possible, healing may not follow. Hermansdorfer and Kleinman (Abstract 8–9) report good results in a small series when a tear from the base of the ulna styloid is repaired. This rationale is scientifically supported by the experimental findings in Abstract 8–10. An excellent study, it demonstrates the vascularity of the TFCC at its insertion on the ulna and the absence of vessels at the insertion on the distal radius. Of concern, in the clinical study (Abstract 8–9) is the absence of positive findings in the arthrogram, even with a distal radioulnar joint arthrogram. Having to depend on the "trampoline effect" at the time of arthroscopy is unsettling. However, they emphasize the clinical exam, a clear-cut history of trauma, and findings of a bony injury on plain radiographs in most of the patients.—B.P. Simmons, M.D.

Radiolunate Arthrodesis in Rheumatoid Wrist (21 Cases)
Chamay A, Della Santa D (Geneva, Switzerland)
Ann Hand Surg 10:197–206, 1991   8–11

Background.—Resection of the ulnar head may play a role in allowing collapse and translation of the carpus. Radiolunate arthrodesis may prevent this occurrence. The results of this procedure on unstable rheumatoid wrists were evaluated.

Technique.—The major indications for radiolunate arthrodesis are radiocarpal instability combined with either dorsal subluxation of the ulnar head, pain, and synovitis or ulnar drift of the fingers. A longitudinal dorsal approach is used, and the ulnar head is resected. The radiolunate joint is relocated as necessary, then fused and fixed using either a screw or a graft from the resected ulnar head. The lunate is left in neutral orientation or in less than 10 degrees of volar angulation.

Experience.—Twenty-one wrists in 19 patients underwent radiolunate arthrodesis combined with a Darrach procedure; 1 patient did not have ulnar head resection. Preoperatively, all wrists had a carpal collapse pattern—carpal height index was between .37 and .51 and the ulnar translation index between .24 and .40. Postoperatively, 13 wrists were free of pain, and 1 had a painful click. Pain and recurrence were noted in 4 patients. Wrist flexion/extension and ulnar and radial deviation were decreased, whereas forearm rotation was increased. For most patients, motion was satisfactory. Extension averaged 41 degrees, flexion 28 degrees, radial deviation 8 degrees, and ulnar deviation 23 degrees.

Conclusions.—For the rheumatoid wrist, radiolunate arthrodesis with ulnar head resection is an appropriate treatment that stabilizes ulnar transition of the carpus. It does not entirely correct significant deformities, but it inhibits their progression. Range of motion is satisfactory and functional in most patients.

▶ The Chamay procedure, or radiolunate arthrodesis, is a reasonable approach to the wrist in rheumatoid arthritis. Unfortunately, because of the nature of the disease, rarely are the prerequisites present: i.e., ulnar translocation of the carpus or collapse of both, but a relatively intact midcarpal joint. The modest success rate also indicates the progressive nature of the disease. We have found that stabilization of the carpus with this procedure allows maintenance of a good range of motion and stabilizes the carpus quite well.—B.P. Simmons, M.D.

Proximal Row Fusion as a Solution for Radiocarpal Arthritis
Bach AW, Almquist EE, Newman DM (Univ of Washington, Seattle)
J Hand Surg 16-A:424–431, 1991   8–12

Background.—Traumatic arthritis of the carpus often requires wrist arthrodesis; in some cases proximal row carpectomy may be sufficient. A series of patients with painful posttraumatic radiocarpal arthritis treated by radius-scaphoid-lunate arthrodesis were reviewed to evaluate their function and determine whether the procedure caused functional problems in other joints.

Methods.—The patients were 31 men and 5 women treated during a 6-year period. Mean age was 41.5 years, and average follow-up was 2.4 years. All patients had pain, ranging from a few months to 20 years duration as the indication for surgery. Twenty-one had chronic scapholunate separation, and 19 had arthritic changes of the radiocarpal joint. Five patients were treated for Kienböck's disease, and 5 had a history of scaphoid fracture. Standard surgical technique was use of iliac crest bone graft and internal fixation with 3.5- or 4-mm cancellous bone screws. A short arm thumb spica cast was kept in place for 2 months, after which active range of motion was allowed if there was evidence of early union.

Results.—Within 4 months all patients had fusion of the radius to the lunate. Some useful range of motion was obtained in all patients. A second procedure was needed in 2 patients. Revision of the proximal fusion to complete wrist fusion was needed because of pain in 7 patients, all of whom had arthritic changes in the midcarpal joint at the time of the limited fusion. No further operation was needed in the remaining 29 patients. Compared to the other side, average grip strength was 70%, and average wrist flexion and extension arc was 48 degrees. Return to previous employment was possible for 18 patients, including heavy labor in many cases. Wrist problems prevented return to work for 5 patients.

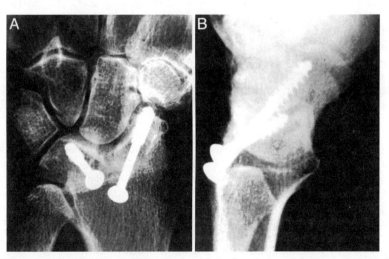

Fig 8–8.—Radiographs 2 years after proximal row fusion for treatment of chronic scapholunate dissociation. No degeneration of the midcarpal joint is seen. The position of the lunate on the lateral view is 0 degrees of extension. The patient had 15 degrees of wrist extension and 20 degrees of wrist flexion. (Courtesy of Bach AW, Almquist EE, Newman DM: *J Hand Surg* 16-A:424–431, 1991.)

Conclusions.—Radioscapholunate fusion can provide a good functional result for patients with radiocarpal arthritis, provided midcarpal arthritis is not present (Fig 8–8). It offers more wrist motion than proximal row fusion, but it is contraindicated by articular damage to the lunate fossa of the distal radius.

▶ Radioscapholunate fusion is one alternative in patients with selective radiocarpal disease where the midcarpal joint is preserved. Certainly, the average range of motion of 48 degrees is valuable. However, the period of immobilization and the reoperation rate, because of either incomplete radioscaphoid fusion or persistent pain, is significant. In these patients, many of whom have had previous surgery, proximal row carpectomy (if the lunate fossa and head of the capitate are preserved) or complete wrist fusion must be considered as well.—B.P. Simmons, M.D.

Functional Ranges of Motion of the Wrist Joint
Ryu J, Cooney WP III, Askew LJ, An K-N, Chao EYS (Mayo Clinic and Found, Rochester, Minn)
J Hand Surg 16-A:409–419, 1991   8–13

Background.—It has only recently become possible to evaluate normal wrist motion during activities. The biaxial electrogoniometer is an electromechanical linkage method that provides real-time analog data acquisition of biplanar joint motion that is reliable and reproducible with acceptable accuracy.

Methods.—Using a biaxial wrist electrogoniometer, the pattern of wrist motion during selected activities of daily living were evaluated in 40 normal participants. The amount of wrist flexion and extension and radial and ulnar deviation were measured simultaneously while performing 7 "palm placement" activities and 24 functional activities involving personal care and hygiene, diet and food preparation, and selected important work functions such as writing, driving, telephone use, hammering, using a screwdriver, and turning a key or door knob.

Results.—The average maximum range of wrist motion was 60 degrees of extension to 78 degrees of flexion and 21 degrees of radial deviation to 38 degrees of ulnar deviation. For personal care and hygiene, wrist motion from 42 degrees of extension to 54 degrees of flexion and from 40 degrees of ulnar deviation to 15 degrees of radial deviation was required (Fig 8–9). For diet and food preparation, wrist motion from 42 degrees of extension to 37 degrees of flexion and 40 degrees of ulnar deviation to 12 degrees of radial deviation was needed (Fig 8–10). To perform all 24 functional tasks, a minimal wrist motion of 60 degrees of extension, 54 degrees of flexion, 40 degrees of ulnar deviation, and 17 degrees of radial deviation was required. The majority of these activities

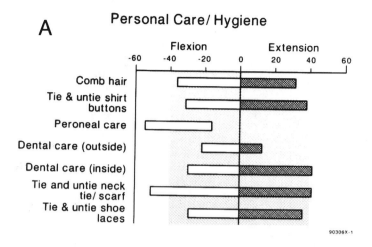

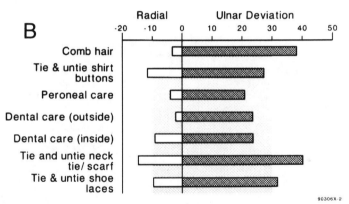

Fig 8–9.—Range of wrist motion required during personal care and hygiene activities. **A,** extension-flexion. **B,** ulnar-radial deviation. The *grey striped area* represents 70% of the maximum motion (40 degrees extension, 40 degrees flexion, 10 degrees radial deviation, and 30 degrees ulnar deviation). (Courtesy of Ryu J, Cooney WP III, Askew LJ, et al: *J Hand Surg* 16-A:409–419, 1991.)

could be achieved with 70% of the maximal range of wrist motion (40 degrees each of flexion and extension, 30 degrees of ulnar deviation, and 10 degrees of radial deviation).

Conclusions.—These findings provide normal standards for the functional range of motion of the wrist. Ulnar deviation and extension are the most important positions for wrist activities. Wrist motion of 40 degrees of extension, 40 degrees of flexion, and a total of 40 degrees of radial–ulnar deviation is required to perform the majority of activities of daily living.

▶ This interesting study concludes that more wrist motion is necessary for functional activities than previously was thought to be necessary. It is remark-

Diet/Food Preparation

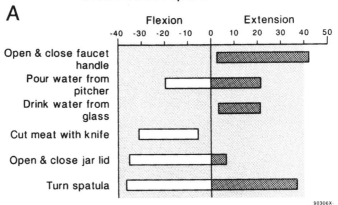

A

90306X-

Diet/Food Preparation

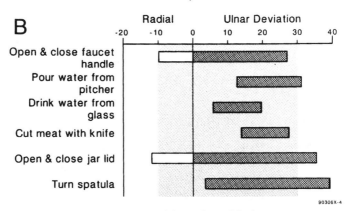

B

90306X-4

Fig 8–10.—Range of wrist motion required during diet and food preparation activities. **A,** extension-flexion. **B,** ulnar-radial deviation. (Courtesy of Ryu J, Cooney WP III, Askew LJ, et al: *J Hand Surg* 16-A:409–419, 1991.)

able how well patients adapt to a fused wrist, but attempts to find a better wrist arthroplasty should continue.—B.P. Simmons, M.D.

Analysis of Scaphoid Fracture Displacement by Three-Dimensional Computed Tomography

Nakamura R, Imaeda T, Horii E, Miura T, Hayakawa N (Nagoya University, Japan)
J Hand Surg 16-A:485–492, 1991   8–14

Background.—Because of overlapping carpal shadows and the 3-dimensional structure of the scaphoid, it has been difficult to appreciate the

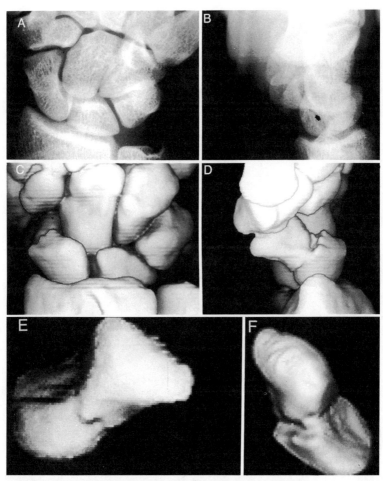

Fig 8–11.—Volar type offset is observed. **A,** posteroanterior film with the wrist in maximum ulnar deviation. No displacement was noticed. **B,** lateral radiograph indicates volar offset of the distal fragment; however, it was not easy to interpret. **C,** posteroanterior three-dimension CT (3DCT) suggests the existence of displacement; however, the details of displacement could not be appreciated well on this view. **D,** lateral 3DCT indicates clearly that the distal fragment overhung in the volar direction to the proximal fragment (volar type). This displacement was not evident on the lateral radiograph. **E,** reconstruction of the scaphoid after all other structures were eliminated from the anteroposterior 3DCT. The fracture lines ran a straight course on both the volar and the medial aspects of the scaphoid. **F,** axial top view of the 3DCT image clearly demonstrates pronation of the distal fragment. (Courtesy of Nakamura R, Imaeda T, Horii E, et al: *J Hand Surg* 16-A:485–492, 1991.)

true pattern of scaphoid fracture displacement with current radiographic and tomographic methods.

Methods.—Scaphoid fracture displacement was analyzed by 3-dimensional computed tomography (3DCT) using a high-resolution CT scanner in 25 patients. Fourteen views of the bony surface structure in each patient were reconstructed using an image editor to eliminate all images

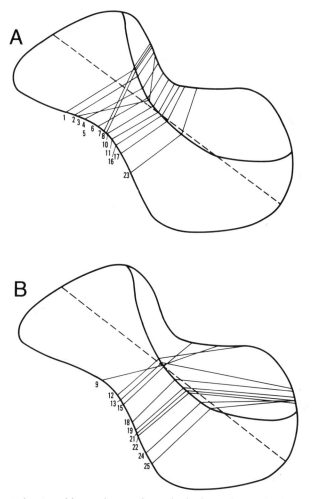

Fig 8–12.—Volar view of fracture lines on the scaphoid. The numbers in the illustration represent the individual case numbers. **A,** volar type: fracture lines run transversely in the distal third or the waist of the scaphoid. **B,** dorsal type: fracture lines lie in the waist or in the proximal third of the scaphoid. The direction of the fracture lines on the volar surface run transversely; however, fracture lines on the medial surface run horizontally through to the dorsal horizontal fracture line. (Courtesy of Nakamura R, Imaeda T, Horii E, et al: *J Hand Surg* 16-A:485–492, 1991.)

other than the scaphoid. The orientation of fracture lines on the volar and dorsal surfaces of the scaphoid, the direction of the offset, the presence of humpback deformity, and the rotatory displacement of the fracture were determined.

Results.—Scaphoid fracture displacement was readily detected and distinct in 3DCT images as compared with plain radiographs. Two different types of offset of the distal fragment relative to the proximal fragment were observed on 3DCT—the volar type and the dorsal type. In the volar type, the distal fragment overhung in the volar direction relative to the proximal segment and frequently was accompanied by humpback deformity and axial rotation (Fig 8–11). In the dorsal type, the distal fragment slipped dorsal on the proximal fragment and commonly was accompanied by humpback deformity. The volar type frequently was associated with fractures of the distal third or waist of the scaphoid, whereas the dorsal type was observed more frequently with proximally located fractures (Fig 8–12). Furthermore, the volar type frequently was associated with transverse or vertical fracture lines on both the volar and dorsal surfaces of the scaphoid, whereas the dorsal type was associated with horizontal fracture lines. All 18 fractures with an offset on radiography showed either volar or dorsal type offset on 3DCT, whereas the offset observed on 3DCT in 5 fractures was not detected on radiography. None of the measurements on radiography correlated with the direction of fracture line or the offset type.

Conclusions.—Three-dimensional CT is a useful tool in the evaluation of scaphoid fracture displacement. The 2 types of offset observed, the volar type and the dorsal type, correlate well to the fracture site and direction of fracture line.

▶ This study graphically demonstrates the usefulness of advanced imaging techniques in evaluation of scaphoid fractures. With increasing evidence that fracture displacement is an important decision-making factor in the treatment of acute scaphoid fractures and with the weak correlation between plain films and 3DCT scans. CT scans have to be considered seriously in evaluating scaphoid fractures.—B.P. Simmons, M.D.

Magnetic Resonance Imaging to Assess Vascularity of Scaphoid Non-unions

Perlik PC, Guilford WB (Walter Reed Army Med Ctr, Washington, DC; The Orthopaedic Hosp of Charlotte; Carolina Med Ctr, Charlotte, NC)
J Hand Surg 16-A:479–484, 1991   8–15

Background.—Current traditional methods of assessing bone vascularity are unreliable. Magnetic resonance imaging (MRI) has become useful in the evaluation of musculoskeletal disorders and may be particularly rewarding in the evaluation of avascular necrosis.

Methods.—In a prospective analysis, MRI was performed in 10 patients with radiographic evidence of scaphoid nonunions in an attempt to predict accurately scaphoid vascularity. The MRI scans were compared to plain radiographs, tomograms, and the operative assessment of punctate bleeding by the surgeon. The diagnostic accuracy of each test was determined relative to histologic findings on bone specimens obtained from the proximal pole.

Findings.—Histological examination revealed avascular bone consistent with ischemic necrosis in 7 specimens and viable bone in 3. The MRI scans accurately predicted scaphoid viability in all 10 patients (Fig

8–13), in contrast with diagnostic errors in 6 of 10 plain radiographs, 1 of 7 tomograms, and 2 of 10 surgical assessments.

Conclusions.—These findings indicate that MRI can accurately predict the vascularity of the ununited scaphoid. With further follow-up of these patients, the healing ability of the avascular scaphoid nonunions may be answered.

▶ Similar to Abstract 8–14, hopefully, this new imaging technique will eventually allow the surgeon to predict more accurately the outcome of surgery. This is a small series and does not report the incidence of union. Although not the goal of the study, that correlation will be necessary to assess the value of this expensive technique.— B.P. Simmons, M.D.

Compression Syndromes in Reflex Sympathetic Dystrophy
Grundberg AB, Reagan DS (Iowa Methodist Med Ctr, Des Moines)
J Hand Surg 16-A:731–736, 1991   8–16

Background.—Reflex sympathetic dystrophy (RSD) can cause profound disability and seems to worsen by some active process. Many patients with associated compression syndromes are resistant to treatment; decompression of the affected nerves may give dramatic improvement. The outcomes of treatment of patients with RSD and compression syndromes were evaluated.

Patients.—All 93 patients with RSD were treated initially with active exercises and intramuscular injection of long-acting methylprednisolone. Twenty-two failed to improve or got worse. There were 16 women and 6 men (average age, 65 years); 10 were retired, 4 were homemakers, and 3 did industrial work. The precipitating cause was injury in 18 patients and operation in 4; the most common injury was Colles' fracture. Rest pain was present in 20 patients, night pain in 16, and pain with motion in all. Twenty-one had numbness and tingling, and 21 had swelling. Underlying carpal tunnel syndrome was present in all patients; in addition, 5 had cubital tunnel syndrome, 1 had ulnar tunnel syndrome, and 1 had a herniated cervical disk. Surgical decompression was done an average of 12 weeks after onset, with systemic long-acting methylprednisolone administered intraoperatively and at 2-week intervals postoperatively if needed. Average follow-up was 22 months.

Results.—Proximal interphalangeal (PIP) joint motion improved an average of 41 degrees. All patients had relief of motion and night pain, and rest pain was eliminated in 19 and mild in 3. Grip strength improved an average of 23 pounds. Swelling was improved in all patients and eliminated in 13.

Conclusions.—Patients with resistant RSD also may have compression syndromes, which must be treated to optimize treatment of RSD. Nerve decompression relieves most pain, including night and motion pain, and this

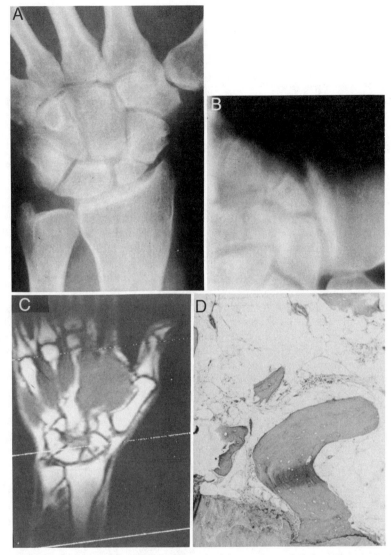

Fig 8–13.—Man, aged 26 years, sustained a scaphoid fracture 8 years before presentation. **A,** plain radiograph shows nonunion. Vascularity of the fragments was believed to be normal. **B,** tomogram of the wrist incorrectly interpreted as avascular necrosis of the proximal pole. **C,** single coronal MR scan (TE31, TR500) shows near normal signal of proximal pole, suggesting normal vascularity. **D,** histologic section shows normal marrow contents and viable bone. (Hematoxylin-eosin; original magnification, ×200). (Courtesy of Perlik PC, Guilford WB: *J Hand Surg* 16-A:479–484, 1991.)

is highly gratifying to patients. Significant PIP motion can be gained, frequently in the first few weeks, but in some patients up to 6 months later.

▶ Reflex sympathetic dystrophy can be an untoward result of an injury or a surgical procedure and can be enormously trying for both the patient and the treating physician. The authors correctly indicate that entrapment neuropathies may be involved in the complex pathophysiology; despite one's reluctance to perform surgery in an already-compromised extremity, decompression is indicated.—B.P. Simmons, M.D.

Muscle Injury Induced Beneath and Distal to a Pneumatic Tourniquet: A Quantitative Animal Study of Effects of Tourniquet Pressure and Duration
Pedowitz RA, Gershuni DH, Schmidt AH, Fridén J, Rydevik BL, Hargens AR (Univ of California, San Diego; University of Umeå, Sweden; Gothenberg University, Sweden; NASA Ames Research Facility, Moffett Field, Calif)
J Hand Surg 16-A:610–621, 1991   8–17

Background.—The use of a pneumatic tourniquet may result in neuromuscular injury, causing postoperative weakness, edema, stiffness, dysesthesia, or pain, which may be wrongly attributed to surgical trauma or lack of patient motivation. In the past, recommendations for "safe" tourniquet times were based mainly on studies of ischemia distal to the tourniquet. In a rabbit model, skeletal muscle injury induced beneath and distal to a pneumatic tourniquet was analyzed quantitatively.

Methods.—Pneumatic tourniquets were applied to the hindlimbs of New Zealand white rabbits for 1, 2, or 4 hours at cuff inflation pressures of 125, 200, or 350 mm Hg. Two days later, ^{99m}Tc pyrophosphate uptake and correlative histologic findings were used to assess tissue damage. The contralateral limbs served as controls.

Results.—On staining with Evans blue dye, no discoloration was noted in muscles from animals undergoing compression for 1 hour,

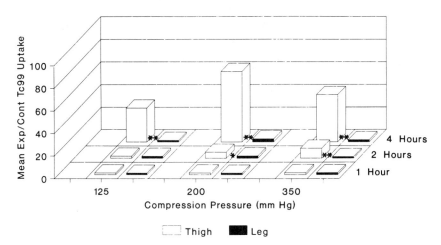

Fig 8–14.—Muscle injury induced beneath (thigh) and distal (leg) to a pneumatic tourniquet applied for various pressures and durations. The ^{99}Tc uptake ratios were statistically significantly increased in all groups (ratios >1). Thigh uptake was significantly greater than leg uptake in the higher pressure and longer duration groups (*$P < .05$; **$P < .01$, paired t tests). (Courtesy of Pedowitz RA, Gershuni DH, Schmidt AH, et al: *J Hand Surg* 16-A:610–621, 1991.)

whereas obvious discoloration was noted in thigh muscles of animals undergoing compression for 2 or 4 hours. All groups showed increased ^{99m}Tc uptake. Uptake ratios were greater in the thigh than in the leg in animals that underwent 2 hours of compression at 200 and 350 mm Hg and in all animals undergoing 4 hours of compression (Fig 8–14). On 2-way analysis of variance, tourniquet time, cuff pressure, and the combination of these variables had significant effects in the compressed thigh. In the leg, tourniquet time and the interaction term were significant, but cuff pressure was not. There were few histologic abnormalities in the 1-hour groups. Thigh muscles compressed for 2 hours at 125 mm Hg showed some fiber necrosis and cellular infiltration but no central nuclei or hyaline degeneration. Those compressed for 2 hours at the higher pressures frequently had fiber necrosis, sometimes regional necrosis, and signs of hyaline degeneration. Severe focal and regional necrosis were noted in the thigh muscles of all animals undergoing 4 hours of compression. In the legs, the most severe changes after 2 hours were occasional focal fiber necrosis and a local inflammatory response. More severe abnormalities were present after 4 hours, but these were variable.

Conclusions.—Muscle injury caused by tourniquet compression results from a complex interaction between tourniquet pressure and duration. The lowest possible pressure should be used, but injury can still occur with longer compression times. Significant injuries can occur at inflation pressures and times commonly used in practice; use of low pressures can be facilitated by wide or limb-shaped tourniquets or direct determination of the minimal pressure needed to occlude blood flow.

▶ This important study emphasizes the deleterious effect of direct pressure on muscle and nerve; previous studies have emphasized injury distal to the tourniquet. Certainly, every effort needs to be made to use the shortest tourniquet time possible at the lowest pressure. If possible, the use of 2 tourniquets on the proximal extremity, each only being used for 1 hour, will still give 2 hours of tourniquet control and minimize injury.—B.P. Simmons, M.D.

Prosthetic Silicone Scaphoid Strains: Effects of Intercarpal Fusions
Toby EB, Glisson RR, Seaber AV, Urbaniak JR (Duke Univ, Durham NC)
J Hand Surg 16-A:469–473, 1991   8–18

Background.—Reactive synovitis occurs in three fourths of patients after placement of a scaphoid implant. A trial was conducted to determine whether shielding from stress and subsequent strain across the prosthesis by partial intercarpal arthrodesis prevents this particular synovitis.

Methods.—Strains within a silicone scaphoid prosthesis were measured in 5 fresh upper extremities through a functional range of motion under loaded conditions in both the nonfused wrist and the wrist with capitate-lunate (C-L) and capitate-hamate-lunate-triquetral (C-H-L-T) intercarpal fusions.

Results.—Average compressive strains were reduced by 18.4% by D-L fusions and by 28.5% by C-H-L-T fusions. Similarly, tensile strains were reduced by 10.8% by C-L fusions and by 26.3% by C-H-L-T fusions. With partial fusions, there were no reductions in strains in radial deviated wrist positions and in a position of extension.

Conclusions.—Modest reductions in strains across a silicone scaphoid implant can be achieved with partial intercarpal fusions. However, this effect is position-dependent and may not be sufficient to prevent the formation of particulate synovitis.

▶ The incidence of Silastic synovitis in the carpus has been reported to be as high as 50% after the use of carpal bone implants. Intercarpal fusion has been proposed as a means of adequately shielding the implant. Toby et al. demonstrate that, at most, a scaphoid implant has only a 28.5% "shield." Although it still needs to be seen whether this may be sufficient to avoid Silastic synovitis, this editor would still avoid carpal bone implants if at all possible.—B.P. Simmons, M.D.

Acute and Chronic Ischemia of the Hand: Pathophysiology, Treatment, and Prognosis

Jones NF (Univ of Pittsburgh)
J Hand Surg 16-A:1074–1083, 1991   8–19

Background.—There has been little attention in the literature to long-term follow-up of patients with acute and chronic ischemia of the hand, perhaps because they are managed by many different specialists. Prophylactic surgical intervention might improve prognosis for patients with se-

TABLE 1.—Causes of Ischemia of the Hand

Etiologic factor		*No. of cases*
Atherosclerosis/Buerger's disease		9
Renal vascular disease ± diabetes		8
Connective tissue disorders		19
Scleroderma	15	
Systemic lupus erythematosus	2	
Mixed connective tissue disease	1	
Wegener's ganulomatosis	1	
Meningococcal septicemia		2
Polycythemia		1
Intravenous drug injections		2
Carcinoma of the lung		1
Radial artery cannulation		3
Vibration		3
Embolus		2
	Total	50

(Courtesy of Jones NF: *J Hand Surg* 16-A:1074–1083, 1991.)

TABLE 2.—Pathophysiologic Mechanisms Producing
Ischemia

Mechanism		No.	%
Emboli		3	6
Vasospasm		5	10
"Sludging"	4		
		14	28
Thrombosis	10		
Occlusive disease alone		13	26
Occlusive disease with associated vasospasm or external compression		15	30

(Courtesy of Jones NF: *J Hand Surg* 16-A:1074–1083, 1991.)

vere Raynaud's phenomenon, digital ulceration, or incipient gangrene, but the indications are imprecise.

Methods.—Fifty consecutively treated patients with acute and chronic ischemia of the hand were investigated during a 4-year period. Forty-four patients were monitored prospectively by a standard protocol after systemic investigation; the rest were reviewed retrospectively. Twenty-seven were female and 23 male; their ages ranged from 9 to 74 years. There were 30 chronic and 20 acute cases. The systematic examination included palpation of pulses, Allen testing, Doppler ultrasound, digital plethysmography, and angiography.

Results.—A specific cause of ischemia was identified in 49 patients, the most common being connective tissue disorders (Table 1). The mechanisms of ischemia included occlusive disease associated with vasospasm or external compression, thrombosis or "sludging," occlusive disease alone, vasospasm alone, and emboli (Table 2). Emergency treatment with intraarterial streptokinase, intravenous heparin, or dextran 40 and continuous stellate ganglion blocks were required in 10 patients. Radial artery thrombosis necessitated emergency microsurgical revascularization in 3 patients. Chronic ischemia was managed with nifedipine, 30–60 mg/day, and pentoxifylline, 1,200 mg/day. Of the patients with chronic digital ischemia, 14 had microsurgical revascularization, and 7 had digital sympathectomy as prophylactic procedures. Eighteen amputations were required for end-stage gangrene, and incidence of recurrent digital ulcerations was 20%. Six patients died during follow-up, 5 of myocardial infarction.

Conclusions.—Immediate diagnosis, best accomplished with the pencil Doppler probe and emergency angiography, is essential in acute ischemia of the hand. Unfortunately, microsurgical revascularization is only palliative, because the underlying arteriopathy generally will progress in the vein grafts as well as in the remaining digital arteries.

▶ This is an excellent review of an uncommon problem that is extremely difficult to treat. Chronic ischemia, not only because of the potential for tissue loss but also because of the severe pain, can be overwhelmingly disabling. Until now, surgery has rarely been thought to be beneficial. Although 18 patients eventually required amputation and 20% had recurrent digital ulcerations, the success rate, especially in terms of pain relief, is sufficiently high to consider the surgical alternatives.—B.P. Simmons, M.D.

Surgery of the Spastic Thumb-in-Palm Deformity
Matev I (Institute of Orthopaedics and Traumatology, Sofia, Bulgaria)
J Hand Surg 16-B:127–132, 1991   8–20

Background.—Treatment of the spastic thumb-in-palm deformity has been controversial in the past 60 years. An experience with the surgical treatment of this deformity was described.

Methods.—A total of 61 patients with cerebral palsy were treated in the past 20 years at 1 center. Patients were 20 females and 41 males aged 6–40 years. Forty-eight patients were 11–25 years of age. Follow-up after surgery for 56 patients was 2–15 years. The surgical procedure involved lengthening of the long flexor of the thumb, proximal thumb intrinsic release, and augmentation of abduction-extension of the thumb. Bone-stabilizing procedures were not done.

Results.—The results of surgery were considered very good in 18 patients, good in 28, fair in 6, and poor in 4. In very good results, the deformity was corrected and the thumb did not remain in the palm when the patient moved the hand and fingers; a normal grip and pinch were achieved. In patients with good results, the deformity was corrected, and the grip was good. However, in pinch, the thumb pulp touched the lateral aspect of the index finger. In patients with fair results, the deformity was partially corrected, and in those with poor results, there was no improvement.

Conclusions.—A good and lasting result in the treatment of spastic thumb-in-palm deformity can be achieved without using bone stabilizing procedures. When this deformity is seen in conjunction with pronation and flexion contractures of the forearm and of the wrist and fingers, respectively, these other contractures must be treated first.

▶ Correction of the thumb-in-palm deformity is one of the most difficult corrections to achieve in the spastic hand. Matev's classification emphasizes findings on the physical exam to help in preoperative planning. Correctly, he emphasizes avoidance of "bone-block" procedures in abduction.—B.P. Simmons, M.D.

9 Trauma and Amputation

Introduction

Treatment of trauma by orthopedic surgeons is very well represented in the literature again this year. The trend toward reporting results in meaningful functional terms, rather than merely reporting the number of cases that healed or had complications, is continuing. In the next few years, all areas in orthopedics and other branches of medicine will be required to demonstrate the effectiveness, particularly the cost-effectiveness, of treatment. Many papers in this year's selection address the success and cost-effectiveness of immediate or early treatment of severe injuries. Interest continues in establishing guidelines for salvage versus immediate amputation of high-energy injuries of the tibia, and the advantages of prolonged salvage attempts are now being questioned in the upper extremity as well. The relatively recent surge of interest in pelvic and acetabular reconstruction created a need for long-term functional outcome studies, which are now beginning to appear. They will have to demonstrate successful outcomes and the cost-effectiveness of these complex, highly technical, and often prolonged operations. From all indications, very early and aggressive anatomical skeletal reconstruction and soft tissue management of high-energy injuries appear to be among the most cost-effective programs in surgery. An underlying reason for this effectiveness is that the average trauma patient is between 32 and 35 years of age, a population that potentially has more than 30 years of productive working life remaining. Future clinical studies will be needed to compare functional results of treatment protocols and the ability of patients to return to work with the cost of treatment.

This year's papers have been divided into 8 sections: General Traumatology, Pelvic and Acetabular Fractures, Amputation Topics, Stimulation of Healing, Soft Tissue Management, Rehabilitation, Complications, and, finally, New Technology and Implant Designs.

Sigvard T. Hansen, M.D.

General Traumatology

Initial Management of Open Fractures Sustained in the M1 Aircraft Disaster

Learmonth DJA, Martindale JP, Rowles JM, Tait GR, Kirsh G, Sheppard I, the Nottingham, Leicester, Derby and Belfast (NLDB) Study Group (Leicester Royal Infirmary, England; Derbyshire Royal Infirmary, England; Queen's Medical Center, Nottingham, England; Queen's University of Belfast, Northern Ireland)
Injury 22:207–211, 1991
9–1

Background.—A large number of passengers survived the M1 crash at the East Midlands airport on January 8, 1989. Of a total of 126 passengers and crew, there were 87 initial survivors, and 83 who lived until hospital admission. The initial management of the many open fractures sustained in the crash is documented. Early results of treatment were evaluated, and injuries were correlated with the crash damage.

Patients.—Twenty-eight of the survivors sustained a total of 40 open fractures. Nineteen of the fractures were classified as grade 3, 16 as grade 2, and 5 as grade 1. Thirty-four involved the lower limb, with 15 identified as fractures of the tibial diaphysis. None of the open fractures was splinted or dressed at the crash site during the first hour. At the hospital all patients received an antibiotic, and their fractures were placed in temporary splints and covered with sterile dressings soaked in povidone-iodine solution. The mean time between the moment of the crash and surgical treatment was 6.25 hours.

Results.—Despite the violence of the injuries and contamination from soil at the crash site, the incidence of wound infection (15%), delayed wound healing (7.5%), and skin flap necrosis (7.5%) was comparable to that of other series. There were 2 hospital deaths among the patients with open fractures, both the result of severe chest injuries.

Conclusion.—The overall results of the treatment of open fractures were satisfactory despite the severity of the injuries. This success can be attributed to the fact that 3 major hospitals were near the crash site, and survivors were dealt with as quickly as possible by senior surgical and anesthetic staff.

▶ Interesting for its account of a large number of orthopedic injuries sustained by air-crash survivors, this retrospective review also reports a much higher incidence of primary closure of open wounds than would be recommended in North American trauma centers. Of 40 open fractures, only 3 significant infections occurred that might be attributed to closure. Three other infections occurred in 1 patient whose wounds had been left open, but this patient died of chest complications. An account of such a disaster emphasizes the need for highly skilled, regionally dispersed trauma teams to maximize the survival and long-term functional outcomes of victims.— S.T. Hansen, M.D.

Forecasting of the Course and Outcome of Shock in Severe Mechanical Traumas

Nazarenko GI, Mironov NP (Central Institute of Traumatology and Orthopedics, Moscow)
Clin Orthop 266:27–33, 1991   9–2

Background.—The ability to predict the course and outcome of shock in severe mechanical trauma would help physicians make decisions about the treatment of such patients. Anatomical and functional data alone are not highly correlated with the real and forecasted outcomes of shock. The use of a dynamic forecasting technique which would incorporate data obtained during a fixed period, would be a better approach.

Methods.—Multifactorial regression models were developed using data from 933 patients with polytrauma and shock. These models of course and outcome had a high predictive value. A two-part data sheet was designed to provide a rating system predicting the duration of shock in surviving patients and the life span of patients who eventually die. Some of the factors considered in the development of the rating system were systemic hemodynamics, hematocrit number, blood density, arteriovenous difference in oxygen saturation, and rectocutaneous temperature gradient.

Conclusions.—The method described allows a correct assessment of shock outcome in 87% of patients. It also permits a tentative determination of shock duration in patients who survive and of the life span of patients who eventually die. Forecasting through this method allows physicians to determine necessary parameters under any conditions and in any emergency which is crucial during a mass influx of patients.

▶ A very complex and interesting approach for determining the triage and prognosis of severely injured patients is described in this study. The Moscow method, which evaluates systemic hemodynamics using a rating system correlated to a scale plotting arterial pressure against pulse rate, is very interesting when compared with pulmonary (Swan-Ganz) catheterization and other standard high-tech methods.—S.T. Hansen, M.D.

Early Orthopedic Intervention in Burn Patients With Major Fractures

Dossett AB, Hunt JL, Purdue GF, Schlegel JD (Univ of Texas, Dallas)
J Trauma 31:888–893, 1991   9–3

Background.—The appropriateness of surgically treating concurrent orthopedic trauma in burn patients is controversial. Major fracture management in a burn unit was evaluated.

Patients.—A group of 101 patients was treated for major fractures and burn injuries during a 10-year period. Twenty-eight patients with 34 fractures underwent early operative fixation. The patients had a mean TBSA burn of 20%. Ten fractures were open, and 24 were closed. Three fourths of the patients underwent a definitive orthopedic procedure within 24 hours of burn. Intramedullary nails were used in 13 patients; ORIF was used in 15. External fixation was used in 3 patients and percutaneous fixation was used in 4 patients. Ten patients had burns overlying the fracture site. In these patients, the surgical incision was made through burned tissue. Four occurred in patients with open fractures.

Results.—The 2 orthopedic complications that occurred were a nonunion of a femoral neck fracture and angulation of a tibial plateau fracture. The nonorthopedic complications were pulmonary in 5 patients, wound in 4, cellulitis in 2, neurologic in 2, gastrointestinal in 1, bacteremia in 1, and amputations in 6. No wound infections occurred in any of the orthopedic incisions. Four patients in the series died.

Conclusions.—The goal of orthopedic management in burn victims is to achieve early reduction to permit optimal wound care and early patient mobility. A team approach is mandatory for patient selection and treatment.

▶ Unfortunately, this study is not as effective as a prospective or randomized study would have been in proving the value of the protocol and in resolving the controversy surrounding fracture management in burn patients. However, it does demonstrate that open reduction can be carried out in burn patients without harboring significant concerns about wound infection. Clearly, internal fixation of fractures is as beneficial for decreasing pain, enhancing mobility, and facilitating management of soft tissues in patients with burns as it is in patients with multiple injuries.—S.T. Hansen, M.D.

Evaluation and Treatment of Atlas Burst Fractures (Jefferson Fractures)
Kesterson L, Benzel E, Orrison W, Coleman J (Univ of New Mexico, Albuquerque; Louisiana State Univ, Shreveport)
J Neurosurg 75:213–220, 1991   9–4

Background.—Several large series of atlas burst fractures have been reviewed recently but they have not concentrated on diagnosis and treatment of atlas ring burst fractures (Jefferson fractures).

Methods.—Seventeen patients aged 4 to 28 years with the diagnosis of Jefferson fracture were treated at 1 center between 1982 and 1989. All complained of cervical or occipital pain, or both, after sustaining trauma. Only 1 patient showed a neurologic deficit. Routine radiographic evaluation consisted of plain radiographs, including open-mouth anteroposterior views, and CT scans; findings were confirmed by conventional tomography. Stable Jefferson fractures were treated with external immobilization. Unstable injuries occurred in 4 patients. They were treated first with early operative fixation with occiput–C2 wiring and fusion and then with external immobilization with a Minerva jacket.

Results.—All 14 patients available for follow-up for at least 1 year had reduced pain, and the single patient with a neurologic deficit returned to normal. Three patients with unstable Jefferson fractures had no complaints of restricted cervical movement at 1 year after surgery. The fourth patient had an associated type II odontoid fracture, and, after an occiput–C2 fusion, died of pulmonary complications related to associated injuries. The most common concurrent upper cervical spine fracture was a type II odontoid fracture, seen in all patients with unstable Jefferson fractures, including the sole patient with a neurologic deficit.

Conclusions.—Stable Jefferson fractures can be treated effectively without complications with Minerva jackets or rigid collar stabilization. Diagnosis of this injury may be difficult or delayed as a result of absence of neurologic deficits and concern about associated injuries. An adequate open-mouth anteroposterior x-ray examination of the atlantoaxial articulations is usually pathognomonic for the diagnosis.

▶ The authors present both a good retrospective review of 17 patients treated at Louisiana State University for Jefferson's fractures and a review of Jefferson's original paper. The proposed treatments, based on anatomy and cadaver studies, make a good case for occipital–C2 fusion for significantly unstable fractures. Although the recommended surgery was demonstrated to be quite safe, the risks of conservative treatment in unstable cases were discussed only theoretically. Similarly, the amount of functional disability in patients after occipital–C2 fusion was only discussed in potential terms but was not evaluated.—S.T. Hansen, M.D.

Mediastinal Widening Associated With Fractures of the Upper Thoracic Spine
Bolesta MJ, Bohlman HH (Case Western Reserve Univ; VA Med Ctr, Cleveland)
J Bone Joint Surg 73-A:447–450, 1991   9–5

Background.—When chest radiography of trauma victims reveals widening of the mediastinum, aortic injury is usually diagnosed. Any mediastinal structures or the thoracic spine might be injured, but because traumatic disruption of the aorta is the most serious of these injuries, immediate diagnosis and treatment may be necessary for survival of the patient. Incomplete traumatic disruption of the aorta may result in paraplegia or paraparesis caused by ischemia of the spinal cord, but similar clinical and radiographic findings may result from a fracture of the upper thoracic spine. Three patients in major motor-vehicle accidents each with a widened mediastinum and a paraparesis or a paraplegia who had initial erroneous diagnoses of disruption of the aorta were described.

Case Report 1.—Girl, 17, had subjective paresis of the left lower extremity and 4 fractured ribs. Results of aortic arteriography were normal at initial evaluation. Because of persistent thoracic pain and weakness of the left leg at 3 months after the injury, this patient was seen by an orthopedic surgeon. His impression of the leg weakness was that it was attributable to a psychological stress reaction. Continuing pain in the upper thorax at 20 months after injury prompted the patient to consult another orthopedic surgeon who found a burst fracture of the third thoracic vertebra with 53 degrees of kyphosis in radiograph. There were a few slight neurologic deficits. A thoracic myelogram with a CT scan revealed compression of the anterior aspect of the spinal cord by a fragment of the fractured vertebra. A transthoracic decompression of the spinal cord and a posterior arthrodesis of the spine without correction of the kyphosis resulted in absence of symptoms or neurologic deficits 7 years later.

Case Report 2.—Man, 22, had a fracture of the left tibia and a laceration of the galea aponeurotica at initial evaluation. Results of neurologic examination and chest radiograph were normal. The galeal laceration was sutured, and the tibial fracture was repaired. Postoperatively, diminished motor function in the left leg and hypoesthesia on the right were noted. At that time, radiography showed a burst fracture at the fourth thoracic vertebra and mediastinal widening;

an aortogram was normal, but a myelogram showed a complete block at the fourth thoracic level. Transthoracic decompression of the spinal cord, insertion of bone grafts in the fourth thoracic vertebra, and a posterior arthrodesis of the spine resulted in complete neurologic recovery and absence of complaints referable to the spine 2 years postoperatively.

Case Report 3.—Man, 23, was brought to an emergency room with paraplegia. Radiographs showed persistent mediastinal widening even after repair of fractured ribs and sternum; arteriography showed an intact aorta. Radiographs of the thoracic spine, confirmed with CT, showed a fracture-subluxation of the fifth and sixth thoracic vertebrae. A complete paraplegia caudad to the thoracic fracture remained.

Conclusions.—Whenever mediastinal widening is noted on radiographs of trauma victims, fracture of the thoracic spine should be included in the differential diagnosis. Such a fracture may be difficult to visualize on standard lateral radiographs, and in obese patients CT or MRI may be needed.

▶ This article presents an excellent discussion of differential diagnosis between aortic injuries and upper thoracic spine fractures with mediastinal widening.— S.T. Hansen, M.D.

Orthopaedic Trauma in Men: The Relative Risk Among Drinkers and the Prevalence of Problem Drinking in Male Orthopaedic Admissions

Chick J, Rund D, Gilbert M-A (Royal Edinburgh Hospital, Scotland; Ohio State Univ, Columbus; The Royal Infirmary, Edinburgh)
Ann R Coll Surg Eng 73:311–315, 1991   9–6

Background.—Acute ethanol intoxication is clearly related to traumatic injury. A standardized interview was administered to patients admitted to the orthopedic wards of one hospital after an accident resulting in significant orthopedic trauma to define the frequency with which problem drinkers are admitted to such a service.

Methods.—The 369 men admitted to the acute orthopedic ward were asked about their accident, their alcohol intake, and alcohol-related problems in the past 2 years. The results of this interview were compared with data from men participating in a community survey.

Results.—The risk of orthopedic admission was increased in drinkers consuming 21 units of alcohol per week or more compared with those drinking less than this amount in men aged 31–50 years. Thirty-four percent of the orthopedic patients met a criterion for problem drinking based on self-reported alcohol consumption or medical and social problems associated with alcohol, or both. Thirteen percent of the patients thought that alcohol contributed to their accident. According to the interviewer's evaluation, alcohol contributed to the accident of 19% of the patients; 76% of these patients were classifiable as problem drinkers. Twenty-six patients said the accident had made them consider changing their drinking habits.

Conclusions.—The estimate that 19% of these admissions are alcohol-related is probably low. Problem drinkers on an orthopedic ward can be identified and may benefit from referral to a counseling service.

▶ The authors make an excellent preliminary attempt to investigate the role of alcohol in trauma. The incidence of alcohol-related injury, which is a major public health concern, no doubt has been underreported here.—S.T. Hansen, M.D.

Treatment of Ipsilateral Fractures of the Distal Femur and Femoral Shaft
Wood EG, Savoie FH, Vander Griend RA (Univ of Mississippi Med Ctr, Jackson; Univ of Florida, Gainesville)
J Orthop Trauma 5:177–183, 1991   9–7

Background.—Fractures involving both the femoral shaft and distal femur (intercondylar or supracondylar) are rare and may require a combination or a modification of fixation techniques. The incidence, treatment options, problems, and outcome of patients with this combination fracture were evaluated.

Patients and Methods.—The 13 patients with combination fractures treated from 1981 to 1987 comprised 4% of all patients with femoral fractures. Of the 12 men and 1 woman (average age, 35), 11 had additional injuries. Nine distal femur fractures were intra-articular. Fixation techniques included plate fixation with a long blade plate used to treat both fractures or separate plates for the supracondylar and shaft fractures. In 3 patients an interlocking nail was used with distal interlocking screws placed as lag screws. One patient was treated with Ender nails.

Results.—Although 2 patients required additional surgical procedures to achieve union, all fractures united after 12–104 weeks. The average total arc of knee motion was 90 degrees, with knee flexion ranging from 85 degrees to 125 degrees and extension from 0 to a 10 degree extension lag. Although no patient was asymptomatic after 18–96 months of follow-up, 10 resumed their preinjury functional level.

Conclusions.—Treatment of this rare injury pattern requires meticulous preoperative planning to determine the best method of stabilization. Priority should be given to restoration of the articular surface and alignment of the distal femur. No single method appears suitable for all patients. Although intramedullary nailing is the preferred method of fixation for femoral shaft fractures, most intra-articular distal femur fractures cannot be stabilized using current interlocking techniques, and plate fixation of the shaft fracture may be necessary in these cases.

▶ A difficult problem is discussed, and functional outcomes are evaluated in this thoughtful retrospective review. The authors emphasize meticulous preoperative planning, use of available technology, and restoration of the articular surface of the distal femur—all good advice. Not mentioned specifically but equally important are the use of biologic soft tissue reduction techniques to preserve all possible blood supply to the bone and the anatomical realignment of the femoral shaft.—S.T. Hansen, M.D.

The Effect of Concomitant Chondral Injuries Accompanying Operatively Reduced Malleolar Fractures

Lantz BA, McAndrew M, Scioli M, Fitzrandolph RL (Univ of Arkansas, Little Rock; Vanderbilt Univ, Nashville; Texas Tech Univ, El Paso, Tex)
J Orthop Trauma 5:125–128, 1991   9–8

Background.—In the treatment of malleolar fractures, the best clinical results are achieved when an anatomical reduction is obtained and maintained until the fractures are healed. However, despite anatomical surgical reduction and stable fixation, ankle pain or tibiotalar arthrosis, or both, have occurred. This might be caused by unrecognized injuries to the cartilaginous surfaces of the tibiotalar joint. The effects of concomitant chondral injuries associated with reduced malleolar fractures were examined.

Methods.—Sixty-three patients with isolated closed melleolar fractures underwent open reduction and internal fixation using standard AO methods between 1984 and 1987. In each patient, the entire talar dome was inspected during surgery. Fractures were type A in 7 patients, type B in 37, and type C in 19. Forty-nine percent of patients had injuries to the talar dome cartilage. These injuries ranged from mild scuffing to free osteochondral fragments.

Results.—At an average of 25 months after surgery, 25 patients were available for assessment. Thirteen complained of pain, 8 of whom had talar dome chondral injuries. Overall, patients with talar dome chondral injuries had poorer results, including poorer functional status and ankle range of motion.

Conclusions.—The incidence of injury to the cartilage surface of the talus associated with malleolar fractures is 49%. The prognosis of patients with these injuries occurring together is much worse than of those with fracture alone. Surgeons should inspect the tibiotalar joint of every surgically treated malleolar fracture and débride it if necessary.

▶ An important but often overlooked step in the treatment of ankle fractures is discussed in this paper. Recognizing a cartilaginous injury is important not only for making an accurate prognosis but also for removing loose pieces of cartilage and possibly drilling subchondral bone when indicated.—S.T. Hansen, M.D.

Immediate Multiple Osteosynthesis in Polytrauma

Costa P, Giancecchi F, Tartaglia I, Fontanesi G (Arcispedale S. Maria Nuova, Reggio Emilia, Italy; Instituto Ortopedico Rizzoli, Bologna, Italy)
Ital J Orthop Traumatol 17:187–198, 1991   9–9

Background.—Increasing high-energy injuries have made polytrauma more of a concern. Polytrauma is defined as 2 or more lesions that can affect the course of circulatory and respiratory function. A series of patients underwent immediate treatment not only of open fractures but also of closed musculoskeletal lesions.

Patients.—Thirty patients with multiple injuries seen in 1983–1988 underwent 2 or more fixations of fractures of the pelvis or long bone. They were chiefly men aged 30–40 years; a majority were injuried in motor vehicle accidents. The patients had a total of 109 fractures, 82 involving the long bones. In addition, there were 8 pelvic and 7 spinal fractures not associated with cord injury.

Methods.—All bony injuries except for spinal fractures and some pelvic fractures were stabilized in a single-stage emergency operation, using various methods of fixation such as external fixators, intramedullary nails, and plates. Nine fasciotomies were carried out, and 8 dislocations were immediately reduced. All patients received intravenous antibiotics and general anesthesia. Assistive functional rehabilitation was carried out postoperatively.

Results.—Substantial improvement was evident with this approach to polytrauma in terms of healing, functional recovery, and the resumption of usual social and occupational activities. Five patients had delayed union of long-bone fractures; and 2 had nonunion, but only 1 further surgical intervention was required to correct these problems except for 1 patient with infected nonunion. Both open and closed fractures healed quickly when fixed with interlocking intramedullary nails. There were 3 early infections, 5 deep venous thromboses, and 2 nonfatal embolic events.

Conclusions.—Immediate surgery is technically easier and relieves pain, as well as lowering the risk of embolism. Nursing care is greatly facilitated. Immediate mobilization promotes normal ventilation and joint motion as well as circulatory stability. The methods of osteosynthesis used should assure stability as well as being minimally aggressive and rapidly applicable.

▶ This excellent review from Bologna, encompassing 6 years' experience using aggressive modern traumatology protocols for early skeletal fixation, parallels the experience in North America. External skeletal fixation was used frequently, and interlocked intramedullary nailing has been gaining favor more recently.—S.T. Hansen, M.D.

Timing of Osteosynthesis of Major Fractures in Patients With Severe Brain Injury

Hofman PAM, Goris RJA (University Hospital, Nijmegen, The Netherlands)
J Trauma 31:261–263, 1991   9–10

Background.—Early osteosynthesis of major fractures decreases the risk of fat embolism, sepsis, and adult respiratory distress syndrome in multiply injured patients, but it is not generally accepted as a primary goal when severe brain injury is present. At 1 center, a policy was developed in which early operative stabilization of major fractures was achieved in such patients after CT study of the brain and optimal stabilization of vital functions.

Patients.—Among 58 consecutive patients seen in 1982–1986 who had a Glasgow Coma Scale score of 7 or less at admission, 15 had osteosynthesis on the day of injury for unstable vertebral, pelvic, or femoral fractures or grade 2 or grade 3 compound tibial fractures (group A). The other 43 patients either had no major fracture or were not treated operatively within 24 hours of injury.

Results.—The mean duration of surgery was 3 hours for group A and 40 minutes for group B. The groups did not differ significantly in the severity of brain injury. Osteosynthesis prolonged the mean stay in the intensive care unit from 9 to 19 days, but the mean hospital stay was similar for both groups. Two of 15 patients in group A and 20 of 43 patients in group B died.

Conclusions.—Major fractures adversely affect the outcome in patients with severe brain injury. A fatalistic approach to these patients is not warranted. The outcome after early osteosynthesis is better than would be expected from the neurologic state at admission.

▶ Even though it is retrospective and nonrandomized, this paper offers very important and interesting information. It addresses a problem common to all major trauma centers—whether to anesthetize brain-injured patients for prolonged surgery to perform osteosynthesis. This institution has a long history of recommending early osteosynthesis in polytrauma and emphasizing the need for assisted respiration and full oxygenation of patients under anesthesia. Their protocols for brain-injured patients also include administering high doses of barbiturates and performing intracranial pressure monitoring. Prospective randomized studies may be needed before this practice can be confidently recommended, but strong evidence is presented that early osteosynthesis in brain-injured patients improves both survival and the final neurologic outcomes. More important, the authors indicate that major fractures can produce a lower rating on the Glasgow Coma Scale on initial evaluation than the severity of brain injury actually warrants, a situation that can lead to undue pessimism regarding eventual recovery and to possibly withholding treatment from patients who, in fact, have a reasonably good prognosis with aggressive treatment.—S.T. Hansen, M.D.

Plating of the Fibula: Its Potential Value as an Adjunct to External Fixation of the Tibia
Morrison KM, Ebraheim NA, Southworth SR, Sabin JJ, Jackson WT (Med College of Ohio, Toledo)
Clin Orthop 266:209–213, 1991   9–11

Objective.—The effect of plating the fibula (in conjunction with external tibial fixation) in interfragmental motion was examined in an experimental model of grade III open tibial fracture with associated fibular fracture.

Methods.—Both legs of 5 fresh anatomical specimens were evaluated. Control extremities had a Vidal-Hoffman external fixation applied in a unilateral biplanar manner using 5-mm half pins. A 2-cm segment of middiaphyseal tibia was removed with a 1-cm segment of the fibular. In the other extremities, the fibula was fixed with a 6-hole AO small fragment standard plate. Fragment motion was assessed using 3-dimensional photographic techniques.

Results.—The preparations with a fibular plate were substantially stiffer than control preparations on axial loading (average 2.2 times stiffer). On testing torsional response, some specimens with fibular plate were more stiff than controls, but the difference in peak torque was not great.

Conclusions.—In patients with tibial fracture with a segmental defect, plating the injured fibular may lessen subsequent morbidity. At least partial weight-bearing may be feasible immediately after operative repair; this may be especially helpful to patients with multiple injuries.

▶ This paper very appropriately stresses the importance of fibular fixation to supplement stabilization of severe tibial injuries. The fibula has the capacity to maintain normal alignment and length during treatment of the tibial defect, even when limited weight-bearing is applied. The benefits of this technique are reflected in functional treatment of the foot and promotion of increased circulation.—S.T. Hansen, M.D.

The Role of Supplemental Lag-Screw Fixation for Open Fractures of the Tibial Shaft Treated With External Fixation

Krettek C, Haas N, Tscherne H (Hannover Medical School, Germany)
J Bone Joint Surg (Am) 73-A893–897, 1991   9–12

Objective.—The value of supplemental lag-screw fixation of open tibial shaft fractures was examined in 97 patients having 99 such fractures, which were treated by unilateral external fixation.

Treatment.—All patients had débridement and external fixation of their injuries with a Monofixateur. Fifty-five fractures also had lag-screw fixation using 3.5-mm AO/ASIF cortical-bone screws. A single screw was employed in 29% of fractures. In 34 instances, the fracture was fixed directly with lag-screws.

Patients.—The 2 treatment groups were similar in age, fracture site, and the severity of associated injuries. Most of the fractures resulted from high-energy trauma in a motor-vehicle or motorcycle accident.

Results.—Lag-screw fixation did not shorten the time to healing or decrease the occurrence of delayed union. Rates of malunion, pin loosening, infection, and osteomyelitis were comparable in the 2 treatment groups. Cancellous bone grafting was done more than twice as often when lag-screw fixation was used, but refracture was more prevalent in this group. Five of 6 refractures resulting from minor trauma occurred in patients having lag-screw fixation.

Conclusion.—Supplemental lag-screw fixation of open tibial shaft fractures has no apparent advantage and, in this series, was associated with a greater risk of refracture and a more frequent need for bone grafting.

▶ The authors attempt to answer a long-held question regarding the risk/benefit ratio of using intrafragmental screws in open fractures to supplement external skeletal fixation. The alignment can be held with screws, but potential risks are associated with their use: the incidence of infection may increase, callus formation may decrease, and soft tissue may become detached from bone. The risks and the benefits of both appear to be minimal, but the increased incidence of refracture seems to indicate that screws should not be used except when they are very important for alignment. In this case, onlay bone grafting performed in the area of the interfragmental screw should preclude later refracture.—S.T. Hansen, M.D.

Additional Readings

The following articles are recommended to the reader:

Lee C, Woodring JH: Unstable Jefferson variant atlas fractures: An unrecognized cervical injury. *AJNR* 12:1105–1110, 1991.

Zanasi R, Franceschini R, Romano P, et al.: Intramedullary osteosynthesis. 2. Küntscher nailing in fractures of the tibia. *It J Orthop Traumatol* 16:203–213, 1990.

Sanders R, Swiontkowski M, Rosen H, et al: Double-plating of comminuted, unstable fractures of the distal part of the femur. *J Bone Joint Surg* 73-A:341–346, 1991.

Leung KS, Shen WY, So WS, et al: Interlocking intramedullary nailing for supracondylar and intercondylar fractures of the distal part of the femur. *J Bone Joint Surg* 73-A:332–340, 1991.

McLaren AC, Blokker CP: Locked intramedullary fixation for metaphyseal malunion and nonunion. *Clin Orthop* 265:253–260, 1991.

Wu C-C, Shih C-H, Zee Z-L: Subtrochanteric fractures treated with interlocking nailing. *J Trauma* 31:326–333, 1991.

Wiss DA, Brien WW, Becker V: Interlocking nailing for the treatment of femoral fractures due to gunshot wounds. *J Bone Joint Surg* 73-A:598–606, 1991.

Hovius SER, Hofman A, van Urk H, et al: Acute management of traumatic forequarter amputations: Case reports. *J Trauma* 31:1415–1419, 1991.

O'Donnell D, Gunn J: Hypercalcaemia and nephrolithiasis following multiple fractures. *J Bone Joint Surg* 73-B:174, 1991.

Pelvic and Acetabular Fractures

▶ ↓ Because interest in the aggressive treatment of pelvic and acetabular fractures has increased in the past 10 years, these papers are listed separately from the General Traumatology section.—S.T. Hansen, M.D.

Improved Outcome With Early Fixation of Skeletally Unstable Pelvic Fractures
Latenser BA, Gentilello LM, Tarver AA, Thalgott JS, Batdorf JW (Univ of Nevada, Las Vegas)
J Trauma 31:28–31, 1991   9–13

Background.—Early fixation is of value in the management of long-bone fractures, but its value in treating unstable pelvic fractures is much less clear. The outcome after routine early fixation was compared with that after standard treatment of unstable pelvic fractures.

Methods.—A total of 37 consecutive patients were seen in 1981–

1988. The first 18 patients were seen in 1981–1984, when early fixation was not used routinely (group 1). Subsequently, all patients had pelvic stabilization unless they were too unstable to tolerate surgery (group 2). The 2 groups were well matched demographically and for severity of injury and type of fracture. Early pelvic stabilization was carried out in 4 patients in group 1 and in 8 patients in group 2.

Results.—The duration of hospital stay was more than one-third shorter for patients in group 2 having early operative stabilization. Almost three fourths of group 2 was discharged home, compared with just more than half of group 1. Sixty percent of the earlier patients were confined to bed or a wheelchair for 6 months or longer, as compared with only 16% of the later patients.

Conclusions.—Early fixation of skeletally unstable pelvic fractures may lessen the need for transfusion and lead to fewer complications as well as decreasing mortality. In addition, early fixation limits pain and increases mobility, reducing the duration of hospitalization.

▶ This retrospective study comparing reasonably similar groups is representative of treatment cost and functional outcome of pelvic fractures. Patients with unstable pelvic fractures who were not treated with early fixation required more blood and had longer hospital stays, more complications, longer disability, and a lower survival rate than those treated with early fixation. This type of study should be extended into a randomized clinical trial, possibly in a multicenter effort. However, in view of these results and what we know about traumatology, it may be impossible to intentionally randomize patients with unstable pelvic fractures into a group receiving delayed fixation or no fixation.—S.T. Hansen, M.D.

Displaced Acetabular Fractures: Long-Term Follow-Up

Kebaish AS, Roy A, Rennie W (Maisonneuve-Rosemont Hospital, Montreal; Univ of Montreal; University of Manitoba, Winnipeg, Canada)
J Trauma 31:1539–1542, 1991   9–14

Background.—Anatomical restoration of the joint space is accepted as the best approach to displaced acetabular fractures, but many believe that skeletal traction provides comparable results. The long-term results of surgery and nonoperative treatment of acetabular fractures were compared.

Methods.—Of 136 patients seen in 1980–1987 with acetabular fractures, 115 had displaced fractures, and 90 were available for follow-up for 2–8 years (mean, 4 years 9 months). Thirty-one patients were managed by skeletal traction, 1 by closed manipulation under anesthesia, and 4 by bed rest alone. The other 54 patients were operated on an average of 10 days after injury. Osteosynthesis was with interfragmentary screws and contoured plates.

Results.—Injury severity scores were comparable in the 2 treatment groups. The long-term outcome was excellent or good in 74% of operated patients; only 9% had a poor outcome. In the nonoperated group, 58% of patients had an excellent or good outcome, and 22% had poor results. There were no operative deaths, but postoperatively 4 patients had deep venous thrombosis, with 2 cases of pulmonary embolism. There was 1 deep infection. Avascular necrosis of the femoral head developed in 2 operated patients and in 1 unoperated patient. Heterotopic ossification developed more often after surgical treatment.

Conclusions.— Open reduction and internal fixation lessen the hospital stay for patients with displaced acetabular fractures. Good results are achieved in a large majority of patients gaining anatomical or near-anatomical reduction. Skeletal traction can relieve pain but does not reduce the fracture anatomically.

▶ This study is also retrospective and nonrandomized, but it presents a good review of the results of open reduction vs. nonoperative treatment of patients with acetabular fractures. Because complications are common with acetabular reductions, the results achieved by experienced and inexperienced surgeons also are compared. The authors conclude realistically that experienced surgeons elected to perform open reduction much more frequently with appropriate indications than did inexperienced surgeons. A new acetabular fracture score developed by the authors indicated that anatomical or near-anatomical reductions, whether open or closed, achieved good or excellent results almost 3 times as often as inadequate reductions. Complication rates were very acceptable in the hands of experienced surgeons, even though the rates were not overwhelmingly high even in inexperienced hands. The paper speaks strongly for treating these patients in trauma centers, where surgeons experienced in the latest techniques are available.— S.T. Hansen, M.D.

Additional Reading

The following articles are recommended to the reader:

Ben-Menachem Y, Coldwell DM, Young JWR, et al: Hemorrhage associated with pelvic fractures: Causes, diagnosis, and emergent management. *AJR* 157:1005–1014, 1991.

Ganz R, Krushell RJ, Jakob RP, et al: The antishock pelvic clamp. *Clin Orthop* 267:71–78, 1991.

Kaempffe FA, Bone LB, Border JR: Open reduction and internal fixation of acetabular fractures: Heterotopic ossification and other complications of treatment. *J Orthop Trauma* 5:439–445, 1991.

Stocks GW, Gabel GT, Noble PC, et al: Anterior and posterior internal fixation of vertical shear fractures of the pelvis. *J Orthop Res* 9:237–245, 1991.

Ebraheim NA, Coombs R, Hoeflinger MJ, et al: Anatomical and radiological considerations in compressive bar technique for posterior pelvic disruptions. *J Orthop Trauma* 5:434–438, 1991.

Webster GD, Ramon J: Repair of pelvic fracture posterior urethral defects using an elaborated perineal approach: Experience with 74 cases. *J Urol* 145:744–748, 1991.

Leighton RK, Waddell JP, Bray TJ, et al: Biomechanical testing of new and old fixation devices for vertical shear fractures of the pelvis. *J Orthop Trauma* 5:313–317, 1991.

Amputation Topics

The Influence of Smoking on Complications After Primary Amputations of the Lower Extremity

Lind J, Kramhøft M, Bødtker S (County Hospital in Hillerød, Denmark)
Clin Orthop 267:211–217, 1991   9–15

Background.—Recovery from amputation requires long periods of hospitalization, and reamputation does occur. Postoperative complications often occur. No one has examined the effect of cigarette smoking on postoperative wound-healing complications. Outcomes in smoking and nonsmoking amputees were compared.

Methods.—One hundred thirty-seven patients undergoing 165 above-the-knee or below-the-knee amputations were examined retrospectively. Forty-four patients smoked cigarettes, 30 smoked cheroots, and 3 smoked a pipe. Eighty-eight patients did not smoke. On average, the 77 smokers were younger than the nonsmokers at the time of surgery.

Results.—Amputation level did not differ between the 2 groups. The below-the-knee to above-the-knee amputation ratio was 2:1. Cigarette smokers had a risk of infection and reamputation 2.5 times higher than in cheroot smokers or nonsmokers. The cigarette smokers smoked during the healing phase. Also, cigarette smokers tended to inhale.

Conclusions.—Inhaling cigarette smoke results in a high concentration of nicotine that compromises the cutaneous blood flow velocity and increases the risk of microthrombi formation. Amputees should not smoke cigarettes during the healing phase. Preferably, patients should break the habit 1 week before surgery as this is the requisite time for the process of coagulation and the fibrinogen level to normalize and for free radicals to be eliminated.

▶ The negative effects of cigarette smoking on the peripheral circulation are documented in this excellent study and are related to wound-healing complications in amputations. Coincidentally, this study demonstrates that amputations occur at an earlier age in cigarette smokers. Of course, both observations seem obvious to clinicians involved with these cases, but they have not been documented previously.—S.T. Hansen, M.D.

Joint Moment and Muscle Power Output Characteristics of Below Knee Amputees During Running: The Influence of Energy Storing Prosthetic Feet

Czerniecki JM, Gitter A, Munro C (Univ of Washington, Seattle; Seattle VA Med Ctr, Seattle)
J Biomechanics 24:63–75, 1991   9–16

Background.—Below-knee amputation increases metabolic energy demand during ambulation. A new class of prosthetic feet—"energy-storing" feet— has been designed to better approximate the normal biomechanics of the foot and ankle, thereby reducing metabolic energy consumption. The effect of energy-storing feet on lower extremity joint moments, muscle power outputs, and mechanical energy characteristics in young patients after unilateral below-knee amputation was examined.

Methods.—Five normal participants and 5 amputees running at 2.8 ms^{-1} were analyzed. Stance phase joint moments, muscle power outputs, and mechanical energy characteristics were determined. The amputees used 3 different prosthetic feet—the solid ankle cushion heel (SACH) foot and 2 energy-storing feet, the Seattle and the Flex.

Results.—While wearing the SACH foot, amputees had major changes in the distribution and magnitude of muscle power output and muscle work. The total work done by the lower extremity was reduced, and the hip extensors became the main source of energy absorption and generation. In normal participants, the ankle plantarflexors were the main energy generators, and the knee extensors were the main energy absorbers. Also in the amputees, the eccentric and concentric knee extensor power outputs were decreased, and an abnormal concentric knee flexor power output was seen immediately after heel contact. In 4 amputees, energy-storing feet resulted in improved power output and mechanical work characteristics of the lower extremity. The energy-storing prosthetic foot generated 2–3 times more energy than the SACH foot. With the Flex footk amputees had a more normal pattern and magnitude of hip and knee extensor muscle work. However, the fifth amputee had increased abnormalities with the energy-storing foot. The amount of energy restored relative to the energy absorbed by the prosthetic feet was greater with the energy-storing foot than with the SACH foot.

Conclusions.—The power output pattern of the lower extremity is substantially different from normal in amputees wearing a conventional prosthetic foot. The wearing of an energy-storing prosthetic foot, especially the Flex, reduced the magnitude of the abnormalities that occurred with the conventional foot in 4 of 5 persons tested.

▶ A good methodology of newer prosthetic foot designs is presented in this study. In spite of advances in this area, there is room for improvement, and different models of prostheses are needed for patients with different functional requirements.—S.T. Hansen, M.D.

Bilateral Lower Limb Amputee Rehabilitation: A Retrospective Review
Torres MM, Esquenazi A (Temple Univ, Philadelphia)
West J Med 154:583–586, 1991   9–17

Background.—Although functional status is routinely appraised in medical rehabilitation, a recent literature review found no reports of functional outcomes after bilateral lower limb amputation. Patients' functional results after bilateral lower limb amputation were documented.

Methods.—Sixty-one patients with bilateral lower limb amputations included 41 men and 20 women (mean age, 61.5 years) admitted to a regional amputee rehabilitation program. Of these, 41 patients were functionally assessed on discharge and at 1 and 3 months after discharge. The remaining 20 were not included in the analysis because they were transferred to acute care or lost to follow-up.

Results.—Seventy-seven percent of the patients were discharged home. For all levels of amputation, the average length of hospital stay was 24 days. At the time of discharge, most patients had attained a level of limited household walking, except for those with bilateral above-knee amputations. At the 3-month follow-up, all patients showed significant functional improvement. Most had achieved a household level of ambulation. Ten remained independent at wheelchair functional levels.

Conclusions.—Patients undergoing bilateral lower limb amputations deserve a comprehensive rehabilitation program to achieve and maintain the goal of limited household walking. Further research should focus on the role that concurrent disease plays in determining the appropriateness for prosthetic management, cost-effectiveness, and the long-term benefits of attaining the highest possible functional level.

▶ The authors discuss a problem that is becoming increasingly common. Fortunately, the prospects for rehabilitation after bilateral lower limb amputations are not as bleak as is often thought. With good surgical technique, postoperative care, modern prostheses, and comprehensive rehabilitation, patients who lose part of both lower limbs can now attain a functional outcome.—S.T. Hansen, M.D.

Limb Salvage *Versus* Traumatic Amputation: A Decision Based on a Seven-Part Predictive Index
Russell WL, Sailors DM, Whittle TB, Fisher DF Jr, Burns RP (Univ of Tennessee, Chattanooga)
Ann Surg 213:473–481, 1991   9–18

Background.—The decision to amputate or attempt to salvage a severely injured extremity often is complex because of the multiple systems involved in the injury. Despite the cooperative efforts of several surgical specialties, some limbs may eventually require amputation after months of reconstructive procedures. Variables that might predict outcome in a severely traumatized extremity with arterial compromise were investigated.

Patients.—During a 5-year period, 67 patients (70 limbs) were treated at 1 institution for major lower extremity arterial injury. Salvage was possible in 51 limbs; 19 limbs sustained primary (11), secondary (6), or functional (2) amputation. The average patient age was 32 years. Variables examined included the mechanism of injury, the type of arterial and nerve injury, associated injuries, the time of injury to operative repair, and the order of repair.

Results.—Blunt injuries carried a higher amputation rate (51%) than penetrating trauma (3%). Patients with crush/avulsion injuries had a high rate (82%) of amputation. Variables not predictive of limb salvage include the presence or absence of shock, the time of injury to operative repair, or the order of vascular and orthopedic repair. The absence of pedal pulses on arrival was associated with a poor outcome. All patients in the amputated group had peripheral nerve injuries. The degree of total injury to the extremity was more important in predicting amputation than was the level at which arterial injury occurred.

Conclusions.—A limb salvage index, a scoring system based on warm ischemia time and the extent of injury sustained by the arteries, nerves, bone, skin, muscle, and deep veins, can be a valuable objective tool for evaluation of patients with severely traumatized extremities. All patients requiring amputation had a limb salvage index score of 6 or greater.

▶ The authors offer a new scoring system for severe limb injuries in an attempt to predict functional limb salvage. Like other such scoring systems, this one is also most pertinent for severe blunt injuries in the tibia. The authors very correctly indicate that the most significant factors predictive of amputation are large amounts of tissue injury, including nerve, bone, and muscle injury, and warm ischemia lasting more than 6 hours. The age of the patients in this series averages 32 years, and the effects of shock and delayed treatment and the existence of concurrent illness did not significantly influence their outcomes.— S.T. Hansen, M.D.

Type III Tibial Fractures in the Elderly: Results of 23 Fractures in 20 Patients
Ritchie AJ, Small JO, Hart NB, Mollan RAB (The Ulster Hospital, Belfast; Queen's University of Belfast)
Injury 22:267–270, 1991   9–19

Introduction.—Severe open fractures of the tibia present particular management problems. The decision whether to attempt salvage or proceed to amputation often is difficult. A review of elderly patients with type III fractures of the tibia was undertaken to determine factors associated with successful salvage.

Patients.—A group of 20 patients had 23 fractures. When first seen, 8 patients were in their 60s, 11 were in their 70s, and 1 was 84 years of age. Management evolved during the treatment period (1974–1988) and included internal fixation, external fixation, fasciocutaneous flaps, muscle flaps, and free tissue transfer.

Results.—The overall amputation rate was 47.5%. The total inpatient duration for those undergoing primary vs. secondary amputation (14.6 vs. 18 weeks) was not significantly different. Independent walking was achieved by all patients at periods ranging from 21 days to 2.5 years after operation. Bony union in the limb salvage group was achieved between 3 months and 2.5 years. The use of internal fixation and muscle flaps was associated with a higher rate of amputation. In patients with bilateral fractures outcome was related to the classification of each fracture rather than to age or other injuries.

Conclusion.—Findings in this small series of patients suggest that age alone is not necessarily a contraindication to limb salvage in type III fractures of the tibia. Attempts at salvage may not unduly delay final discharge.

▶ The question of amputation vs. limb salvage in elderly patients is addressed in this retrospective study. The prevailing assumption is that patients in this age group are less likely to heal severe injuries and that more of them would be better served by immediate amputation than would young patients. The type of internal fixation used to stabilize the fractures was not always identified, but those mentioned included tibial plates, external skeletal fixators, and nonreamed locking nails, all currently preferred devices for type III fractures. The study's limitations were recognized by the authors. For reasons that were not explained and that remain unclear, the hospital times for immediate and delayed amputations were similar. Amputation in the elderly is an important topic that needs prospective studies, an analysis of cost-effectiveness, and an analysis of functional outcome. These factors should then be related to precise grading of the injuries and overall pre- and post-injury health and function of the patients.—S.T. Hansen, M.D.

Outcome of Complex Vascular and Orthopedic Injuries of the Lower Extremity
Alexander JJ, Piotrowski JJ, Graham D, Franceschi D, King T (Cleveland Metropolitan Gen Hosp)
Am J Surg 162:111–115, 1991   9–20

Background.—Patients with complex vascular and orthopedic injuries of the lower extremity have high rates of chronic disability and amputation. In an attempt to determine potential risk factors for limb loss and disability, patients with injury of the lower extremity involving open long-bone fractures and evidence of limb-threatening ischemia were examined.

Patients.—The group included 32 patients, 26 males and 6 females (mean age, 27.4 years). Most (91%) had experienced blunt trauma resulting from automobile, motorcycle, or industrial accidents or falls. Two patients were injured by shotgun blasts, and 1 was injured by a propeller. Major soft-tissue defects were seen in 21 patients. Fifteen had remote injuries, including closed head trauma. Arterial reconstruction was completed in 20 patients before definitive orthopedic treatment.

Results.—One patient died as a result of remote injury and sepsis. Nine patients (28%) required amputation, and 13 (56%) of those whose limbs were salvaged experienced chronic morbidity. Two had continued pain, 1 had cold intolerance, 4 had persistent infection with nonunion of fracture, and 6 complained of chronic sensory or motor deficits. Amputation was not related to patient age, trauma characteristics, delay, or method of repair. The most significant factor associated with amputation was infection, which was not prevented by the perioperative use of antibiotics.

Conclusion.—For many potentially salvageable extremities, a poor outcome is related to either nerve injury or infection. Early amputation is recommended for patients with significant nerve disruption. Delayed amputation significantly extended the total period of hospitalization. Infection may be limited by adequate wound débridement, intravenous antibiotics, and early wound coverage.

▶ In this retrospective look at type IIIC fractures, the authors noted a significant rate of early amputation (28%) and a high rate of functional and neurologic deficit (56%) in salvaged limbs. A very noteworthy finding was that infection, which is predictive of unsuccessful limb salvage, was not significantly affected by the use of perioperative antibiotics nor did the use of antibiotics affect the rate of amputations. The clearest indication for early amputation was determined to be neural disruption, and, in contrast to Abstract 9–19, delayed amputation significantly increased hospital time. When salvage was attempted, extensive débridement, appropriate skeletal stabilization, and early wound coverage were performed.—S.T. Hansen, M.D.

Continuous Postoperative Regional Analgesia by Nerve Sheath Block for Amputation Surgery—A Pilot Study
Fisher A, Meller Y (Soroka Medical Center; Ben Gurian University of the Negev, Beersheva, Israel)
Anesth Analg 72:300–303, 1991   9–21

Background.—Efforts to relieve established phantom limb pain with a wide variety of treatment have been disappointing. A simple way to prevent immediate postoperative pain and long-term pain after limb amputation would be of great value. A prospective trial was done to assess continuous postoperative regional analgesia (CPRA) by nerve sheath block for lower limb amputation achieved by continuous infusion of local anesthetic agent directly into the transected nerve sheath.

Methods.—Eleven patients with ASA physical status III or IV undergoing above- or below-knee amputations were included. At the time of exposure of the sciatic or posterior tibial nerve trunks, a catheter was introduced directly into the transected nerve sheath for continuous infusion of .25% bupivacaine at a rate of 10 mL/hr for 72 hours. For comparison, a retrospective control group of 20 patients who had received only parenteral narcotic analgesics on demand after lower limb amputation also were examined.

Results.—The mean morphine equivalent requirement in the CPRA and control groups were 2.1 and 15.9 mg after below-knee amputation and 0 and 28.1 mg after above-knee amputation. Overall, these means were 1.4 and 18.4 mg, indicating a highly significant reduction in narcotic analgesic requirement in the CPRA group. Follow-up of the patients treated by CPRA indicated a total absence of phantom pain. Two died after 2 months; follow-up for the remaining 9 patients was more than 1 year. Two patients reported occasional paresthesia, which did not bother them.

Conclusions.—Continuous postoperative regional analgesia appears to be a promising way to prevent immediate postoperative and long-term pain after limb amputation. With CPRA, there is a reduced need for postoperative narcotic analgesics. Further trials are planned.

▶ The authors present an excellent preliminary study of a technique that is also being explored at other centers. The continuous regional block not only prevents early severe postoperative pain after major amputations but also frequently reduces late postoperative pain—both very worthwhile goals. The technique requires further investigation but appears to be very promising.— S.T. Hansen, M.D.

Additional Reading

The following articles are recommended to the reader:

Gottschalk FA: Amputation as alternative management in severe limb trauma. *Complications in Surg* April 1991, pp 41–46.

Roessler MS, Wisner DH, Holcroft JW: The mangled extremity: When to amputate? *Arch Surg* 126:1243–1249, 1991.

Netz P, Olsson E, Ringertz H, et al: Functional restitution after lower leg fractures: A long-term followup. *Arch Orthop Trauma Surg* 110:238–241, 1991.

Lerner RK, Esterhai JL, Polomono RC, et al: Psychosocial, functional, and quality of life assessment of patients with posttraumatic fracture nonunion, chronic refractory osteomyelitis, and lower extremity amputation. *Arch Phys Med Rehabil* 72:122–126, 1991.

Robertson PA: Prediction of amputation after severe lower limb trauma. *J Bone Joint Surg* 73-B:816–818, 1991.

Topper AK, Fernie GR: An evaluation of computer aided design of below-knee prosthetic sockets. *Prosthet Orthot Int* 14:136:142, 1990.

Torres-Moreno R, Saunders CG, Foort J, et al: Computer-aided design and manufacture of an above-knee amputee socket. *J Biomed Eng* 13:3–9, 1991.

Michaels JA: The selection of amputation level: An approach using decision analysis. *Eur J Vasc Surg* 5:451–457, 1991.

Pinzur MS, Perona P, Patwardhan A, et al: Loading of the contralateral foot in peripheral vascular insufficiency below-knee amputees. *Foot Ankle* 11:368–371, 1991.

Pohjolainen T: A clinical evaluation of stumps in lower limb amputees. *Prosthetics and Orthotics International* 15:178–184, 1991.

Harrington IJ, Lexier R, Woods, JM, et al: A plaster-pylon technique for below-knee amputation. *J Bone Joint Surg* 73-B:76–78, 1991.

Pinzur MS: Sciatic nerve block for residual limb pain following below-knee amputation. *Contemp Orthop* 22:290–292, 1991.

Fiddler DS, Hindman BJ: Intravenous calcitonin alleviates spinal anesthesia-induced phantom limb pain. *Anesthesiology* 74:187–189, 1991.

Stimulation of Healing

▶ ↓ Stimulation of healing is an important and productive area of research. A trend is noted toward autogenous bone graft and autogenous-substitute materials to enhance direct bone grafting and away from electric stimulation. The newer methods are compatible with anatomical internal fixation and theoretically result in the most anatomical and functional outcomes. It is clearly recognized that the most cost-effective and functional outcomes result when union is achieved in a minimal amount of time and some degree of function is maintained. Prolonged treatment that does not allow ongoing function leads to muscle atrophy, joint stiffness, and markedly higher costs of treatment. The cost of treatment must include the amount of time a patient is away from work and normal activities.—S.T. Hansen, M.D.

Multicenter Trial of Collagraft as Bone Graft Substitute

Cornell CN, Lane JM, Chapman M, Merkow R, Seligson D, Henry S, Gustilo R, Vincent K (Hosp for Special Surgery, New York)
J Orthop Trauma 5:1–8, 1991   9–22

Background.—Because autogenous bone grafts are limited in supply and have harvest-associated morbidity, substitute substances have been sought. In a prospective, randomized, multicenter trial, Collagraft, a synthetic bone-graft substitute, was compared with autogenous cancellous bone for achieving osseous union in long-bone fractures.

Materials and Methods.—Collagraft is a mixture of porous calcium phosphate granules, .5–1 mm in diameter, composed of about 65% hydroxyapatite and 35% tricalcium phosphate, and highly purified fibrillar collagen, 95% type I and 5% type III. Included were 267 patients with long-bone fractures for which bone grafting had been recommended. Fractures were grafted using autogenous cancellous graft harvested from the iliac crest in 128 patients and using Collagraft mixed with autogenous marrow in 139 patients. Patients were examined at intervals to 24 months; radiographs were assessed by an independent, blinded, nonbiased radiologist.

Results.—Patients in the Collagraft group had a significantly shorter mean operative time than patients in the control group. No significant differences between groups in healing, analgesic use, or limitations in activities of daily living caused by the fracture site were seen in radiographic assessments. There were 12 overall wound healing complications in the Collagraft group and 20 in the control group, including infections of the fracture sites in the Collagraft group and 13 in the control group. The overall fracture healing complication rate was 8.1% for the Collagraft group and 6% for the control group.

Conclusions.—Collagraft is as safe and effective as autogenous cancellous bone for the treatment of acute long-bone fractures and significantly shortens operative time. No noticeable adverse effects have been associated with the use of Collagraft, but additional analysis is needed to determine the long-term effects of residual hydroxyapatite on bone remodeling.

▶ A synthetic bone-graft substitute was compared to autogenous bone graft in an excellent multicenter prospective trial. This type of study is most effective for providing a definitive answer to a specific question—in this case, is bone-graft substitute as effective as autogenous bone in enhancing union in long-bone fractures? A major criticism of the study, recognized by the authors, is absence of a third group of patients in whom bone grafting was not done. This criticism, however, was not particularly pertinent to the study. It appears that the authors have demonstrated that Collagraft is as effective as autogenous bone and that this material also decreases operative time and patient morbidity. Further long-term studies using more patients are needed to confirm these findings. Should future studies determine that Collagraft is as safe and effective as autogenous bone, the cost-effectiveness of the technique will have to be determined.—S.T. Hansen, M.D.

Autogeneic Bone Marrow and Porous Biphasic Calcium Phosphate Ceramic for Segmental Bone Defects in the Canine Ulna
Grundel RE, Chapman MW, Yee T, Moore DC (Univ of California, Davis)
Clin Orthop 266:244–258, 1991   9–23

Background.—Autogeneic bone marrow has several drawbacks as a graft for bony defects. Pure marrow is difficult to handle and provides no immediate mechanical stability. Thus composite grafts composed of marrow and other materials have been developed. The value of a porous biphasic hydroxyapatite–calcium phosphate ceramic as a modifier and extender of an autogeneic marrow graft was assessed.

Methods.—The ceramic was manufactured from high-purity tricalcium phosphate. Two forms of the ceramic were used, the first a cylindrical block and the second a granular ceramic composed of particles created by crushing samples of the block form. Twenty adult mongrel dogs were surgically treated to create diaphyseal defects in the left ulnae. The animals were randomly divided into 4 groups according to treatment. Three dogs received no graft, 5 received autogeneic bone marrow alone, 6 received ceramic in block form shaped into a hollow cylinder mixed with the marrow, and 6 other dogs received grafts with a mixture of 50% bone marrow and 50% granular ceramic.

Results.—All animals were fully weight-bearing by 1 week and had no apparent disability. There were no infections at the incision site, nor mechanical failures of the fixation. Roentgenographic analysis showed that all dogs with granular ceramic grafts had mineralized callus formation by 4 weeks. Stable union occurred in all but 1 of the ulnae in this group. Significant callus formation was seen in 4 dogs with block ceramic implants by 4 weeks and in 1 such dog by 8 weeks. The remaining dog in this group failed to show callus formation by 24 weeks. Only 3 dogs in the block group had solid union. Defects united in all 5 dogs grafted with autogeneic bone marrow, whereas the 3 dogs with no implant had nonunions.

Conclusions.—Bone marrow alone was quite effective, but the liquid nature of the material makes it difficult to handle and inappropriate for many types of fracture reconstructions. The addition of granular ceramic improves the handling characteristics of the graft material and accelerates healing.

▶ In this experimental study, bone grafting was used for structural support, not for stimulation of healing. Segmental defects occur commonly in high-energy trauma, and healing them is an important area of study. To date, block ceramic is less effective than granular ceramic. Although the nature of the defect in this study did not require additional stability, it might be required in another situation. Clinically, granular graft is commonly used in addition to structural graft in an effort to attain the best of both worlds. Future studies are needed in this area.—S.T. Hansen, M.D.

Residual Functional Deficit After Partial Fibulectomy for Bone Graft
Anderson AF, Green NE (Vanderbilt Hosp, Nashville)
Clin Orthop 267:137–140, 1991   9–24

Background.—The fibular is often used to reconstruct skeletal defects in long bones. However, little is known about the long-term effects of fibulectomy on the donor leg. The residual functional deficit caused by partial fibulectomy was documented through clinical and instrumented examinations.

Methods.—Ten patients underwent partial fibulectomy for bone-graft reconstruction between 1968 and 1985. Six had wide tumor resection in the upper extremities. Four had bone grafting of an atrophic nonunion of the upper extremity. The interval between surgery and final assessment ranged from 3 to 20 years (mean, 7 years).

Results.—In many patients, the donor leg remained mildly symptomatic. Excision of the middle one third of the fibula resulted in residual weakness. However, the mild discomfort, residual weakness, and laxity were not judged to be significant enough to discontinue the transplantation of large segments of the fibula.

Conclusions.—Even though the donor site often remains mildly symptomatic, the fibula remains an excellent source of bone graft for reconstructing skeletal defects in long bones. The functional deficit may be minimized through postoperative therapy that emphasizes muscular strength.

▶ There is a very important study about donor-site morbidity after the addition of large structural grafts. The authors believe that the advantages of fibular grafting override the relatively mild morbidity and chronic symptomology experienced by the 10 patients in this study group. In my experience, patients occasionally experience much more serious symptoms, including complete foot drop. I agree that technical precision and good rehabilitation are indicated for fibulectomy but believe that other sources of bone should be used whenever possible.—S.T. Hansen, M.D.

Autologous Marrow Injection as a Substitute for Operative Grafting of Tibial Nonunions
Connolly JF, Guse R, Tiedeman J, Dehne R (Univ of Nebraska, Omaha; VA Med Ctrs, Omaha)
Clin Orthop 266:259–270, 1991   9–25

Background.—Animal studies demonstrate the osteogenic properties of stromal or stem cells of bone marrow, but marrow has not been widely used as an osteogenic source. Percutaneous marrow injections were used as a substitute for operative bone grafting in patients with nonunion.

Methods.—In 1984–1988, 20 patients with nonunited tibial fractures were treated a median of 14 months after injury. They mostly had Gustilo-Anderson type III open fractures that had failed to unite despite multiple attempts. Bone grafts had been tried in 9 instances. Marrow was harvested by needle aspiration from the pelvis, usually the posterior iliac wing, and injected percutaneously into the site of nonunion under fluoroscopic control. Most procedures were done on an outpatient basis under general anesthesia.

Results.—Of the 20 fractures, 18 healed after marrow injection combined with adequate immobilization. Intramedullary nailing was more reliable than external cast immobilization. Union took place a median of 6 months after treatment. Persistent infection responded to drainage and sequestrectomy. Draining skin defects healed spontaneously once the fracture united. Use of too large a needle produced prolonged burning pain in 1 patient.

Conclusion.—Currently, marrow mixed with a demineralized bone matrix carrier is used when nonunion is associated with a large defect. Marrow injection provides a reliable and renewable source of osteogenic stem cells.

▶ This excellent clinical study demonstrates a method of obtaining the benefit of autogenous bone stimulation while markedly decreasing the morbidity and complications associated with open autologous grafting. This technique may be carried out in conjunction with intramedullary nailing, and the authors point out the benefits of using both techniques together.—S.T. Hansen, M.D.

Lipid Extraction Enhances Bank Bone Incorporation: An Experiment in Rabbits
Aspenberg P, Thorén K (Lund University Hospital, Sweden)
Acta Orthop Scand 61:546–548, 1990   9–26

Rationale.—Conventional frozen bank bone carries a risk of viral contamination. Its preparation may be time-consuming, and most of the implant consists of dead marrow cells that must be eliminated by the recipient. A trial in rabbit skeletal defects was conducted to determine whether a reduction in necrotic soft tissue by lipid extraction might facilitate incorporation of frozen allogeneic cancellous bone.

Methods.—Some implants were extracted with chloroform/methanol after harvesting from a previously placed titanium chamber filled with cancellous bone. After processing, the donor bone was transferred to an empty chamber in another rabbit. Bony ingrowth was estimated using ^{99m}Tc-MDP and ^{45}Ca.

Results.—Activities of Ca and Tc-MDP were higher in defatted implants; median increases were 70% and 40%, respectively. Histologic analysis confirmed an association between the degree of ^{99m}TC-MDP activity and high bone-forming activity in most areas of the specimens.

Conclusions.—Simple defatting may significantly lessen some of the disadvantages of ordinary bank bone when used in total hip revision surgery. Treatment of bank bone with fat solvents and high-pressure irrigation may promote more rapid bony incorporation of the graft.

▶ This very interesting study describes the preparation of bank bone, which promises to become less antigenic and more effective. Since the advent of AIDS, I suspect that bone substitutes will eventually replace bank bone, but this process may be well worth a larger trial.— S.T. Hansen, M.D.

Additional Reading

The following articles are recommended to the reader:

Tiedeman JJ, Connolly JF, Strates BS, et al: Treatment of nonunion by percutaneous injection of bone marrow and demineralized bone matrix: An experimental study in dogs. *Clin Orthop* 268:294:302, 1991.

Horisaka Y, Okamoto Y, Matsumoto N, et al: Subperiosteal implantation of bone morphogenetic protein adsorbed to hydroxyapatite. *Clin Orthop* 268:303–312, 1991.

Hall MB, Vallerand WP, Thompson D, et al: Comparative anatomic study of anterior and posterior iliac crests as donor sites. *J Oral Maxillofac Surg* 49:560–563, 1991.

Todd BD, Reed SC: The use of bupivacaine to relieve pain at iliac graft donor sites. *Int Orthop* 15:53–55, 1991.

Sakai K, Doi K, Kawai S: Free vascularized thin corticoperiosteal graft. *Plast Reconstr Surg* 87:290–298, 1991.

Jaffe KA, Morris SG, Sorrell RG, et al: Massive bone allografts for traumatic skeletal defects. *S Med J* 84:975–982, 1991.

Thakur AJ, Patankar J: Open tibial fractures. Treatment by uniplanar external fixation and early bone grafting. *J Bone Joint Surg* 73-B:448–451, 1991.

Moed BR, Budorick TE, Smith DJ Jr, et al: The effect of autogenous bone graft application on wound contamination. *J Orthop Trauma* 5:465–468, 1991.

O'Keefe RM, Riemer BL, Butterfield SL: Harvesting of autogenous cancellous bone graft from the proximal tibial metaphysis: A review of 230 cases. *J Orthop Trauma* 5:469–474, 1991.

Soft Tissue Management

Why the Denervated Gastrocnemius Muscle Flap Should Be Encouraged
Pico R, Lüscher NJ, Rometsch M, de Roche R (Klinic für Wiederherstellende Chirurgie der Universität, Basel, Switzerland)
Ann Plast Surg 26:312–324, 1991   9–27

Background.—The superiorly based, denervated gastrocnemius muscle flap provides an aesthetically excellent and functionally good cover for defects of the upper third of the calf, including the knee, and lower third of the thigh. The stability of wound closure and condition of the involved bone were analyzed during a 1-year follow-up of patients undergoing coverage of a soft tissue defect with a gastrocnemius flap.

Methods.—Forty-one consecutive muscle and musculocutaneous gastrocnemius flaps were assessed. Thirty-six patients (88%) were available for reexamination. Mean follow-up was 36 months, with a minimum of 12 months.

Results.—At examination all skin defects and the incidental concomitant osteomyelitis had healed completely. However, 40% of the patients needed second operations. Half had a functional deficiency, and one fifth had lost sensation in some areas. After surgery with musculocutaneous flaps, all of the patients had sensory loss of the saphenous nerve. Peripheral edema also occurred more often than after surgery with a simple muscle flap. Muscle flaps with residual innervation had more secondary wound breakdown and more contraction pain because of spasms.

Conclusions.—The best functional and aesthetic results are achieved with denervated muscle flaps covered by a split-thickness skin graft. The use of denervated, pure muscle flaps has several advantages. Early wound dehiscence is avoided because there is no muscle contraction, no pain is associated with contraction, and a better cosmetic result is produced.

▶ Various gastrocnemius muscle flaps, including musculocutaneous flaps, innervated muscle flaps, and denervated muscle flaps are compared in this excellent paper. The best results, in terms of persisting coverage with the least complications, clearly occurred with denervated muscle flaps. This straightforward technique is very useful and can easily be done by trauma surgeons because it does not require microsurgery or other specialized skills, but it is probably underused.— S.T. Hansen, M.D.

Treatment of Chronic Traumatic Bone Wounds: Microvascular Free Tissue Transfer: A 13-Year Experience in 96 Patients
May JW JR, Jupiter JB, Gallico GG III, Rothkopf DM, Zingarelli P (Massachusetts Gen Hosp, Boston)
Ann Surg 214:241–252, 1991

9–28

Background.—Chronic traumatic bony wounds continue to be difficult to treat. Microvascular free tissue transfer in patients with chronic traumatic bone wounds was examined during a 13-year period.

Patients.—A total of 97 microvascular free tissue transfers were performed for soft tissue reconstruction in 96 patients aged 11–66 years after bone débridement for chronic traumatic bone wounds. The mean period of chronic bone exposure and drainage was 40 months (range, 6 weeks to 41 years). Mean follow-up was 77 months.

Results.—During follow-up, 96% of patients had complete wound closure with a lack of drainage after débridement and free tissue transfer. Ninety percent of patients were ambulatory without assistance; 5% had amputation. Twenty-three percent needed subsequent segmental bone defect reconstruction in the lower extremity after infection eradication.

Conclusions.—The freedom of débridement provided by the almost unlimited microsurgical free tissue wound closure method is associated with a very good chance of successful long-term wound management in patients with chronic traumatic bony wounds. The findings from this 13-year trial support this conclusion.

▶ An extremely thoughtful review of free tissue transfers in a special group of patients with chronically infected traumatic bony wounds is presented in this long-term study. These wounds were clearly distinct from chronic hematogenous osteomyelitis, and the treatment demonstrated a high rate of success. Débridement of all devitalized bone was, of course, the basis of the procedure and nowadays might be facilitated with laser Doppler flowmetry. The selection criteria appear to have been correct in most cases, and the possibility of achieving a functional limb after a successful procedure was analyzed carefully. However, the majority of the cases were tibial injuries, and more than 20 of these were type III, type IV, or type V injuries, which are associated with a predictable delay in ambulation for a year or longer. As always, a cost-benefit analysis of these prolonged salvage attempts must be done in view of the excellent function that can be attained with modern below-knee prosthetic limbs in young posttrauma patients. This paper contains a very complete bibliography and is essential reading for surgeons interested in limb salvage.— S.T.Hansen, M.D.

A Comparison of the Effects of Skin Coverage and Muscle Flap Coverage on the Early Strength of Union at the Site of Osteotomy After Devascularization of a Segment of Canine Tibia

Richards RR, McKee MD, Paitich CB, Anderson GI, Bertoia JT (University of Toronto; St Michael's Hospital, Toronto)
J Bone Joint Surg 73-A:1323–1330, 1991   9–29

Background.— Muscle flap coverage promotes the return of blood flow to devascularized segments of canine tibia and also enhances repair within the bone segment. Muscle flaps are widely used clinically, but their effect on the strength of bony union is uncertain.

Methods.— The effects of coverage with skin and muscle on return of strength were examined at a canine tibial osteotomy site after interposition of a 2-cm devascularized autogenous graft. The bone was fixed with a plate. Tibias were tested to failure 8 and 12 weeks postoperatively. Muscle coverage entailed rotating the tibialis muscle to cover the segment of devascularized tibia.

Results.— Maximum bending load and the amount of energy absorbed to failure increased significantly 8–12 weeks postoperatively when a muscle flap was used for coverage. Bending stiffness at 8 weeks was significantly greater than when only skin was used.

Conclusions.— Muscle flaps are superior to local skin coverage alone when a devascularized segment of autogenous bone is interposed in a canine tibial defect. Under optimal conditions, covering dysvascular or devascularized tibial bone with muscle tissue may promote solid bony union.

▶ Our clinical impression that the increased vascular contribution of a muscle flap has a positive effect on the rate and strength of bone healing underneath it is backed up in this excellent research protocol. This type of research, in addition to functional outcome studies with cost comparisons in human patients, is needed to justify our use of expensive high-tech procedures.—S.T. Hansen, M.D.

The Timing of Flap Coverage, Bone-Grafting, and Intramedullary Nailing in Patients Who Have a Fracture of the Tibial Shaft With Excessive Soft-Tissue Injury
Fischer MD, Gustilo RB, Varecka TF (Hennepin County Med Ctr, Minneapolis)
J Bone Joint Surg 73-A:1316–1322, 1991   9–30

Objective.—How treatment of soft tissue injury influences the occurrence of complications was examined in a series of 43 patients seen in 1980–1987 with type IIIB open fractures of the tibial shaft.

Methods.—All patients had a salvageable limb and lacked major vascular injury that required repair. Twenty-three of the patients had other injuries. The soft tissue injury was débrided immediately after admission and at 2- to 3-day intervals as necessary. Twenty-four patients received a muscle flap for soft tissue coverage (12 a free flap and 12 a local muscle rotation flap). The other wounds were allowed to granulate and were covered with split-thickness skin.

Results.—Two free flaps failed and 2 local rotation flaps sloughed partially. Patients with early muscle flap coverage were hospitalized for a shorter period than the others and had infection less often. Patients who underwent bone grafting after the wound had re-epithelialized had early infection less often than those with an open or draining wound. The time to union was shorter in the former patients. Almost half of the patients who had delayed intramedullary nailing with reaming had infection.

Conclusions.—Early soft tissue coverage, within 1–2 weeks of injury, enhances the outcome of bone grafting in patients with tibial shaft fractures. Secondary bony reconstruction is a less complicated procedure when the soft tissue injury is well healed.

▶ The obvious problem with this retrospective study is that the patient groups may not be totally comparable. However, the overall sophistication of the authors and of the study itself would indicate that the conclusions are probably quite valid. The experience of other trauma centers also indicates that early soft tissue closure and delayed bone grafting is the most desirable treatment for these injuries. Moreover, delayed reamed intramedullary fixation, especially after initial external skeletal fixation, is very risky in a type IIIB tibial injury. The consensus for treatment of high-grade tibial fractures calls for thorough initial débridement and stabilization with external skeletal fixation or nonreamed locked nailing followed by soft tissue coverage at 5–7 days. Cancellous bone grafting is performed between 3 and 6 postoperative weeks, assuming that the soft tissue envelope is clean and the patient is healthy. Otherwise, bone grafting is delayed for at least 3 weeks after soft tissue integrity is obtained. The overall rate of serious complications is very high with grade IIIB fractures; serious infections develop in approximately half of these patients and 12% come to amputation, even in the hands of experts! It is also important to note that these patients usually have been given cephalosporin and aminoglycosides, a fact that once again demonstrates that antibiotics have little effect in preventing infection in high-energy injuries. This paper should also be essential reading for those who would prefer to attempt salvage in high-grade tibial fractures.—S.T. Hansen, M.D.

Additional Reading

The following articles are recommended to the reader:

Brunner WG, Spencer RF: Posterior tibial nerve neurotmesis complication a closed tibial fracture. A case report. *S Afr Med J* 78:607–608, 1990.
Hoekman P, Van de Perre P, Nelissen J, et al: Increased frequency of infection after open reduction of fractures in patients who are seropositive for human immunodeficiency virus. *J Bone Joint Surg* 73-A:675–679, 1991.
Knottenbelt JD: Low initial hemoglobin levels in trauma patients: An important indicator of ongoing hemorrhage. *J Trauma* 31:1396–1399, 1991.
Downey DJ, Omer GE, Moneim MS: New Mexico rattlesnake bites: Demographic review and guidelines for treatment. *J Trauma* 31:1380–1386, 1991.
Piza-Katzer H, Balogh B: Experience with 60 inferior rectus abdominis flaps. *Br J Plastic Surgery* 44:438–443, 1991.

Rehabilitation

A Study of Function and Residual Joint Stiffness After Functional Bracing of Tibial Shaft Fractures
Pun W-K, Chow S-P, Fang D, Ip F-K, Leong JCY, Ng C (University of Hong Kong)
Clin Orthop 267:157–163, 1991   9–31

Background.—Although functional bracing permits early mobilization of joints, joints do not always recover complete range of motion. Little is known about the degree of improvement in range of motion of joints after functional bracing is discontinued. A patient series was reexamined regularly to investigate the recovery of joint motion and function.

Methods.—Ninety-eight diaphyseal tibial fractures in 97 patients were treated with custom-made functional braces. All patients were older than 14 years of age. Follow-up averaged 1.9 years; 53 patients were observed for more than 2 years.

Results.—Most patients did not have full range of motion in the ankle and subtalar joints when the brace was removed after the fracture healed. The stiffness lessened with time, but many patients still had residual joint stiffness. At an average follow-up of 1.9 years, 68% had normal ankle motion. Sixty percent had normal inversion and eversion of the hind foot. In patients observed for more than 2 years, 75.5% had normal ankle motion, and 71% had normal inversion and eversion of the foot. The incidence of residual joint stiffness in the knee joint was small, with a clinically insignificant amount of stiffness. The incidence of ankle and subtalar joint stiffness was high among patients with an abnormal walking pattern after fracture healing.

Conclusions.—Early joint mobilization in functional bracing appears to offer a distinct advantage in reducing the incidence of joint stiffness. This is particularly important in the ankle and subtalar joints, as stiffness commonly occurs in these joints in patients with an abnormal walking pattern. Recovery of joint motion was satisfactory for the knee joint and full extension returned.

▶ A simple retrospective study of a single technique, this paper is valuable primarily for a look at the natural history of ankle and subtalar stiffness after immobilization of a tibial fracture. Historical controls from other papers may not be particularly valid, but, certainly, it is well known that significant stiffness occurs in these joints after prolonged casting. Functional bracing decreases stiffness. Range of motion in the joints continues to improve for 2–3 years after casting, and failur to regain motion is associated with persisting symptoms and limping. The authors were unable to correlate stiffness to factors such as fracture type or the length of treatment, leaving the cause of stiffness unclear in patients treated with functional bracing. Partial deep posterior compartmental syndromes or tethering of the muscles to the fracture line in deep compartments are possible causes. Otherwise, stiffness no doubt relates to individual patient characteristics. This explanation may be valid in that the patients in the study are Chinese, and the characteristics of their connective tissue may be different from those of whites or blacks. For example, it is apparent in our region that Native Americans are less susceptible to stiffness from immobilization than whites are. A fact that was not stated in the study but that is related to persistent symptoms and stiffness is that functional range of motion in the subtalar joint is necessary for normal gait. The need for postoperative function and protection of these joints may itself be an indication for reamed or non-reamed locked intramedullary nailing in many tibial fractures. The authors point out that, even with optimal functional bracing, only 75% of patients attained normal ankle motion, and 70% had normal inversion and eversion 2 years postoperatively.—S.T. Hansen, M.D.

Continuous Passive Motion Versus Immobilization: The Effect on Post-traumatic Joint Stiffness
Namba RS, Kabo JM, Dorey FJ, Meals RA (Wadsworth VA Med Ctr; Univ of California, Los Angeles)
Clin Orthop 267:218–223, 1991   9–32

Background.—Joint stiffness often complicates the management of intra-articular fractures long after bony healing has occurred. A series of experiments was done to provide biomechanical evidence for the efficacy of continuous passive motion in maintaining joint function in stabilized articular injuries.

Methods.—An intra-articular injury was created in the ankles of 10 rabbits by Steinmann pin penetration. On each animal, 1 limb was immobilized and the other was placed in a continuous passive motion machine for 3 weeks. Joint stiffness was quantified before injury and after 3 weeks of treatment with an arthrograph. Hind limb volumes also were noted before injury and were monitored weekly using a water-displacement method.

Results.—In immobilized limbs, joint stiffness increased 2.6 times compared with preinjury levels. Joint stiffness did not differ significantly between preinjury values and values in ankles treated with continuous passive motion. The posttraumatic difference between limbs treated with continuous passive motion and immobilized limbs was very significant. Continuous passive motion did not affect limb swelling.

Conclusions.—Immobilization is clearly detrimental to joint function. However, inappropriate doses of motion after injury may be worse. Further research is needed to determine appropriate speeds, forces, and duration before motion machines can be applied intelligently in clinical situations.

▶ Rabbits were used to evaluate continuous passive motion in posttraumatic rehabilitation. Because postoperative care of internally fixed supracondylar femoral fractures often includes continuous passive motion and because this modality is being used increasingly in other joints as well, its cost must be justified. Continuous passive motion was first used after total knee replacements, where it was useful but did not always significantly improve the final range of motion. The study is preliminary and the model may be imperfect, but indications are strong that continuous passive motion is very effective in posttraumatic joint rehabilitation.—S.T. Hansen, M.D.

Complications

Compartment Syndrome After Low-Velocity Gunshot Wounds to the Forearm

Moed BR, Fakhouri AJ (Henry Ford Hosp, Detroit; Wayne State Univ, Detroit)
J Orthop Trauma 5:134–137, 1991   9–33

Background.—Gunshot injuries to the upper extremity may cause a compartment syndrome, a relationship that has not been documented in the literature. Retrospective analysis was done to assess the incidence of compartment syndrome and the associated risk factors after low-velocity gunshot wounds to the forearm.

Methods.—One hundred twenty-seven patients with 131 low-velocity gunshot wounds to the forearm were treated at 1 center between 1980 and 1988. There was no bony injury in 71 extremities; 60 extremities were fractured. Compartment syndrome was diagnosed on the basis of tissue pressure measurements or clinical assessment, or both. Univariate analysis and a multivariate stepwise logistic regression were used to assess potential risk factors, including fracture location, displacement, comminution, and the number of radiographically determined metallic foreign bodies in the wound.

Results.—Thirteen extremities (10%) were diagnosed with a compartment syndrome. The only risk factor for the development of the syndrome was fracture location. In all 9 cases of compartment syndrome in fractured forearms, the fractures were comminuted. Highly displaced fractures had an incidence of compartment syndrome of 35%, whereas nondisplaced and minimally and moderately displaced fractures had incidences of 6%, 22%, and 0, respectively.

Conclusions.—Patients with low-velocity gunshot wounds to the forearm are at risk of having a compartment syndrome. Physicians must keep a high index of suspicion to prevent untoward consequences. Patients with this injury should be monitored closely, especially those with a fracture of the proximal third of the forearm.

▶ The incidence of gunshot wounds is on the increase in our emergency departments and is even epidemic in some. This paper is a very timely reminder that we must not become complacent about low-velocity gunshot wounds. Proximal-third comminuted forearm injuries are most susceptible to related complications.—S.T. Hansen, M.D.

Acute Compartment Syndrome: Effect of Dermotomy on Fascial Decompression in the Leg

Cohen MS, Garfin SR, Hargens AR, Mubarak SJ (Univ of California, San Diego)
J Bone Joint Surg 73-A:287–290, 1991   9–34

Background.—Prompt release of the fascia is necessary in acute compartment syndrome, but the length of the dermotomy necessary for adequate decompression in the lower extremity is uncertain. There have been reports in which skin continued to cause compression after fasciotomy through short incisions.

Patients.—The effect of the length of the skin incision was examined in 8 patients with posttraumatic compartment syndrome in the lower limb. All 8 had painful limb swelling and a palpably tense compartment. Distal hypesthesia usually was present. Intracompartmental pressures exceeded 30 mm Hg.

Technique.—All affected compartments were initially released through 8-cm skin incisions. After pressure measurements indicated equilibrium, the anterolateral incision was enlarged 2 cm at a time until readings showed no further change. Posteromedial incisions were enlarged only if the posterior compartment pressure approached 30 mm Hg.

Results.—Mean compartment pressure decreased from 48 mm Hg to 25 mm Hg after limited fascial release. Pressure remained greater than 30 mm Hg in 9 of 29 compartments. Incisions were extended to an average of 16 cm in these instances, and the mean final compartment pressure was 13 mm Hg, representing significant further decompression.

Conclusions.—Limited skin incisions may preclude a thorough reduction in compartment pressure. The present findings support the use of both intraoperative compartment pressure measurements and generous skin incisions.

▶ This very important paper was written by a group with extensive experience investigating compartmental syndromes. I have seen numerous failures of treatment of compartmental syndromes caused by inadequate skin incisions. The skin is occasionally the primary restrictive envelope in a compartmental syndrome in the foot.—S.T. Hansen, M.D.

Additional Reading

The following articles are recommended to the reader:

Almekinders LC: Gradual closure of fasciotomy wounds. *Orthop Rev* 20:82–84, 1991.

Rööser B, Bengtson S, Hägglund G: Acute compartment syndrome from anterior thigh muscle contusion: A report of eight cases. *J Orthop Trauma* 5:57–59, 1991.

Koval KJ, Clapper MF, Brumback RJ, et al: Complications of reamed intramedullary nailing of the tibia. *J Orthop Trauma* 5:184–189, 1991.

Quiñones-Baldrich WJ, Chervu A, Hernandez JJ, et al: Skeletal muscle function after ischemia: "No reflow" versus reperfusion injury. *J Surg Res* 51:5–12, 1991.

Cambria RA, Anderson RJ, Dikdan G, et al: Leukocyte activation in ischemia–reperfusion injury of skeletal muscle. *J Surg Res* 51:13–17, 1991.

Rubin B, Tittley J, Chang G, et al: A clinically applicable method for long-term salvage of postischemic skeletal muscle. *J Vasc Surg* 13:58–68, 1991.

New Technology and Implant Designs

Polyacetal Rod Fixation of Fractures in Osteoporotic Bone: A Preliminary Report

Ryan MD (Royal North Shore Hospital, Sydney, Australia)
J Bone Joint Surg 73-B:506–508, 1991   9–35

Introduction.—Diaphyseal fractures in osteoporotic bone are difficult to treat successfully by nonoperative means. Plaster casts may result in joint stiffness and prolonged traction in loss of bone and muscle mass. Promising results have been obtained with intramedullary rods manufactured from polyacetal.

Methods.—Polyacetal rods were used in the treatment of 14 closed fractures in 13 patients. Ten of the patients were women (average age, 77 years). Nine femora and 5 tibiae were fixed, using nails that were 440 mm in length and 14–17 mm in diameter. With 6 of the fractures, some form of supplementary external support was used for 4–8 weeks.

Results.—At an average follow-up of 26 months, no rod had broken. Thirteen fractures united primarily, and 1 required bone grafting. No infections occurred. Radiographs revealed the formation of abundant periosteal callus.

Conclusion.—The pliability of polyacetal rods allows them to be introduced into osteoporotic bones without further comminution. The pliable rods can be locked with cortical bone screws without the need of jigs or radiographic control. In this small group of patients, all of whom weighed 75 kg or less, none of the implants broke.

▶ A very interesting idea is presented for treatment of femoral shaft fractures in elderly patients with osteoporotic bone. These patients differ from the usual trauma patients in several respects: they usually sustain oblique or spiral fractures and have very large medullary canals and soft bone. Because they are not always treated in trauma centers that have special equipment, targeting devices, and surgeons experienced in standard interlocked nailing, this device deserves further study. The long-term performance of the rod in marrow canals will be of great interest.—S.T. Hansen, M.D.

Internal Fixation With a Self-Compressing Plate and Lag Screw: Improvements of the Plate Hole and Screw Design. 1. Mechanical Investigation
Klaue K, Perren SM, Kowalski M (AO/ASIF Foundation, Davos, Switzerland)
J Orthop Trauma 5:280–288, 1991   9–36

Background.—Self-compressing plates with oval holes and special drill guides have been used for many years. Recently, the advantages of lag-screw interfragmentary compression inserted through the plate have been demonstrated. Such screws often are inserted on an incline toward the fracture plane for better efficiency. However, inclined screws placed into oval holes undergo a displacement toward the fracture. A new plate and screw interaction, resulting from efforts to improve the effect of this technique, was examined.

Methods.—Conventional, fully threaded and shank screws were used. The plate was a straight conventional bone plate with a rectangular cross-section and elongated holes flared along the long axis toward the upper and lower surfaces. The plate design permits plate tensioning in both directions along the axis with no locking effect. An experimental device consisting of a tension transducer hinged with a 2-hole segment of a plate was also used. The tensile force on the plate from the conventional lag screw through plate technique was measured in 21 cadaveric humeri.

Results.—There was a substantial loss of compression force exerted by the plate when the fully threaded screw, applied as a lag screw, was tightened onto the dynamic compression plate hole. Compression was measured after tightening the screw inserted in the loading position of the self-compressing plate hole and after tightening the lag screw. The difference between the 2 screws' compression values was significant. Plate tension achieved with the new plate after the compression screw was tightened after the usual plate-tensioning screw was tightened varied between 900 and 1,360 N after the fully threaded screw was driven home and between 1,200 and 1,630 N after the oblique compression screw was tightened. When compression exerted by the screw on cadaveric bone was tested, there was a loss of effective compression by the screw wherever the fully threaded screw was used. All lag screws apparently generated enough compressive force. However, the effective lag force generated is probably not sufficient for stable fixation clinically. The shank screw gave a much more reliable transmission of the lag force onto the opposite fragment.

Conclusions.—When physicians select internal fixation as a treatment method, they should follow certain principles. The devices used should be easy to handle and tolerant of a small degree of misuse. The implants should be versatile, with a wide range of applications. Finally, their implantation should require minimal additional disturbance of the injured tissues so that surgical dissection is minimized and recovery of normal function in adjacent joints is facilitated.

▶ This paper describes the features of an improved plate, but it is more noteworthy for its investigation of the intended and actual effects of plates and screws on bone.—S.T. Hansen, M.D.

Internal Fixation With a Self-Compressing Plate and Lag Screw: Improvements of the Plate Hole and Screw Design. 2. In Vivo Investigations
Klaue K, Kowalski M, Perren SM (AO/ASIF Foundation, Davos, Switzerland)
J Orthop Trauma 5:289–296, 1991   9–37

Background.—Lag screws can cause a great amount of holding power between fragments. However, the biologic implementation of those mechanical effects has to be demonstrated. A mechanically improved design of bone plate and screw was compared with conventional plate fixation in vivo.

Methods.—Forty-one sheep were selected for the study on the basis of matching tibia shape and size. A standardized osteotomy was done. The animals were killed 56 days after implantation. Clinical, radiologic, and microscopic assessments were done.

Results.—Five of the sheep had to be excluded from the experiment because of early fractures. On radiologic assessment, the osteotomies without callus formation showed a narrow band of radiolucent bone at the osteotomy site. Histologically, there was complete remodeling at the osteotomy site.

Conclusions.—This new system of compression plates and screws provides a more versatile and efficient compression method with a limited surgical approach. Previous in vitro mechanical tests showed that the principles were conclusive, and these in vivo findings indicate that interfragmentary remodeling occurs more rapidly than with standard techniques.

▶ A companion to Abstract 9–36, this study presents the results of testing the newly designed plate in vivo. Again, the paper emphasizes related topics of great importance, for example, methods of plate insertion causing minimal surgical trauma. Protection of the blood supply to bone during stabilization has been a major issue in traumatology for the past several years. The discussion of the 6 types of plate fixation contains a great deal of information about bone healing and plate fixation.—S.T. Hansen, M.D.

Additional Reading

The following articles are recommended to the reader:

Saragaglia D, Tourne Y, Montbarbon E, et al: L'ostéosynthèse des fractures de l'avant-bras par plaque P.C.D. "petit fragments" de l'instrumentation A.O.: A propos de 283 plaques vissées. *J Chir (Paris)* 128:3–7, 1991.

Claudi BF, Oedekoven G: "Biologische" osteosynthesen. *Chirurg* 62:367–377, 1991.

Rosson J, Murphy W, Tonge C, et al: Healing of residual screw holes after plate removal. *Injury* 22:383–384, 1991.

Murphy CP, D'Ambrosia R, Dabezies EJ: The small pin circulator fixator for proximal tibial fractures with soft tissue compromise. *Orthopedics* 14:273–280, 1991.

Murphy CP, D'Ambrosia R, Dabezies EJ: The small pin circular fixator for distal tibial pilon fractures with soft tissue compromise. *Orthopedics* 14:283–290, 1991.

Rosson JW, Petley GW, Shearer JR: Bone structure after removal of internal fixation plates. *J Bone Joint Surg* 73-B:65–67, 1991.

Henley MB, Monroe M, Tencer AF: Biomechanical comparison of methods of fixation of a midshaft osteotomy of the humerus. *J Orthop Trauma* 5:14–20, 1991.

Daum WJ, Patterson RM, Cartwright TJ, et al: Comparison of cortical and cancellous screw pull-out strengths about the posterior column and sacroiliac joint. *J Orthop Trauma* 5:34–37, 1991.

Subject Index

A

Acetabular
  cups, retrieved, polyethylene wear from, 178
  dysplasia after Pavlik harness in congenital hip dislocation, 22
  fracture (*see* Fracture, acetabular)
  rim syndrome and hip dysplasia, 155
Acetabuloplasty
  pericapsular, triradiate cartilage premature closure complicating, 21
Acetaminophen
  in knee osteoarthritis, 125
Acromioclavicular
  dislocation, surgery outcome, 56
  joint injuries in sport, 109
Acromionectomy
  total, 20 year review, 70
Acrylic
  cementation in bone tumors, aggressive benign, 301
Adductors
  posterior transfer, in children with cerebral palsy, 5
Adolescence
  low back pain in athletes during, 12
  spondylolisthesis during, symptomatic isthmic low-grade, natural history of, 11
Aged
  shoulder disorders, 65
  tibial fracture, type III, 362
Aircraft disaster
  M1, open fracture initial management in, 345
Akin double osteotomy
  chevron, for hallux valgus correction, 279
Akin procedure
  results analysis, 273
Allograft
  massive retrieved human, observations on, 305
  vs. autograft for benign lesions in children, 302
Alvik's glenoplasty
  for humeroscapular dislocation, 59
Amputation
  analgesia by nerve sheath block after, 364
  below knee, running and prosthetic feet, 359
  lower extremities
    bilateral, rehabilitation, 360
    smoking complicating, 358

Syme's, indications for, and fibular deficiency, 14
  traumatic, vs. extremity salvage, 361
Analgesia
  after amputation by nerve sheath block, 364
  of morphine, intraarticular, after knee arthroscopy, 93
Anesthesia
  brachial plexus, interscalene, hemidiaphragmatic paresis in, 83
  epidural, in deep vein thrombosis in total hip arthroplasty, 171
  general vs. regional, as risk for deep vein thrombosis after hip surgery, 170
Angiogenin
  for neovascularization of meniscus (in rabbit), 118
Ankle
  arthrodesis (*see* Arthrodesis, ankle)
  deformity, correction, preoperative Ilizarov frame construction for, 18
  fracture (*see* Fracture, ankle)
  impingement, anterolateral, arthroscopy in, 270
  instability, lateral, Evans procedure results in, 268
  ligament injuries, grade III, early mobilization, 270
  mortise stability in Weber C fracture, syndesmotic fixation, 262
  MRI of, 271
  physeal injury, long-term follow-up, 279
  talonavicular joints and, talocalcaneal fusion in, 281
Anti-inflammatory drugs
  nonsteroidal, stopped before elective surgery, 166
Antibiotic
  in arthroplasty infection, acute, 151
  in osteomyelitis, bioabsorbable delivery system, 122
  in prosthetic joint infections, chronic, 151
  resistance of staphylococci, biomaterial-adherent coagulase-negative and -positive, 188
Antigen
  matched graft transplant, meniscus cartilage after, 118
Anulus
  tears and disc degeneration (in sheep), 222
Arm
  position in rotator cuff repair, 77

Arteries
popliteal, injuries, in knee fracture and
dislocation after blunt trauma, 96
Arthritis
of elbow, after trauma, total
replacement, 81
osteoarthritis (*see* Osteoarthritis)
radiocarpal, fusion in, 330
rheumatoid (*see* Rheumatoid arthritis)
Arthrodesis
ankle
with Calandruccio frame and
bimalleolar onlay graft, 267
with internal screw fixation, 265
in lumbar spondylolisthesis with spinal
stenosis, and decompression, 237
radiolunate, in rheumatoid wrist, 330
shoulder, rigid internal fixation, 80
spinal
with pedicle screw-plate fixation, 251
in spinal canal enlargement in cervical
spondylotic myelopathy, 205
subtalar, with bone graft and fixation in
myelomeningocele, in children, 6
triple, in adults, 268
Arthrography
of rotator cuff degenerative lesions, 46
Arthroplasty
hip (*see* Hip arthroplasty)
infected, acutely, local antibiotics in,
151
Keller resection, experience with, 274
knee (*see* Knee arthroplasty)
revision, ultrasound tool cement
removal in, 181
shoulder
in humeral fracture, 78
total, vs. hemiarthroplasty in glenoid
resurfacing, 79
Arthroscopy
of ankle impingement, anterolateral,
270
for distension in frozen shoulder, 68
in inflammatory joint diseases with
synovectomy, 114
knee
intraarticular morphine analgesia
after, 93
in knee osteoarthritis for
debridement, 125
in polyethylene wear in total knee
arthroplasty, 149
subacromial decompression for chronic
impingement of shoulder, 70
Arthrosis
hip joint, quality of life before and after
arthroplasty in, 185
Articular cartilage (*see* Cartilage, articular)

Aseptic
necrosis in football after hip
subluxation, 110
Aspirin
in deep vein thrombosis after total hip
replacement prevention, 168
Athletes
during adolescence, low back pain of, 12
in overhand sports, shoulder
reconstruction, anterior
capsulolabral, 58
Atlantoaxial
instability presenting as cerebral and
cerebellar infarcts in children, 8
Atlas
burst fracture, evaluation and
treatment, 348
Autograft
vs. allograft for benign lesions in
children, 302
Avascular
necrosis of femoral head, natural
history, 189

B

Back
low back injury, occupational, after
lumbar laminectomy for disc
degeneration, 226
pain
low (*see* Low back pain)
lumbar pathology in, 224
in lumbar spine in middle aged
women, 229
psychometric instruments in, 227
Bacteremia
bone and joint infections due to
Staphylococcus aureus, 121
Bacteria
counts in operating rooms, ultraviolet
radiation vs. ultra-clean air
enclosure, 119
cultures, positive, from clean orthopedic
operations, 120
Barlow test
hip stability in newborn and, 25
Bean-shaped foot
cuneiform osteotomy and cuboid
osteotomy in, 17
Benign lesions
in children, autograft vs. allograft, 302
Biceps
tendon
brachii, dislocation, and bicipital
groove dysplasia, 65
dislocation, MRI of, 49

Bicipital
groove dysplasia and biceps brachii
tendon dislocation, 65
Bimalleolar onlay graft
in ankle arthrodesis, 267
Bioabsorbable
delivery system for antibiotics in
osteomyelitis, 122
Biomaterial
adherent to Staphylococci, antibiotic
resistance of, 188
Birth palsy, brachial plexus (*see* Brachial
plexus birth palsy)
Block
nerve sheath, for analgesia after
amputation surgery, 364
Blood
autologous, postoperative collection and
reinfusion in total knee
arthroplasty, 133
loss after total knee replacement,
tourniquet release and continuous
passive motion in, 132
Bone
bank bone incorporation, lipid
extraction enhancing (in rabbit), 369
calvarial, response to cyclic biaxial
mechanical strain (in rat), 193
deficiency in total knee arthroplasty,
metal wedge augmentation, 130
disease, metastatic, in breast cancer,
prognostic indicators, 306
endosteal, after cement removal, 181
Ewing's sarcoma of (*see* Ewing's
sarcoma of bone)
femoral, resorption and stem stiffness
after porous-coated total hip
arthroplasty (in dog), 157
formation, heterotopic, after
uncemented total hip arthroplasty,
indomethacin for, 165
graft (*see* Graft, bone)
growth, longitudinal, and hypertrophic
chondrocyte volume in growth
plates, 38
imaging in painful prosthetic joint, 112
infections due to *Staphylococcus aureus*,
121
loss
from femur after total hip
arthroplasty, 158
predicting fragility fractures in
women, 197
morphogenesis in replicas of
hydroxyapatite from calcium
carbonate of coral, 195
Paget's disease of, familial aggregation,
191

regenerate, histomorphometry in limb
lengthening by Ilizarov method, 40
tissue transformation into, practical
application, 194
tumors
aggressive benign, cryosurgery and
acrylic cementation in, 301
for femur, prosthetic replacement,
303
wounds, chronic traumatic,
microvascular free tissue transfer
in, 371
Brachial plexus
anesthesia, interscalene,
hemidiaphragmatic paresis in, 83
birth palsy
persistent, 1
surgery of, 3
microsurgery in children, 2
palsy with rotator cuff tear and
shoulder dislocation, 62
Bracing
functional, in tibial shaft fracture, joint
stiffness after, 374
Brain
injury, osteosynthesis of major fractures
in, 353
Breast
cancer, metastatic
bone disease in, prognostic indicators,
306
bone-only, 307
Bristow procedure
failed, complications of, 61
Bunionette
osteotomy for
chevron metatarsal, 275
longitudinal diaphyseal, with soft
tissue repair, 277
Burns
fracture in, major, early orthopedic
intervention, 347

C

Calandruccio frame
in ankle arthrodesis, 267
Calcaneus
fracture (*see* Fracture, calcaneal)
Calcium
carbonate exoskeletons of coral, bone
morphogenesis in replicas of
hydroxyapatite from, 195
phosphate ceramic in ulnar bone defects
(in dog), 367
supplement in osteoporosis prevention,
postmenopausal, 200

Calvaria
bone cell response to cyclic biaxial
mechanical strain (in rat), 193
Cancer
metastases (*see* Metastases)
Cannula
for decompression and lumbar
discectomy, failures and
complications, 244
Capsular
release in rotator cuff repair, 77
Carpal
intercarpal fusion in prosthetic silicone
scaphoid strains, 341
tunnel syndrome
occupational, 319
surgery, vibration exposure in, and
recovery after surgery, 321
Cartilage
articular
changes after meniscal lesions (in
rabbit), 117
regeneration after chondral shaving
and subchondral abrasion (in
rabbit), 115
formation, new, synthetic polymers as
template for, 190
knee joint, in inflammatory diseases,
synovectomy in, 114
meniscus, after graft transplant, 118
triradiate, premature closure
complicating pericapsular
acetabuloplasty, 21
Cast
with elbow extended in forearm
fracture in children, 32
Cells
Langerhans', histiocytosis chemotherapy
in children, 299
Cement
extraction technique in revision total
hip arthroplasty, 180
removal
endosteal bone after, 181
ultrasound tool, in revision
arthroplasty, 181
Cementation
acrylic, in bone tumors, aggressive
benign, 301
Cemented
prosthesis in total hip replacement, 185
Ceramic
calcium phosphate, in ulnar bone
defects (in dog), 367
hydroxyapatite coating of hip
prosthesis, 176
intervertebral disc replacement in
cervical disc lesion, 208

Cerebellar
infarct, atlantoaxial instability
presenting as, in children, 8
Cerebral
infarct, atlantoaxial instability
presenting as, in children, 8
palsy
gait analysis in ambulatory children,
7
rhizotomy and, follow-up with gait
analysis, 4
spastic, Green transfer in, 8
transfer of adductors in, posterior, in
children, 5
Cervical
disc lesion, artificial ceramic
intervertebral disc replacement in,
208
dislocation, closed reduction with
traction in, 211
injuries, traumatic distractive flexion,
posterior wiring in, 212
myelopathy, spondylotic, spinal canal
enlargement with arthrodesis in,
205
stenosis and morphometry in football
players, 213
Chemotherapy
in fibromatosis, aggressive, in children,
299
in histiocytosis, Langerhans' cell, in
children, 299
Chevron
Akin double osteotomy for hallux
valgus correction, 279
metatarsal osteotomy for bunionette,
275
Chiari's
osteotomy in Perthes' disease, 29
Children
atlantoaxial instability presenting as
cerebral and cerebellar infarcts, 8
benign lesions, autograft vs. allograft,
302
brachial plexus microsurgery, 2
cerebral palsy
gait analysis in ambulatory child, 7
posterior transfer of adductors in, 5
childhood tumor radiotherapy, leg
length discrepancy after, 13
clubfoot relapse correction with Ilizarov
apparatus, 19
condylar fracture, lateral, late surgery,
32
fibromatosis, aggressive, chemotherapy,
299
forearm fracture, cast with elbow
extended, 32

histiocytosis, Langerhans' cell,
  chemotherapy, 299
low back pain and disk degeneration, 12
myelomeningocele, subtalar arthrodesis,
  bone graft and fixation in, 6
osteosarcoma, 295
physeal injuries, partial growth arrest
  after, MRI of, 37
sarcoma
  osteogenic, incidence and survival
    rates, 294
  soft tissue, of extremities,
    nonrhabdomyosarcoma, 296
spondylolisthesis, symptomatic isthmic
  low-grade, natural history, 11
supracondylar fracture, displaced,
  transarticular fixation, 31
Volkmann's ischemic contracture,
  muscle transplant in, 34
Chiropractic services
use study, 242
Chondral
  injuries in malleolar fracture operatively
    reduced, 352
  shaving, articular cartilage regeneration
    after (in rabbit), 115
Chondrocytes
  hypertrophic, volume of, and
    longitudinal bone growth in growth
    plates, 38
  synthetic polymers seeded with, as
    template for new cartilage
    formation, 190
Chondroitinase ABC
  for nucleolysis of disc (in rabbit), 246
Chondrolysis
  in football player after hip subluxation,
    110
Clavicle
  fracture of mid-shaft, non-union, 52
  pseudarthrosis, congenital, surgery of, 35
Clubfoot
  deformity, residual, cuneiform
    osteotomy and cuboid osteotomy
    in, 17
  relapse correction with Ilizarov
    apparatus in children, 19
Cobalt-alloy heads
  corrosion at interface on titanium-alloy
    stems, 163
Collagraft
  as bone graft substitute, 366
Compartment syndrome
  dermotomy in fascial decompression in
    leg and, 377
  of foot (*see* Foot, compartment
    syndrome)
  in gunshot wounds to forearm, 376

Compression
  syndrome in reflex sympathetic
    dystrophy, 338
Computed tomography
  in cervical stenosis and morphometry,
    213
  of disc herniation
    lumbar, after myelography, 238
    thoracic, 217
  in patellar tendinitis, 94
  three-dimensional, in scaphoid fracture
    displacement, 334
Condyle
  femur (*see* Femur, condyle)
  fracture, lateral, late surgery in children,
    32
  medial, osteonecrosis of, survival in
    total knee arthroplasty, 143
Consent
  informed, for surgery, patients' recall of
    preoperative instruction for, 172
Contracture
  Volkmann's ischemic, in children,
    muscle transplant for, 34
Cooling pad
  after total knee arthroplasty, 134
Coral
  calcium carbonate exoskeletons, bone
    morphogenesis in replicas of
    hydroxyapatite from, 195
Corticosteroids
  injection into facet joints for low back
    pain, 241
Cost
  of arthroplasty, hip and knee, 145
Cruciate ligament
  anterior
    deficient knee, 100
    Leeds-Keio replacement, results, 104
    reconstruction, proprioception and
      function after, 103
    reconstruction, thigh muscle electrical
      stimulation after, 106
    reconstruction with patellar tendon
      graft, 101
    reconstruction with patellar tendon
      graft and tenodesis, 102
    rupture, knee function after
      treatment, 99
  injuries of knee, MRI of, 105
  posterior, tear repair results, 107
  retention and substitution in total knee
    arthroplasty, 128
Cryopreserved
  allograft transplant, meniscus cartilage
    after, 118
Cryosurgery
  in bone tumors, aggressive benign, 301

Cuboid
    osteotomy, closing wedge, in residual
        clubfoot deformity, 17
Cuneiform
    osteotomy, opening wedge medial, in
        residual clubfoot deformity, 17

D

Darrach procedure
    technique redefined and long-term
        follow-up, 325
Debridement
    of rotator cuff tears, superior humeral
        dislocation after, 72
Dermotomy
    in fascial decompression in leg, and
        compartment syndrome, 377
Disc
    cervical, lesion, artificial ceramic
        intervertebral disc replacement in,
        208
    degeneration
        anulus tears (in sheep), 222
        and low back pain in children, 12
        lumbar laminectomy for, in
            occupational low back injury, 226
    herniated
        lumbar, myelographic diagnosis, CT
            after, 238
        thoracic, CT of, 217
    nucleolysis with chondroitinase ABC (in
        rabbit), 246
    rupture, mechanism of, 220
Discectomy
    lumbar
        and decompression with cannula,
            failures and complications, 244
        peridural fibrosis after, 240
Dislocation
    acromioclavicular, surgery outcome, 56
    biceps tendon
        brachii, with bicipital groove
            dysplasia, 65
        MRI of, 49
    cervical, closed reduction with traction
        in, 211
    hip (see Hip dislocation)
    humeroscapular, Alvik's glenoplasty for,
        59
    humerus, superior, after rotator cuff
        tear decompression and
        debridement, 72
    knee, 95
        blunt trauma causing, popliteal artery
            injuries in, 96
    radial head, 64

    shoulder (see Shoulder dislocation)
DNA
    content prognostic in soft tissue
        sarcoma, 298
Double crush hypothesis
    nerve compression model for, 204
Drinkers
    male, orthopedic trauma in, 350
Dupuytren's disease
    relation to work and injury, 323
Dynamometer
    Cybex II Isokinetic, in shoulder strength
        analysis, 67
Dysplasia
    acetabular, after Pavlik harness in
        congenital hip dislocation, 22
    epiphyseal, multiple, shoulder in, 84
    hip (see Hip dysplasia)
Dystrophy, reflex sympathetic (see Reflex
    sympathetic dystrophy)

E

Elbow
    arthritis after trauma, total replacement,
        81
    instability, posterolateral rotatory, 63
    replacement, capitellocondylar total, in
        rheumatoid arthritis, 82
    synovectomy in rheumatoid arthritis,
        results, 83
Elderly (see Aged)
Electrical stimulation
    nerve, after total knee arthroplasty, 134
    of thigh muscles after cruciate ligament
        reconstruction, 106
Embolism
    pulmonary, after total hip replacement,
        heparin to prevent, 169
Endosteal
    bone after cement removal, 181
Energy
    storing prosthetic feet and running, 359
Epicondylitis
    medial, surgery of, 69
Epidural
    anesthesia and deep vein thrombosis in
        total hip arthroplasty, 171
Epiphysis
    dysplasia, multiple, shoulder in, 84
    femoral (see Femur, epiphysis)
Evans procedure
    in ankle instability, lateral, results, 268
Ewing's sarcoma
    of bone
        combined modality treatment,
            long-term follow-up, 286

pelvic and sacral, multimodal
therapy, 292
radiotherapy, twice-a-day, local
control and function after, 290
radiotherapy
limited-volume, failure patterns after,
287
local treatment results, 289
Exercise
in osteoporosis prevention,
postmenopausal, 200
Extremities
lengthening by Ilizarov method,
histomorphometry of regenerate
bone in, 40
lower
amputation (*see* Amputation, lower
extremities), 358
fascial decompression, dermotomy in,
and compartment syndrome, 377
injuries to, complex vascular and
orthopedic, 363
salvage vs. traumatic amputation, 361
sarcoma, soft tissue,
nonrhabdomyosarcoma, in
children, 296

F

Facet
joints, corticosteroid injections into, for
low back pain, 241
Falls
hip fracture due to, in women, 196
Fascial
decompression in leg dermotomy in,
and compartment syndrome, 377
Feet (*see* Foot)
Femur
bone loss from, after total hip
arthroplasty, 158
bone resorption and stem stiffness after
porous-coated total hip
arthroplasty (in dog), 157
components in hip arthroplasty,
cemented, failure of, 161
condyle
osteochondral allograft of, 90
osteochondral fragment stability (in
dog), 91
osteonecrosis, course and
radiographic changes, 89
distal, prosthetic replacement in bone
tumors, 303
epiphysis, capital
necrosis of, and medial approaches to
hip (in piglet), 26

slipped, intertrochanteric corrective
osteotomy in, 28
slipped, single vs. double pin fixation
for, 27
fracture (*see* Fracture, femur)
graft in hip arthroplasty, revision, 184
head, necrosis, avascular, natural
history, 189
prosthesis, hydroxyapatite-coated,
bonding of, 177
stems, hydroxyapatite-coated, 175
Fenestration
in lumbar stenosis, central, 234
Fibrocartilage, triangular (*see* Triangular
fibrocartilage complex)
Fibromatosis, aggressive
chemotherapy in children, 299
radiotherapy of, 300
Fibrosis
peridural, after lumbar laminectomy
and discectomy, 240
Fibula
centralization failure in tibial
longitudinal deficiency, congenital,
15
deficiency and Syme's amputation
indications, 14
plating in tibial fracture, 354
Fibulectomy
for bone graft, functional deficit after, 368
Flap
coverage of tibial shaft fracture, timing
of, 372
gastrocnemius muscle, denervated,
discussion of, 370
muscle, for coverage of osteotomy site
in devascularized tibia (in dog),
372
pedicles and free muscle flaps in chronic
infected hip arthroplasty wounds,
182
Foot
bean-shaped, cuneiform osteotomy and
cuboid osteotomy in, 17
compartment syndrome
after calcaneal fracture, 257
management, 257
deformities, correction, preoperative
Ilizarov frame construction for, 18
MRI of, 271
prosthetic, energy storing, and running,
359
to-ground contact forces and plantar
pressure distribution, 282
valgus (*see* Valgus)
Football players
cervical stenosis and morphometry in,
213

Forearm
  fracture (*see* Fracture, forearm)
  gunshot wounds, compartment
    syndrome after, 376
Fracture
  acetabular
    displaced, long-term follow-up, 357
    somatosensory evoked potential
      monitoring in, 186
  ankle
    surgery complications, early, 261
    Weber C, mortise stability after, and
      syndesmotic fixation, 262
  atlas burst, evaluation and treatment,
    348
  calcaneal
    foot compartment syndrome after,
      257
    surgery results, 260
    three dimensional analysis, 264
  clavicle mid-shaft, non-union, 52
  condylar, lateral, late surgery in
    children, 32
  femur
    after knee arthroplasty, total, 153
    distal and shaft, ipsilateral, treatment,
      351
  forearm
    in children, cast with elbow extended,
      32
    osteosynthesis, radioulnar synostosis
      after, 55
  fragility, in women, bone loss
    predicting, 197
  hip, from falls in women, 196
  humerus
    displaced, open reduction and
      internal fixation, 54
    shoulder arthroplasty in, 78
  interphalangeal joint, proximal, pilon,
    315
  Jefferson, evaluation and treatment,
    348
  knee, after blunt trauma, popliteal
    artery injuries in, 96
  major
    in burns, early orthopedic
      intervention, 347
    osteosynthesis in, in brain injury, 353
  malleolar, operatively reduced, chondral
    injuries in, 352
  metacarpal, functional treatment, 317
  open, initial management in M1 aircraft
    disaster, 345
  osteoporotic bone, polyacetal rod
    fixation in, 378
  pelvis, skeletally unstable, early fixation
    outcome, 356

radius
  head, open reduction and internal
    fixation, 54
  unstable, augmented external fixation,
    314
scaphoid
  displacement, three-dimensional CT
    of, 334
  nonunion, vascularity assessment with
    MRI, 337
spine, thoracic, mediastinal widening in,
  349
supracondylar, displaced, transarticular
  fixation in children, 31
tibia
  nonunion, marrow injection
    substituting for graft in, 368
  plafond, open reduction and internal
    fixation results, 256
  plating of fibula in, 354
  shaft, functional bracing of, residual
    joint stiffness after, 374
  shaft, open, lag screw fixation in, 355
  shaft, timing of flap coverage, bone
    graft and intramedullary nailing in,
    373
  type III, in aged, 362
Fragility
  fractures in women, bone loss
    predicting, 197
Frozen
  shoulder, arthroscopic distension, 68

G

Gait
  after quadriceps femoris and hamstring
    muscle contraction, 106
  analysis in cerebral palsy
    in ambulatory child, 7
    rhizotomy and, 4
  high-heel, first metatarsophalangeal
    joint reaction forces during, 278
  in valgus deformities of foot in
    rheumatoid arthritis, 280
Gastrocnemius
  muscle flap, denervated, discussion of,
    370
Glenohumeral
  laxity, capsular venting in, 62
Glenoid
  labrum, evaluation with MRI, 52
  resurfacing, total shoulder arthroplasty
    vs. hemiarthroplasty in, 79
Glenoplasty
  Alvik's, for humeroscapular dislocation,
    59

GM-1 ganglioside
  in motor function recovery after spinal
    cord injury, 210
Gonarthrosis
  knee
    arthroplasty in, tricompartmental vs.
      unicompartmental, 140
    medial, prognosis, 127
    prosthesis for, unicompartmental, 139
Graft
  allograft (*see* Allograft)
  autograft vs. allograft for benign lesions
    in children, 302
  bimalleolar onlay, in ankle arthrodesis,
    267
  bone
    cancellous, in myelomeningocele with
      subtalar arthrodesis and fixation in
      children, 6
    in clavicle mid-shaft fracture
      non-union, 52
    coverage of tibial shaft fracture, 373
    fibulectomy for, functional deficit
      after, 368
    substitute, collagraft as, 366
  femur, in hip arthroplasty, revision, 184
  flap (*see* Flap)
  osteochondral, of femoral condyle, 90
  patellar tendon, in cruciate ligament
    reconstruction, 101, 102
  in tibial nonunion, marrow injection
    substituting for, 368
  transplant, meniscus cartilage after, 118
Green transfer
  in cerebral palsy, spastic, 8
Growth
  arrest, partial, after physeal injuries in
    children, 37
  bone, longitudinal, and hypertrophic
    chondrocyte volume in growth
    plates, 38
  plates, hypertrophic chondrocyte
    volume and longitudinal bone
    growth in, 38
Gunshot wounds
  to forearm, compartment syndrome
    after, 376

H

Hagie
  intramedullary pin in clavicle mid-shaft
    fracture non-union, 52
Hallux
  fusion with metatarsal head excision in
    rheumatoid arthritis, 113

valgus correction with chevron-Akin
  double osteotomy, 279
Hamstring
  muscles, contraction, gait and thigh
    muscle strength after, 106
Hand
  ischemia, pathophysiology, treatment
    and prognosis, 342
Hemiarthroplasty
  vs. shoulder arthroplasty, total, in
    glenoid resurfacing, 79
Hemidiaphragmatic
  paresis in interscalene brachial plexus
    anesthesia, 83
Heparin
  in deep vein thrombosis during total hip
    arthroplasty, 171
  to prevent deep vein thrombosis and
    pulmonary embolism after total hip
    replacement, 169
Herniated disc (*see* Disc, herniated)
Heterotopic
  ossification after total hip arthroplasty,
    radiotherapy to prevent, 166
High-heel gait
  first metatarsophalangeal joint reaction
    forces during, 278
Hip
  arthroplasty
    cemented, fixation and loosening,
      160
    femoral components, cemented,
      failure, 161
    functional improvement and costs,
      145
    infected, chronic, debridement and
      flaps in, 182
    of joint after arthrosis, quality of life
      before and after, 185
    revision, femoral allografts in, 184
  arthroplasty, total
    femoral bone loss after, 158
    heparin and deep vein thrombosis
      during, 171
    heterotopic ossification after,
      radiotherapy to prevent, 166
    modular head-neck components in,
      162
    porous-coated, and stem stiffness in
      femoral bone resorption (in dog),
      157
    range of motion in, 162
    recalcitrant wound, 181
    revision, cement extraction technique
      in, 180
    somatosensory evoked potential
      monitoring in, 187

uncemented, indomethacin for
heterotopic bone formation after,
165
dislocation, congenital
newborn screening and early
treatment, 23
Pavlik harness for, acetabular
dysplasia after, 22
still missed, why, 25
dysplasia, acetabular rim syndrome and,
155
dysplasia, congenital
MRI in, 20
newborn screening and early
treatment, 23
fracture from falls in women, 196
MAXIMA technique, 156
medial approaches to, and capital
femoral epiphysis necrosis (in
piglet), 26
osteoporosis, MRI of, 198, 199
pain in late pregnancy, 199
prosthesis
fixation and loosening, 160
hydroxyapatite ceramic coatings for,
176
McKee-Farrar total, long-term results,
173
measurement with image analysis, 156
modular, corrosion of, 162
replacement, total
cemented, patients under fifty,
long-term follow-up, 183
with cemented, uncemented and
hybrid prostheses, 185
deep vein thrombosis after,
prevention, 168, 169
failed titanium alloy, metal wear and
tissue response in, 179
nerve palsy in, 187
pulmonary embolism after, heparin to
prevent, 169
stability in newborn and Barlow test, 25
subluxation, traumatic, aseptic necrosis
and chondrolysis in football player
after, 110
surgery, deep vein thrombosis after,
general vs. regional anesthesia as
risk in, 170
synovitis, transient, ultrasound of, 39
Histiocytosis
Langerhans' cell, chemotherapy in
children, 299
Hormone
replacement therapy in osteoporosis
prevention, postmenopausal, 200
Humeroscapular
dislocation, Alvik's glenoplasty for, 59

Humerus
dislocation, superior, after rotator cuff
tear decompression and
debridement, 72
fracture (*see* Fracture, humerus)
Hyaluronate
in peridural fibrosis after lumbar
laminectomy and discectomy, 240
Hybrid
prosthesis in total hip replacement,
185
Hydroxyapatite
coating
ceramic, of hip prosthesis, 176
femoral prosthesis, bonding of, 177
femoral stems, 175
of prostheses, 175
porous, bone morphogenesis in replicas
of, 195
Hypertension
venous, in Legg-Perthes disease
pathogenesis, 29
Hypertrophic
chondrocyte volume and longitudinal
bone growth in growth plates, 38
Hypotension
controlled, in deep vein thrombosis in
total hip arthroplasty, 171

I

Ibuprofen
antiinflammatory vs. analgesic dose in
knee osteoarthritis, 125
Ilizarov
apparatus in clubfoot relapse correction
in children, 19
frame construction, preoperative, in
ankle and foot deformity
correction, 18
method for limb lengthening,
histomorphometry of regenerate
bone in, 40
Image
analysis in hip prosthesis measurement,
156
Imaging
bone, in painful prosthetic joint, 112
magnetic resonance (*see* Magnetic
resonance imaging)
Immobilization
joint stiffness after, posttraumatic,
375
Indomethacin
for heterotopic bone formation after
uncemented total hip arthroplasty,
165

Infarcts
  cerebral and cerebellar, atlantoaxial
    instability presenting as, in
    children, 8
Inflammatory
  joint diseases, synovectomy in,
    arthroscopy in, 114
Informed consent
  preoperative instruction for, for surgery,
    patients' recall of, 172
Injury
  relationship to Dupuytren's disease, 323
Instruction
  preoperative, for informed consent for
    surgery, patients' recall of, 172
Intercarpal
  fusion in prosthetic silicone scaphoid
    strains, 341
Interphalangeal joint
  proximal, pilon fracture, 315
Interscalene
  brachial plexus anesthesia,
    hemidiaphragmatic paresis in, 83
Intertrochanteric
  corrective osteotomy in slipped capital
    femoral epiphysis, 28
Intervertebral disc (*see* Disc)
Irradiation (*see* Radiography,
    Radiotherapy)
Ischemia
  of hand, pathophysiology, treatment
    and prognosis, 342
Ischemic
  contracture of Volkmann, in children,
    muscle transplant for, 34

J

Jefferson fracture
  evaluation and treatment, 348
Joint
  acromioclavicular, injuries in sport, 109
  aspiration in painful prosthetic joint,
    112
  facet, corticosteroid injections into, for
    low back pain, 241
  infections due to *Staphylococcus aureus*,
    121
  inflammatory joint diseases,
    synovectomy in, arthroscopy of,
    114
  interphalangeal, proximal, pilon
    fracture, 315
  knee, cartilages in inflammatory joint
    diseases, synovectomy in, 114
  metatarsophalangeal, first, reaction
    forces during high-heel gait, 278

  moment characteristics in below knee
    amputees, 359
  patellofemoral, reflex sympathetic
    dystrophy of, 97
  prosthesis (*see* Prosthesis, joint)
  radioulnar, distal, Sauvé-Kapandji
    procedure as salvage for, 324
  stiffness, continuous passive motion vs.
    immobilization in, 375
  talonavicular, ankle contact, and
    talocalcaneal fusion, 281
  wrist, functional ranges of motion, 332

K

Keller resection arthroplasty
  experience with, 274
Knee
  arthroplasty, infected, follow-up, 150
  arthroplasty, synovitis after,
    metal-induced, radiography of, 152
  arthroplasty, total
    bilateral, cruciate retaining vs.
      cruciate substituting, 128
    blood in, autologous, postoperative
      collection and reinfusion, 133
    bone deficiency in, metal wedge
      augmentation, 130
    femoral fracture after, 153
    polyethylene wear, arthroscopy of,
      149
    primary, subvastus approach, 127
    survival in osteonecrosis of medial
      condyle, 143
    vs. unicompartmental, 139
  arthroplasty, unicompartmental
    diagnostic protocol in, preoperative,
      135
    efficacy, long-term, 136
    survivorship analysis and follow-up,
      137
    vs. total, 139
    vs. tricompartmental, on
      gonarthrosis, 140
  arthroscopy, intraarticular morphine
    analgesia after, 93
  complaints, subjective, visual analog
    scales in, 98
  deficiency, anterior cruciate ligament,
    100
  dislocation, 95
    blunt trauma causing, popliteal artery
      injuries in, 96
  fracture, blunt trauma causing, popliteal
    artery injuries in, 96
  function after cruciate ligament rupture
    treatment, 99

gonarthrosis (*see* Gonarthrosis, knee)
joint cartilages in chronic inflammatory
joint diseases, synovectomy in, 114
kinematics, prosthetic joint line position
in, 131
meniscal and cruciate injuries, MRI of,
105
MRI, high signal in meniscus, 92
osteoarthritis (*see* Osteoarthritis, knee)
osteochondritis dissecans, 108
osteonecrosis, MRI of, 90
replacement, in morbid obesity, 144
replacement, total
blood loss after, tourniquet release
and continuous passive motion in,
132
coronal alignment, 129
Stanmore, survivorship analysis and
confidence intervals in, 142
in tibia metastases, 145
wear production by cycling sliding,
148
Kyphosis
Scheuermann's, vertebral alterations in,
218

L

Labral
capsular complex, MRI of, 51
Lactic acid
oligomer carrying antibiotic in
osteomyelitis, bioabsorbable
delivery system, 122
Lag screw
for internal fixation, with
self-compressing plate, 379, 380
in tibial shaft open fracture, 355
Laminectomy, lumbar
decompressive, in lumbar stenosis, 231
in disc degeneration in occupational low
back injury, 226
peridural fibrosis after, 240
Langerhans' cell
histiocytosis, chemotherapy in children,
299
Leg
length discrepancy after childhood
tumor radiotherapy, 13
(*See also* Extremities, lower)
Legg-Perthes disease
pathogenesis, venous hypertension in,
29
Ligament
ankle, grade III injuries, early
mobilization, 270
cruciate (*see* Cruciate ligament)

Limb (*see* Extremities)
Lipid
extraction enhancing bank bone
incorporation (in rabbit), 369
Low back pain
in athletes during adolescence, 12
chronic, corticosteroid injections into
facet joints for, 241
and disk degeneration in children, 12
Lumbar
back pain, radiographic changes in, in
middle aged women, 229
discectomy (*see* Discectomy, lumbar)
fusion, single-level, with and without
hardware, 253
laminectomy (*see* Laminectomy,
lumbar)
pathology, back pain, occupation and
physical loading in, 224
segmental instability, compression-
traction radiography of, 249
spondylolisthesis with spinal stenosis,
decompression and arthrodesis in,
237
stenosis (*see* Stenosis, lumbar)
vertebral motion segment sagittal
translation, radiography for
measurement, 247
Lumbosacral
segmental motion, instability
measurements in, 248

M

Magnetic resonance imaging
ankle, 271
of biceps tendon dislocation, 49
in cervical stenosis and morphometry, 213
of femoral condyle osteochondral
fragment stability (in dog), 91
foot, 271
for glenoid labrum evaluation, 52
in hip dysplasia, congenital, 20
in hip osteoporosis, 198, 199
knee
high signal in meniscus, 92
meniscal and cruciate injuries, 105
osteonecrosis, 90
of labral-capsular complex, 51
in patellar tendinitis, 94
in physeal injuries in children, with
partial growth arrest, 37
in scaphoid nonunion, vascularity
assessment, 337
of shoulder, 46
sensitivity, specificity and predictive
value, 47

of spinal cord transection, 10
of supraspinatus tendon alterations, 48
Malleolar
  fracture operatively reduced, chondral
    injuries in, 352
Marrow
  injection substituting for graft in tibial
    nonunion, 368
  for ulnar defects (in dog), 367
MAXIMA
  hip technique, 156
McKee-Farrar total hip prosthesis
  results, long-term, 173
Mechanical trauma
  shock in, forecasting course and
    outcome, 346
Mediastinal
  widening in spine fracture, thoracic,
    349
Meniscectomy
  of meniscal lesions, articular cartilage
    changes after (in rabbit), 117
Meniscus
  cartilage after graft transplant, 118
  high signal in, in knee MRI, 92
  in inflammatory joint diseases,
    synovectomy in, 114
  injuries of knee, MRI of, 105
  lesions, articular cartilage changes after
    (in rabbit), 117
  neovascularization with angiogenin (in
    rabbit), 118
Metacarpal
  fracture, functional treatment, 317
Metal
  backed patella, failure of, 146
  induced synovitis, in knee arthroplasty,
    radiography of, 152
  wear in failed titanium alloy total hip
    replacement, 179
  wedge augmentation, in bone deficiency
    in total knee arthroplasty, 130
Metastases
  of bone disease in breast cancer,
    prognostic indicators, 306
  in breast cancer, bone-only, 307
  of cancer, spinal instability secondary
    to, 310
  spine tumor prognosis, scoring system
    for preoperative evaluation, 309
  tibia, total knee replacement in, 145
Metatarsal
  head excision for rheumatoid arthritis
    with hallux fusion, 113
  osteotomy, chevron, for bunionette, 275
Metatarsophalangeal
  joint, first, reaction forces during
    high-heel gait, 278

Microsurgery
  of brachial plexus, in children, 2
Microvascular
  free tissue transfer in chronic traumatic
    bone wounds, 371
Microvasculature
  of triangular fibrocartilage complex,
    329
Model
  nerve compression, for double crush
    hypothesis, 204
Monitoring
  somatosensory evoked potentials (*see*
    Somatosensory evoked potential
    monitoring)
Morphine
  intraarticular, as analgesia after knee
    arthroscopy, 93
Motor
  function recovery after spinal cord
    injury, GM-1 ganglioside in, 210
Muscle
  flap
    in chronic infected hip arthroplasty
      wounds, 182
    coverage of osteotomy site in
      devascularized tibia (in dog), 372
    gastrocnemius, flap, denervated,
      discussion of, 370
  hamstring, contraction, gait and thigh
    muscle strength after, 106
  injury due to pneumatic tourniquet (in
    rabbit), 340
  power output characteristics in below
    knee amputees, 359
  quadriceps femoris, contraction, gait
    and thigh muscle strength after,
    106
  subscapularis, tendon of, rupture,
    features, 75
  thigh
    electrical stimulation after cruciate
      ligament reconstruction, 106
    strength after quadriceps femoris and
      hamstring muscle contraction, 106
  transplant, free vascularized, in
    Volkmann's ischemic contracture in
    children, 34
Myelography
  in disc herniation, lumbar, CT after,
    238
Myelomeningocele
  subtalar arthrodesis, bone graft and
    fixation in, in children, 6
Myelopathy
  cervical spondylotic, spinal canal
    enlargement with arthrodesis for,
    205

N

Nailing
    intramedullary, of tibial shaft fracture,
        373
Necrosis
    aseptic, in football player after hip
        subluxation, 110
    avascular, of femoral head, natural
        history, 189
    of femoral epiphysis, capital, and
        medial approaches to hip (in
        piglet), 26
Neonatal (*see* Newborn)
Neovascularization
    of meniscus with angiogenin (in rabbit),
        118
Nerve
    compression model for double crush
        hypothesis, 204
    electrical stimulation after total knee
        arthroplasty, 134
    palsy with hip replacement, total,
        187
    sheath block for analgesia after
        amputation, 364
    suprascapular, lesions at spinoglenoid
        notch, 110
Newborn
    hip stability and Barlow test, 25
    screening for congenital hip dislocation
        and dysplasia, 23
Nonsteroidal anti-inflammatory drugs
    stopped before elective surgery, 166
Nonunion
    clavicle mid-shaft fracture, 52
    of scaphoid, vascularity assessment with
        MRI, 337
    tibia, marrow injection substituting for
        graft in, 368
Nucleolysis
    of disc with chondroitinase ABC (in
        rabbit), 246

O

Obesity
    morbid, knee replacement in, 144
Occupation
    lumbar pathology in, 224
Occupational
    carpal tunnel syndrome, 319
    low-back injury after lumbar
        laminectomy for disc degeneration,
        226

Orthopedic
    injury, complex, of lower extremity,
        363
    trauma in male drinkers, 350
Ossification
    heterotopic, after total hip arthroplasty,
        radiotherapy to prevent, 166
Osteoarthritis
    knee
        arthroscopic debridement, 125
        ibuprofen vs. acetaminophen in, 125
    rapid destructive, clinical, radiographic
        and pathologic features, 123
Osteoarthropathy
    pustular, differential diagnosis, 85
Osteochondral
    fragment stability of femoral condyle (in
        dog), 91
    graft of femoral condyle, 90
Osteochondritis
    dissecans of knee, 108
Osteogenesis
    imperfecta, surgery functional results,
        elongating and nonelongating rods
        in, 16
Osteogenic sarcoma
    incidence and survival rates of children
        and young adults, 294
Osteomyelitis
    antibiotic in, bioabsorbable delivery
        system, 122
Osteonecrosis
    condyle, medial, survival in total knee
        arthroplasty, 143
    femoral condyle, course and
        radiographic changes, 89
    knee, MRI of, 90
Osteoporosis
    bone in, fracture of, polyacetal rod
        fixation, 378
    of hip, MRI of, 198, 199
    postmenopausal, prevention, 200
Osteosarcoma
    in children, 295
Osteosynthesis
    immediate multiple, in polytrauma, 352
    of major fractures in brain injury, 353
Osteotomy
    Akin double, chevron, for hallux valgus
        correction, 279
    in bunionette, longitudinal diaphyseal,
        with soft tissue repair, 277
    Chiari's, in Perthes' disease, 29
    cuboid, closing wedge, in residual
        clubfoot deformity, 17
    cuneiform, opening wedge medial, in
        residual clubfoot deformity, 17

intertrochanteric corrective, in slipped
capital femoral epiphysis, 28
metatarsal chevron, for bunionette, 275
of tibia, devascularized, union strength
at osteotomy site, skin vs. muscle
flap coverage in (in dog), 372

P

Paget's disease
of bone, familial aggregation, 191
Pain
back (*see* Back pain)
hip, in late pregnancy, 199
low back (*see* Low back pain)
of prosthetic joint, bone scan,
sedimentation rate and joint
aspiration in, 112
Palsy
brachial plexus birth (*see* Brachial
plexus birth palsy)
cerebral (*see* Cerebral palsy)
nerve, with hip replacement, total,
187
Par
interarticularis, stress injury to, SPECT
of, 12
Paresis
hemidiaphragmatic, in interscalene
brachial plexus anesthesia, 83
Patella
metal-backed, failure of, 146
polyethylene components, problems
with, 148
position, prosthetic joint line position
and, 131
tendinitis, ultrasound, CT and MRI of,
94
Patellar
tendon graft in cruciate ligament
reconstruction, 101, 102
Patellofemoral
joint, reflex sympathetic dystrophy of,
97
Pavlik harness
in hip dislocation, congenital,
acetabular dysplasia after, 22
Pediatric (*see* Children)
Pedicle
screw-plate fixation in spinal
arthrodesis, 251
spinal instrumentation, survival, 252
Pelvis
bone Ewing's sarcoma, multimodal
therapy, 292
fracture, skeletally unstable, early
fixation outcome, 356

Pericapsular
acetabuloplasty, triradiate cartilage
premature closure complicating, 21
Peridural
fibrosis after lumbar laminectomy and
discectomy, 240
Peroneus
brevis tendon longitudinal attrition in
fibular groove, 272
Perthes' disease
Chiari's osteotomy in, 29
Physeal injury
of ankle, long-term follow-up, 279
partial growth arrest after, MRI of, in
children, 37
Physical
loading, lumbar pathology in, 224
Pin
fixation, single vs. double, in slipped
capital femoral epiphysis, 27
Hagie intramedullary, modified, in
clavicle mid-shaft fracture nonunion, 52
Plantar
pressure distribution and foot-to-ground
contact forces, 282
Plate
self-compressing, internal fixation with,
with lag screw, 379, 380
Plating
of fibula in tibial fracture, 354
Pneumatic
compression, intermittent, to prevent
deep vein thrombosis after total hip
replacement, 168
tourniquet, muscle injury due to (in
rabbit), 340
Polyethylene
as bearing surface, biomechanical
problems, 178
patellar components, problems with, 148
wear
of acetabular cups, retrieved, 178
in total knee arthroplasty,
arthroscopy of, 149
Polymers
synthetic, and template for new
cartilage formation, 190
Polytrauma
osteosynthesis in, immediate multiple,
352
Popliteal
artery injury in knee fracture and
dislocation after blunt trauma, 96
Postmenopausal
osteoporosis, prevention, 200
Pregnancy
late, hip pain in, 199

Prosthesis
  femur
    in bone tumors, 303
    hydroxyapatite-coated, bonding of,
      177
  foot, energy storing, and running, 359
  for hip replacement, total, cemented,
    uncemented and hybrid, 185
  hip (*see* Hip prosthesis)
  hydroxyapatite coating, 175
  joint
    infections, chronic, suppressive
      antibiotics in, 151
    line position in knee kinematics and
      patellar position, 131
    painful, bone scan, sedimentation rate
      and joint aspiration in, 112
    knee, in gonarthrosis, 139
    silicone scaphoid strains, and
      intercarpal fusions, 341
Pseudarthrosis
  clavicle, congenital, surgery of, 35
Psychometric
  instruments in back pain, 227
Pulmonary
  embolism after total hip replacement,
    heparin to prevent, 169
Putti-Platt surgery
  in shoulder dislocation, recurrent
    anterior, results, 59

Q

Quadriceps
  femoris muscle contraction, gait and
    thigh muscle strength after, 106
  patellar tendon graft in cruciate
    ligament reconstruction, 101
Quality
  of life before and after arthroplasty in
    hip joint arthrosis, 185

R

Radiocarpal
  arthritis, fusion in, 330
Radiography
  in back pain of lumbar spine in women,
    229
  in cervical stenosis and morphometry,
    213
  in femoral condyle osteonecrosis, 89
  in knee arthroplasty metal-induced
    synovitis, 152
  of lumbar segmental instability,
    compression-traction, 249

in lumbar stenosis after fenestration, 234
  in lumbar vertebral motion segment
    measurement of sagittal translation,
      247
  in osteoarthritis, rapid destructive, 123
Radiolunate
  arthrodesis in rheumatoid wrist, 330
Radiotherapy
  of Ewing's sarcoma (*see* Ewing's
    sarcoma, radiotherapy)
  of fibromatosis, aggressive, 300
  for heterotopic ossification after total
    hip arthroplasty prevention, 166
  of tumors, childhood, leg length
    discrepancy after, 13
Radioulnar
  joint, distal, Sauvé-Kapandji procedure
    as salvage for, 324
  synostosis after forearm fracture
    osteosynthesis, 55
Radius
  fracture (*see* Fracture, radius), 54
  head, dislocation and chronic posterior
    subluxation, 64
Reconstruction
  cruciate ligament (*see* Cruciate ligament,
    anterior, reconstruction)
  shoulder, anterior capsulolabral, in
    athletes in overhand sports, 58
Reflex sympathetic dystrophy
  compression syndrome in, 338
  of patellofemoral joint, 97
Rehabilitation
  in lower extremity amputation,
    bilateral, 360
Rheumatoid arthritis
  arthroplasty in, hip and knee, functional
    improvement and costs, 145
  elbow replacement in, capitellocondylar
    total, 82
  elbow synovectomy in, results, 83
  metatarsal head excision in, with hallux
    fusion, 113
  in valgus deformities of foot, gait
    characteristics in, 280
  wrist, radiolunate arthrodesis in, 330
Rod
  elongating and nonelongating, in
    osteogenesis imperfecta surgery
    functional results, 16
  fixation, polyacetal, in osteoporotic
    bone fracture, 378
Rotator cuff
  degenerative lesions, arthrography vs.
    ultrasound in, 46
  repair
    arm position and capsular release in,
      77

functional results and cuff integrity
after, 72
surgery, results, evaluation methods, 74
tear
with brachial plexus palsy and
shoulder dislocation, 62
decompression and debridement,
humeral dislocation after, 72
shoulder surgery for, ultrasound for
follow-up, 73
ultrasound for diagnosis, 45
Running
in below knee amputees, and prosthetic
feet, 359
Rupture
cruciate ligament, knee function after
treatment, 99
disc, mechanism of, 220
tendon of subscapularis muscle,
features, 75

S

Sacral bone: Ewing's sarcoma of,
localized, multimodal therapy, 292
Sarcoma
Ewing's (*see* Ewing's sarcoma)
osteogenic, incidence and survival rates
of children and young adults, 294
soft tissue
DNA content prognostic in, 298
nonrhabdomyosarcoma of
extremities, in children, 296
Sauvé-Kapandji procedure
as salvage for radioulnar joint, 324
Scanning (*see* Imaging)
Scaphoid
fracture (*see* Fracture, scaphoid), 334
strains, prosthetic silicone, and
intercarpal fusion, 341
Scheuermann's
kyphosis, vertebral alterations in, 218
Screw
internal screw fixation in ankle
arthrodesis, 265
lag (*see* Lag screw)
plate fixation, pedicle, in spinal
arthrodesis, 251
Shock
in mechanical trauma, forecasting
course and outcome of, 346
Shoulder
arthrodesis, rigid internal fixation, 80
arthroplasty (*see* Arthroplasty, shoulder)
dislocation
anterior, with rotator cuff tear and
brachial plexus palsy, 62

primary anterior, prognosis in young
adults, 57
recurrent anterior, Putti-Platt
operation results, 59
disorders in aged, 65
in epiphyseal dysplasia, multiple, 84
frozen, arthroscopic distension, 68
impingement, chronic, arthroscopic
subacromial decompression for,
70
MRI of, 46
sensitivity, specificity and predictive
value, 47
reconstruction, anterior capsulolabral,
in athletes in overhand sports, 58
strength analysis with Cybex II
Isokinetic Dynamometer, 67
surgery for rotator cuff tears,
ultrasound follow-up, 73
ultrasound of, 46
Silicone
scaphoid strains, prosthetic, and
intercarpal fusion, 341
Skin
coverage of osteotomy site in
devascularized tibia (in dog), 372
Smoking
complicating lower extremity
amputation, 358
Sodium
hyaluronate in peridural fibrosis after
lumbar laminectomy and
discectomy, 240
Soft tissue sarcoma (*see* Sarcoma, soft
tissue)
Somatosensory evoked potential
monitoring
in acetabular fracture, 186
in hip arthroplasty, total, 187
Sonography (*see* Ultrasound)
Spastic
cerebral palsy, Green transfer in, 8
thumb-in-palm deformity, surgery of,
344
SPECT
of stress injury to pars interarticularis,
12
Spine
arthrodesis with pedicle screw-plate
fixation, 251
canal enlargement with arthrodesis in
cervical spondylotic myelopathy,
205
cervical (*see* Cervical)
cord
injury, motor function recovery after,
GM-1 ganglioside in, 210
transection, MRI of, 10

fracture, thoracic, mediastinal widening
in, 349
instability secondary to metastatic
cancer, 310
instrumentation, pedicle, survivorship
analysis, 252
lumbar (*see* Lumbar)
stenosis with lumbar spondylolisthesis,
decompression and arthrodesis in,
237
tumor prognosis, metastatic, scoring
system for preoperative evaluation,
309
Spinoglenoid
notch, suprascapular nerve lesions at,
110
Spondylolisthesis
lumbar, with spinal stenosis,
decompression and arthrodesis in,
237
symptomatic isthmic low-grade, natural
history, in children and adolescents,
11
Spondylosis
in cervical myelopathy, spinal canal
enlargement with arthrodesis for,
205
Sports
acromioclavicular joint injuries in, 109
Stanmore total knee replacement
survivorship analysis and confidence
intervals in, 142
Staphylococci
antibiotic resistance of biomaterial
adherent to, 188
Staphylococcus aureus
bone and joint infections due to, 121
Stenosis
lumbar
central, fenestration for, radiography
and functional changes after, 234
laminectomy in, decompressive, 231
spine
cervical morphometry and, in football
players, 213
with lumbar spondylolisthesis,
decompression and arthrodesis in,
237
Stiffness
in tibial shaft fracture after functional
bracing, 374
Strain
mechanical, cyclic biaxial, calvarial
bone cell response to (in rat), 193
scaphoid prosthetic silicone, and
intercarpal fusion, 341
Stress
injury to pars interarticularis, SPECT
of, 12

Subacromial
decompression, arthroscopic, in chronic
impingement of shoulder, 70
Subchondral
abrasion, articular cartilage regeneration
after (in rabbit), 115
Subscapularis
muscle tendon, rupture, features, 75
Subtalar
arthrodesis with bone graft and fixation
in myelomeningocele in children, 6
Supracondylar
fracture, displaced, transarticular
fixation in children, 31
Suprascapular
nerve lesions at spinoglenoid notch, 110
Supraspinatus
tendon alterations at MRI, 48
Syme's amputation
indications for, and fibular deficiency,
14
Sympathetic dystrophy, reflex (*see* Reflex
sympathetic dystrophy)
Synostosis
radioulnar, after forearm fracture
osteosynthesis, 55
Synovectomy
elbow, in rheumatoid arthritis, results,
83
open, in inflammatory joint diseases,
arthroscopy in, 114
Synovitis
hip, transient, ultrasound of, 39
metal-induced, in knee arthroplasty,
radiography of, 152

T

Talocalcaneal
fusion and contact in ankle and
talonavicular joints, 281
Talonavicular joint
ankle contact, talocalcaneal fusion on,
281
Tendinitis
patellar, ultrasound, CT and MRI of, 94
Tendon
biceps (*see* Biceps tendon)
patellar, graft, in cruciate ligament
reconstruction, 101, 102
peroneus brevis, longitudinal attrition in
fibular groove, 272
of subscapularis muscle, rupture,
features, 75
supraspinatus, alterations at MRI, 48
Tenodesis
extra-articular, in cruciate ligament
reconstruction, 102

Thigh muscles (*see* Muscle, thigh)
Thrombosis
  deep vein
    after hip surgery, general vs. regional
      anesthesia as risk in, 170
    in hip arthroplasty, total, and
      heparin, 171
    in hip replacement, total, prevention,
      168, 169
  proximal vein, after total knee
    arthroplasty, ultrasound in, 135
Thumb
  in-palm deformity, spastic, surgery of,
    344
Tibia
  devascularized, union strength at
    osteotomy site, skin vs. muscle flap
    coverage (in dog), 372
  fracture (*see* Fracture, tibia)
  longitudinal deficiency, congenital, and
    fibular centralization failure, 15
  metastatic destruction, total knee
    replacement in, 145
Tissue
  transfer, microvascular free, in chronic
    traumatic bone wounds, 371
  transformation into bone, practical
    application, 194
Titanium-alloy
  stems, cobalt-alloy heads corrosion at
    interface on, 163
  total hip replacement, failed, metal wear
    and tissue response in, 179
Tomography, computed (*see* Computed
    tomography)
Tourniquet
  pneumatic, muscle injury due to (in
    rabbit), 340
  release and blood loss after total knee
    replacement, 132
Traction
  in cervical dislocation, 211
  compression radiography of lumbar
    segmental instability, 249
Transfer
  of adductors in children with cerebral
    palsy, 5
Transplantation
  graft, meniscus cartilage after, 118
  muscle, free vascularized, in
    Volkmann's ischemic contracture in
    children, 34
Trauma
  mechanical, shock in, forecasting course
    and outcome, 346
  orthopedic, in male drinkers, 350
  polytrauma, osteosynthesis in,
    immediate multiple, 352

Traumatic
  bone wounds, chronic, microvascular
    free tissue transfer in, 371
Triangular fibrocartilage complex
  microvasculature of, 329
  tears in, chronic peripheral,
    management, 327
Triradiate
  cartilage premature closure,
    complicating pericapsular
    acetabuloplasty, 21
Tumors
  bone (*see* Bone tumors)
  radiotherapy in children, leg length
    discrepancy after, 13
  spine, metastatic, prognosis in, scoring
    system for preoperative evaluation,
    309

U

Ulna
  bone defects, marrow and calcium
    phosphate ceramic for (in dog),
    367
Ultra-clean air enclosure
  vs. ultraviolet radiation, bacteria counts
    in operating rooms, 119
Ultrasound
  cement removal, tool, in revision
    arthroplasty, 181
  of hemidiaphragmatic paresis in
    interscalene brachial plexus
    anesthesia, 83
  in hip synovitis, transient, 39
  in patellar tendinitis, 94
  of rotator cuff degenerative lesions, 46
  in rotator cuff tear
    diagnosis, 45
    shoulder surgery, for follow-up, 73
  of shoulder, 46
  venous, in proximal vein thrombosis
    after total knee arthroplasty, 135
Ultraviolet
  radiation vs. ultra-clean air enclosure,
    bacterial counts in operating
    rooms, 119

V

Valgus
  deformities of feet, in rheumatoid
    arthritis, gait characteristics in,
    280
  hallux, chevron-Akin double osteotomy
    for, 279

Vascularized
muscle transplant in Volkmann's
ischemic contracture in children, 34
Vein
hypertension in Legg-Perthes disease
pathogenesis, 29
proximal, thrombosis after total knee
arthroplasty, ultrasound in, 135
thrombosis (see Thrombosis, deep vein)
ultrasound in proximal vein thrombosis
after total knee arthroplasty, 135
Venting
capsular, in glenohumoral laxity, 62
Vertebra
alterations in Scheuermann's kyphosis,
218
lumbar, motion segment sagittal
translation, radiography for
measurement, 247
Vessels
assessment in scaphoid nonunion, MRI
of, 337
complex injuries of lower extremities,
363
Vibration
exposure and carpal tunnel syndrome
surgery, 321

Visual
analog scales in knee, subjective
complaints, 98
Volkmann's
ischemic contracture, muscle transplant
for, in children, 34

W

Warfarin
in deep vein thrombosis after total hip
replacement prevention,
168
Weber C fracture of ankle
mortise stability after, and syndesmotic
fixation, 262
Wiring
posterior, in cervical injuries, traumatic
distractive flexion, 212
Work
relationship to Dupuytren's disease,
323
Wrist
joint motion, functional ranges, 332
rheumatoid, radiolunate arthrodesis in,
330

Author Index

A

Aalto, T., 238
Ackroyd, C.E., 105
Adam, G., 91
Adams, R.A., 81
Adelaar, R.S., 281
Agren, M., 158
Aichroth, P.M., 108
Akeson, W.H., 90
Alaranta, H., 238
Albrecht-Beste, E., 317
Alexander, I.J., 282
Alexander, J.J., 363
Allan, D.G., 184
Allard, Y., 241
Allon, S.M., 264
Almquist, E.E., 330
Amstutz, H.C., 187
An, K.-N., 332
Anderson, A.F., 368
Anderson, G.I., 372
Andersson, C., 99
Angulo, D.L., 134
Annertz, M., 212
Anthmyr, B.A., 169
Anzel, S.H., 181
Arai, Y., 287
Arand, M., 55
Archibald, D.A.A., 31
Arnoczky, S.P., 329
Arnold, P.G., 181
Aronson, D.D., 5, 6
Ashley, R.K., 1
Askew, L.J., 332
Askin, F.B., 292
Aspenberg, P., 369
Awwad, E.E., 217

B

Bach, A.W., 330
Baker, B.K., 217
Balderston, R.A., 112, 211
Baran, D.T., 158
Barnes, R., 110
Barrat, E., 40
Barrett, D.S., 103
Batdorf, J.W., 356
Baudouin, C.J., 94
Bauer, G., 55, 257
Bauer, H.C.F., 298
Bauer, T.W., 175
Bauza, S., 218
Baxter, D.E., 279
Beach, W.R., 8
Beaudoin, A.J., 281
Beck, P.A., 26
Becker, M.W., 128
Bednar, M.S., 329
Behal, R., 253

Bell, D.F., 63
Bell, S.N., 64
Bellah, R.D., 12
Bengtson, S., 150
Benjamin, J., 262
Bennett, G.L., 268
Bennett, J.B., 80
Bennett, J.T., 29
Bentzon, M.W., 121
Benzel, E., 348
Bereiter, H., 260
Berg, M., 119
Berger, M., 74
Bergman, B.R., 119
Berman, B., 4
Bertoia, J.T., 372
Bhatnagar, M., 8
Bianco, A.J., Jr., 64
Bigliani, L.U., 54
Bini, S.A., 32
Binski, J.C., 267
Black, D.L., 187
Blaha, J.D., 172
Bleck, E.E., 261
Blokker, C.P., 125
Blomgren, G.G.A., 162
Blunn, G.W., 148
Bobyn, J.D., 157
Boden, S.D., 248
Bødtker, S., 358
Boehme, D., 52
Boeree, N.R., 105
Bohlman, H.H., 349
Bohndorf, K., 91
Bohne, W.H.O., 272
Boileau, G., 74
Bolesta, M.J., 349
Bollinger, R.O., 5
Bonamo, J.J., 100
Booth, R.E., Jr., 112
Bortell, D.T., 144
Bos, C.F.A., 23
Bosley, R.C., 70
Bovill, D.F., 1
Boyd, A.D., Jr., 79
Bradford, D.S., 251
Bradley, J.D., 125
Bragdon, C.R., 161
Brandt, K.D., 125
Brandt, L., 212
Breur, G.J., 38
Brick, G.W., 152
Brien, W.W., 171
Brighton, C.T., 193
Brockman, R., 3
Bronson, M.J., 110
Brook, R.H., 242
Brooks, C.E., 157
Brooks, G.G., 199
Brooks, M.T., 287
Brown, D.E., 92
Brown, K., 18
Brugioni, D.J., 302
Bryan, R.S., 81

Bryan, T., 96
Bryant, D.D., III, 15
Bühne, M., 91
Burger, B.J., 23
Burger, J.D., 23
Burgers, A.M.J., 57
Burgers, J.M.V., 289
Burgert, O., Jr., 292
Burke, D.W., 162
Burns, R.P., 361
Butler, M.S., 13

C

Cahalan, T.D., 67
Caillouette, J.T., 181
Campbell, D.C., II, 275
Candlish, S., 34
Cangir, A., 292
Cantor, A., 290
Capelli, A.M., 21
Carette, S., 241
Carlioz, H., 3
Carlow, J.J., 252
Carragee, E.J., 261
Carroll, C., IV, 8
Cash, J.D., 29
Caterini, R., 279
Cauchoix, J., 246
Cervilla, V., 48
Chamay, A., 330
Chan, D., 303
Chan, K.M., 68
Chan, T.W., 49
Chang, F.M., 302
Chao, E.Y.S., 67, 282, 332
Chapman, M., 366
Chapman, M.W., 367
Chard, M.D., 65
Checkoway, H., 319
Chervrot, A., 49
Chesnut, W.J., 135
Chick, J., 350
Chin, A.K., 180
Chiu, G.Y., 196
Choueka, J., 77
Chow, S.-P., 374
Christensen, N.O., 139
Clark, P., 113
Cobb, A.G., 137
Coe, J., 8
Cohen, M.S., 377
Coleman, J., 348
Coleman, W.P., 210
Collatz, M.A., 253
Collier, J.P., 148, 163, 178
Collis, D.K., 183
Colwell, C.W., Jr., 134
Comisel, K., 93
Connelly, C.S., 166
Connolly, J.F., 368
Convery, F.R., 90

Cooke, T.D.V., 278
Cooney, W.P., III, 332
Cooper, D.E., 110
Cornell, C.N., 366
Corpe, R.S., 146
Costa, P., 352
Cotler, J.M., 211
Coughlin, M.J., 277
Covall, D.J., 166
Cram, R., 253
Csongradi, J.J., 261
Cuomo, F., 54
Currie, I.C., 133
Curtis, R.J., Jr., 52
Czerniecki, J.M., 359

D

Dailey, L., 8
Dalinka, M.K., 47, 49
Dandy, D.J., 102
D'Angio, G.J., 13
Danielson, B.I., 11
Dauphinais, L.A., 178
Davenport, K., 151
Davies, S.G., 94
Davis, K.M., 20
De Boer, H.H., 118
DeHaan, J.T., 52
Dehne, R., 368
De Lange, E.E., 199
Delince, P.E., 177
Della Santa, D., 330
Dellon, A.L., 204
Del Pizzo, W., 270
DeLuca, P.A., 7
Denham, R.A., 129
de Roche, R., 370
Desai, K., 108
Dias, J.J., 109
Dick, I.M., 200
Dietz, F.R., 120
DiGioia, A.M., III, 153
DiGiovanni, B.F., 218
Dillingham, M.F., 213
Dorey, F.J., 187, 375
Dorsey, F.C., 210
Dossett, A.B., 347
Dunham, W., 301
Dunst, J., 289
Durnin, C.W., 155

E

Eadie, P., 182
Eaton, R.G., 325
Eberhart, R.E., 325
Ebraheim, N.A., 354
Ecker, M.L., 132
Edholm, C.D., 15
Egerszegi, E.P., 34
Egund, N., 127

Eilert, R.E., 302
Einola, S., 238
Eizember, L.E., 143
El-Khoury, G.Y., 52
Elkins, B.S., 271
Ellman, H., 70
Engh, G.A., 146
Enneking, W.F., 300, 305
Epps, C.H., Jr., 15
Eriksson, B.I., 169
Eschenroeder, H.C., Jr., 199
Eskola, A., 56, 83
Espersen, F., 121
Esquenazi, A., 360
Esterhai, J.L., 47
Etter, C., 256
Evans, D.C., 54
Evans, R.G., 292
Ewald, F.C., 139

F

Fairclough, D.L., 287
Fakhouri, A.J., 376
Fang, D., 374
Faralli, V.J., 132
Faris, P.M., 128, 143
Farnum, C.E., 38
Farsetti, P., 279
Fay, C., 100
Ferkel, R.D., 270, 271
Fertchak, W., 173
Finsterbush, A., 97
Fiore, S.M., 281
Firestone, T., 100
Fischer, M.D., 373
Fischer, S.P., 270
Fisher, A., 364
Fisher, D.F., Jr., 361
Fisher, E.H., III, 26
Fisher, R., 20
Fitzrandolph, R.L., 352
Flandry, F., 98
Flannigan, B.D., 271
Flaster, E., 191
Flatow, E.L., 54
Fleming, B., 101
Fleming, I.D., 296
Fontanesi, G., 352
Fontanesi, J., 287, 296
Fossel, A.H., 231
Found, E.M., 120
Fowler, P.J., 125
Franceschi, D., 363
Franke, J., 19
Frankl, U., 97
Franklin, G.M., 319
Fraser, R.D., 222, 227
Frassica, F.J., 95
Frayssinet, P., 177
Frederick, H.A., 324
Fredriksson, A.-S., 59
Frennered, A.K., 11

Frey, C., 273
Frich, L.H., 78
Fridén, J., 340
Friedman, M.J., 270
Friedman, R.J., 48
Frimodt-Møller, N., 121
Froimson, A.L., 314
Fuchs, W.A., 46
Furlong, R.J., 176

G

Gagnon, J., 241
Galasko, C.S.B., 310
Gallico, G.G., III, 371
Ganz, R., 155, 256
Ganzalez, D., 62
Gärdsell, P., 197
Garfin, S.R., 377
Garneau, R.A., 52
Garnsey, L.A., 292
Garvin, K., 171
Garvin, K.L., 92
Gebhardt, M.C., 295
Geesink, R.C.T., 175
Gehan, E.A., 292
Geisler, F.H., 210
Gentilello, L.M., 356
Gerber, C., 75
Gershuni, D.H., 340
Ghosh, L., 240
Giancecchi, F., 352
Giangarra, C.E., 58
Gibb, T.D., 62
Gibson, A.E., 140
Gilbert, A., 3
Gilbert, M.-A., 350
Gillquist, J., 99
Gilula, L., 292
Girson, M., 10
Gitter, A., 359
Glancy, G.L., 302
Glassman, A.H., 157
Glatstein, E., 286
Glisson, R.R., 341
Glousman, R.E., 58
Gluckman, S.J., 112
Goel, V., 247
Goldstein, S.A., 27
Gondolph-Zink, B., 85
Goorin, A.M., 295
Gorab, R.S., 181
Gordon, S.J., 220
Goris, R.J.A., 353
Goto, H., 157
Grace, D., 113
Graham, C.E., 268
Graham, D., 363
Graham-Pole, J., 290
Green, N.E., 368
Greenough, C.G., 227
Gregg, P.J., 109
Grill, F., 19

Grimer, R.J., 303
Grisso, J.A., 196
Gristina, A., 188
Grogan, D.P., 35
Grönblad, M., 56
Grondin, C., 241
Gronley, J.K., 280
Gross, A.E., 184
Gross, S.B., 193
Grundberg, A.B., 338
Grundel, R.E., 367
Guidera, K.J., 35
Guilford, W.B., 337
Guilhem, A., 177
Guille, J.T., 22
Günther, R.W., 91
Guse, R., 368
Gustilo, R., 366
Gustilo, R.B., 151, 373

H

Haapala, J., 268
Haas, N., 355
Hack, B., 96
Hagberg, M., 321
Haghighi, P., 48
Haimer, E., 93
Haire, T., 161
Hak, D.J., 27
Hansen, S.T., 265
Hardinge, K., 148, 156
Hardy, D.C.R., 177
Hargens, A.R., 340, 377
Harris, M.M., 200
Harris, W.H., 161, 162
Harryman, D.T., 72
Harryman, D.T., II, 62
Hart, N.B., 362
Haug, J., 319
Havránek, P., 37
Hawliczek, R., 289
Hayakawa, N., 334
Hayashi, H., 205
Hayes, F.A., 287
Hazleman, B.L., 65
Hazleman, R., 65
Healy, W.L., 90, 166
Heare, T., 300
Heare, T.C., 290
Heck, D.A., 140
Heddson, B., 127
Hede, A., 117
Hein, G., 19
Helfet, D.L., 186
Heller, E., 16
Henderson, N., 246
Henderson, N.K., 200
Henry, S., 366
Hentz, V.R., 2
Herkowitz, H.N., 237
Herlant, M., 74
Hermansdorfer, J.D., 327

Herz, A., 93
Herzenberg, J.E., 27
Herzog, R.J., 213
Heyer, N., 319
Hilding, S., 45
Hirsh, J., 170
Hissa, E.A., 186
Ho, C.P., 48
Ho, T.-C., 29
Hoborn, J., 119
Hodgson, S.P., 82
Hodler, J., 46
Hoelen, M.A., 57
Hoffer, M.M., 26
Hoffman, K.J., 180
Hoffman, S., 196
Hofman, P.A.M., 353
Hofmann, A.A., 127
Holiday, A.D., Jr., 275
Hølmer, P., 270
Holt, E.S., 265
Homa, D.M., 294
Hontas, R.B., 324
Horii, E., 334
Horowitz, M.E., 286
Hosoya, T., 205
Howe, J.G., 101
Hozack, W.J., 112
Hsu, S.Y.C., 68
Hudson, M., 296
Hughes, J., 113
Hughston, J.C., 98
Hukins, D.W.L., 156
Hunt, J.L., 347
Hunt, J.P., 98
Hurme, M., 238
Hutson, M.M., 172
Hyon, S.-H., 122

I

Iannotti, J.P., 47
Ichimura, K., 208
Ikada, Y., 122
Ilstrup, D.M., 141
Imaeda, T., 334
Inaji, H., 307
Infosino, A., 32
Ingram, R.R., 84
Insall, J.N., 128
Ip, F.-K., 374
Ippolito, E., 279
Isaac, G.H., 178
Ishihara, H., 208
Itoh, T., 208

J

Jackins, S.E., 72
Jackson, W.T., 354
Jahnke, A.H., 1, 51
Jahss, M., 273

James, P., 1
Jantsch, S., 173
Jarvinen, M., 101
Jasty, M., 161
Jeffery, R.S., 129
Jellema, L.M., 218
Jensen, R.E., 148, 163, 178
Jobe, F.W., 58, 69
Johnell, O., 197
Johnson, C., 105
Johnson, K.A., 282
Johnson, M.E., 67
Johnson, P.C., 182
Johnson, R.J., 101
Jones, A.A., 211
Jones, D.A., 25
Jones, N.F., 182, 342
Jones, P.R., 156
Jonsson, B., 145
Joshi, A., 148
Jupiter, J.B., 371
Jürgens, H., 289

K

Kabo, J.M., 375
Kadowaki, T., 189
Kadziolka, R., 249
Kalasinski, L.A., 125
Kälebo, P., 169, 249
Kambin, P., 244
Kamby, C., 306
Kamogawa, M., 198
Kaplan, F., 196
Kaplan, M.J., 101
Kaplan, P.A., 92
Karzel, R.P., 270
Kastenbaum, D.K., 123
Katevuo, K., 238
Katz, B.P., 125
Katz, J.N., 231
Kaukonen, J.-P., 59
Kawano, H., 309
Kay, S.P., 52, 70
Keating, E.M., 143
Kebaish, A.S., 357
Keenan, M.A.E., 280
Kellam, J.F., 54
Kelsey, J.L., 191, 196
Kerr, R., 48
Kesterson, L., 348
Khouri, R.K., 194
Kiefhaber, T.R., 315
Kim, H.K.W., 115
King, G.J.W., 54
King, J.B., 94
King, R.H., 65
King, T., 363
King, T.V., 118
Kinsella, T.J., 286
Kirsh, G., 345
Kish, V.L., 220
Kissane, J.M., 292

Kitaoka, H.B., 275
Kjellin, I., 48
Klapper, R.C., 181
Klaue, K., 155, 379, 380
Kleinman, W.B., 327
Klenerman, L., 113
Kneeland, J.B., 49
Knutson, K., 150
Kokubo, T., 198
Komatsubara, Y., 307
Konradesen, L., 317
Konradsen, L., 270
Koontz, F.P., 120
Korkala, O., 56, 268
Kormano, M.J., 12
Koshino, T., 89
Kotoura, Y., 122
Koudsi, B., 194
Koudstaal, J., 118
Kowalski, M., 379, 380
Koyama, H., 307
Kozakewich, H., 295
Kramhøft, M., 358
Krause, W.R., 281
Kreicbergs, A., 298
Kressel, H.Y., 47
Krettek, C., 355
Kristensen, B., 306
Kruger, D.M., 27
Kruger, L.M., 15
Krushell, R.J., 75, 162
Krygier, J.J., 157
Kumar, S.J., 22
Kummer, F., 77
Kummer, F.J., 273
Kun, L.E., 287
Kurol, M., 45
Kürten, R., 289
Kurz, L.T., 237
Kvitne, R.S., 58

L

Ladin, Z., 106
LaFontaine, M.A., 177
LaGrone, M.O., 274
Lamont, R.L., 5
Lane, J.M., 366
Langer, R., 190
Lantz, B.A., 352
Larson, M.G., 231
Larsson, J., 127
Larsson, S.-E., 145
Lascombes, P., 40
Latenser, B.A., 356
Latimer, B.M., 218
Latulippe, M., 241
Laurencin, C.T., 139
Lavoie, G.J., 184
Lazansky, M.G., 123
Leahey, D., 158
Learmonth, D.J.A., 345
Leatherwood, D.F., II, 193

Leb, R., 314
LeBlanc, J.-M., 77
Lee, C.L., 5
Lee, R., 262
Lehmann, T.R., 247
Lehrberger, K., 93
Lehtonen, J.Y., 59
Lemke, J.H., 52
Lenhart, M.K., 17
Leong, J.C.Y., 374
Lettin, A.W.F., 142
Leutenegger, A., 260
Levinsohn, E.M., 65
Levitsky, K.A., 112
Levy, M.E., 272
Liang, M.H., 231
Lind, J., 358
Lindgren, J.U., 162
Lindstrand, A., 127
Lipson, S.J., 231
Liu, S.-L., 29
Liveson, J.A., 110
Lizler, J., 37
Lo, T.C.M., 166
Lob, G., 257
Lopez, R.A., 62
Lorenz, M., 253
Lotke, P.A., 132
Love, S.M., 35
Lowe, J., 97
Lüscher, N.J., 370

M

McAfee, P.C., 252
McAndrew, M., 352
McBride, I.D., 278
McCarroll, H.R., Jr., 1
McCarthy, C.K., 158
McColl, M.B., 180
McCollough, W.M., 300
McCrae, C.R., 149
McDonald, S., 184
McDonough, J.J., 315
Mace, A.H., Jr., 220
McFarlane, R.M., 323
McHale, K.A., 17
Mächler, G., 257
McIlveen, S.J., 54
McInnes, J.M., 231
Mack, L.A., 72
McKee, M.D., 372
Mackinnon, S.E., 204
McLaren, A.C., 125
McLeod, A., 34
McMahon, J.S., 165
McMahon, J.T., 175
McNamara, J.L., 148
Macnicol, M.F., 104
McQuade, K.J., 62
McQueary, F.G., 137
Maday, M.G., 54
Maislin, G., 196

Majkowski, R.S., 133
Mäkijärvi, J., 268
Makley, J.T., 292
Malarkey, R.F., 267
Malawer, M.M., 301
Maloney, W.J., 161
Manktelow, R.T., 34
Mann, G., 97
Manske, P.R., 8
Marcoux, S., 241
Marcus, R.B., Jr., 290
Marsh, J.L., 120
Martin, D.S., 217
Martindale, J.P., 345
Maslack, M.M., 112
Mast, J.W., 186
Matev, I., 344
Mathiesen, E.B., 162
Matsen, F.A., III, 62, 72
Matsuzaki, 309
Mauldin, D.M., 268
Maussen, J.P.G.M., 28
May, J.W., Jr., 371
Mayer, P.J., 220
Mayo, K.A., 265
Mayor, M.B., 163, 178
Mazurek, R.T., 29
Meals, R.A., 375
Mears, D.C., 182, 264
Mehlhoff, M., 185
Meland, N.B., 181
Melcher, G., 260
Meller, Y., 364
Melzer, C., 73
Membre, H., 40
Mendelhall, N.P., 290
Mendelsohn, D.B., 10
Merkow, R., 366
Merritt, P., 96
Mestdagh, H., 74
Meyer, R.D., 2
Meyer, S., 16
Meyer, W.H., 287
Meyers, M.H., 90
Micheli, L.J., 12
Middleton, D.L., 6
Miller, J.E., 157
Miller, S.R., 54
Milliano, M.T., 131
Million, R.R., 290
Mindell, E.R., 305
Mineo, R., 171
Mintz, L., 149
Mironov, N.P., 346
Misamore, G.W., 46
Miser, J.S., 286
Mitchell, L.A., 279
Mittlmeier, T., 257
Miura, T., 334
Mjöberg, B., 160
Moed, B.R., 376
Moll, F.H., 180
Mollan, R.A.B., 362
Moore, D.C., 367
Moore, T.E., 52

Moran, M.E., 115
Morii, T., 89
Morita, I., 208
Morrey, B.F., 63, 64, 81
Morris, B.A., 134
Morris, R.W., 129, 142
Morrison, K.M., 354
Morscher, E.W., 175
Morton, J., 165
Motohashi, M., 89
Mubarak, S.J., 377
Munro, C., 359
Murdock, L.E., 127
Murphy, L., 278
Müschenich, M., 289
Mutschler, W., 55, 257
Myerson, M.S., 257
Myrvik, Q.N., 188

N

Nachemson, A.L., 11
Nakai, O., 234
Nakamura, R., 334
Nakamura, T., 198
Namba, R.S., 375
Naylor, P.T., 188
Nazarenko, G.I., 346
Neff, J., 292
Nelson, N.L., 92
Nepola, J.V., 52
Nesbit, M.E., 292
Neumann, C.H., 51
Newman, D.M., 330
Newman, J.H., 133
Ng, C., 374
Nielsen, C.F., 212
Nielsen, P.T., 317
Nilsson, B.E., 197
Ninomiya, S., 198
Nishina, T., 189
Niskanen, R.O., 59
Noble, J., 82
Nolte-Ernsting, C., 91
Norman, A., 123
Nurminen, M., 224
Nykvist, F., 238
Nyström, Å., 321

O

Oakeshott, R., 184
Obermann, W.R., 23, 28
O'Brien, L.A., 196
O'Brien, T.S., 20
O'Connor, D.O., 161
Odenbring, S., 127
Odensten, M., 99
O'Driscoll, S.W., 63
Ogden, J.A., 35
Ogilvie, J.W., 251
Ohsaka, S., 309

Ohzono, K., 189
Oka, M., 122
Oka, S., 205
Okada, K., 205
Okutsu, I., 198
Olney, S.J., 278
Ono, K., 189, 307
Ookawa, A., 234
Oppenheim, W.L., 14
Orenstein, E.M., 132
Orrison, W., 348
Osborn, J.F., 176
Østhus, P., 39
Osti, O.L., 222
Ottman, R., 191

P

Paajanen, H.E.K., 12
Pahle, J.A., 114
Pairolero, P.C., 95
Paitich, C.B., 372
Panush, R.S., 166
Parham, D., 296
Parkinson, R.W., 82
Parsons, J.T., 300
Paus, A.C., 114
Peabody, T.D., 280
Peacock, W.J., 4
Peck, N., 319
Pedowitz, R.A., 340
Peltonen, J., 83
Penny, I.D., 104
Perez-Atayde, A.R., 295
Perlik, P.C., 337
Perren, S.M., 379, 380
Perry, C., 151
Perry, J., 280
Perry, J.D., 94
Persson, L., 212
Peter, K., 93
Peters, J.D., 146
Petersen, S.A., 51, 274
Pfeifer, B.A., 166
Philippe, P., 296
Phillips, J., 278
Pico, R., 370
Piotrowski, J.J., 363
Pitt, M., 262
Plaster, R.L., 21, 127
Pohl, K.P., 136
Pollack, M.A., 110
Pollack, S.R., 193
Porat, S., 16
Porter, M.L., 156
Porter, S.S., 187
Pottorff, G., 135
Pournaras, J., 107
Pratt, C.B., 296
Prescher, A., 91
Prévot, J., 40
Price, R.I., 200
Prince, R.L., 200

Prins, M.H., 170
Pritchard, D.J., 292
Pritchett, J.W., 144
Puhl, W., 85
Pun, W.-K., 374
Purdue, G.F., 347

R

Rackemann, S., 102
Radin, E.L., 220
Rahme, H., 45
Rand, J.A., 130, 141
Raney, R.B., Jr., 299
Rang, M., 32
Rao, B.N., 287, 296
Rasmussen, B.B., 306
Rate, W.R., 13
Reagan, D.S., 338
Reckling, F.W., 187
Reddi, H., 194
Redlund-Johnell, I., 25
Reimann, I., 117
Reinholt, F.P., 162
Reiss, B.B., 65
Renfrew, D.L., 52
Rennie, W., 357
Resnick, D., 48
Richards, R.R., 372
Richardson, M.L., 72
Ripamonti, U., 195
Risberg, B., 169
Ritchie, A.J., 362
Ritter, M.A., 143
Roberts, J.A., 31
Roberts, P., 303
Robertson, W.W., Jr., 13
Rock, M.G., 125
Rockwood, C.A., Jr., 52, 61
Roginson, A., 102
Rokkanen, P., 56
Roman, R.J., 315
Romanus, B., 185
Rometsch, M., 370
Rosdahl, V.T., 121
Rosenberg, Z.S., 123
Rosman, M., 18
Roth, J.N., 125
Rothkopf, D.M., 371
Rothman, R.H., 112
Rougraff, B.T., 140
Rowles, J.M., 345
Roy, A., 357
Roye, D.P., Jr., 32
Rozing, P.M., 23, 28, 57
Rubash, H.E., 153
Rubbo, E.R., 22
Rüedi, T., 260
Rund, D., 350
Russell, W.L., 361
Ryan, J., 226
Ryan, M.D., 378
Ryan, S.I., 125

Rydevik, B.L., 340
Ryu, J., 332

S

Sailors, D.M., 361
Saito, M., 189
Saito, S., 189
Salminen, J.J., 12
Salter, R.B., 115
Salvati, E.A., 171
Salzer-Kuntschik, M., 289
Sanders, R.A., 324
Sanfridson, J., 25
Sangeorzan, B.J., 265
Santana, V.M., 296
Santavirta, S., 56
Santelli, E.D., 65
Sauer, R., 289
Saveland, H., 212
Savin, J.J., 354
Savoie, F.H., 351
Scales, J.T., 303
Schaffer, J.L., 244
Schell, M.J., 296
Schepsis, A.A., 106
Schlegel, J.D., 347
Schloo, B., 190
Schmalzried, T.P., 187
Schmidt, A.H., 340
Schmidt, D., 74
Schneider, J., 134
Schoenecker, P.L., 8, 21
Schwaegler, P., 253
Schwägerl, W., 173
Schwartz, A.G., 294
Scioli, M., 352
Scoles, P.V., 218
Scott, R.D., 79, 137, 139, 152
Sculco, T.P., 171
Seaber, A.V., 341
Seidman, D.S., 16
Seitz, W.H., Jr., 314
Seligson, D., 366
Semlitsch, M., 173
Sergay, S., 186
Shaffer, W.O., 247
Shankman, S., 123
Shapiro, J.D., 314
Sharrock, N.E., 83, 171
Shekelle, P.G., 242
Sheppard, I., 345
Sheppard, L., 104
Shirasaki, N., 205
Sidles, J.A., 62
Sim, F.H., 95
Simon, M., 19
Sinha, R., 211
Siris, E.S., 191
Skinhøj, P., 121
Sledge, C.B., 79
Small, J.O., 362
Smith, K.R., Jr., 217

Smith, M., 200
Smith, M.G.H., 31
Smith, R.B., 145
Sneath, R.S., 303
Sneppen, O., 78
Snyder-Mackler, L., 106
Sobel, M., 272
Søjbjerg, J.O., 78
Solari, J., 262
Søndergaard, L., 270
Songer, M.N., 240
Sontag, M.J., 213
Sorvali, T., 268
Southworth, S.R., 354
Sowes, M.F.R., 294
Spencer, D.L., 240
Spindler, K.P., 47
Sponseller, P.D., 8
Spratt, K.F., 247
Staehell, J.W., 95
Stanescu, V., 246
Star, A.M., 211
Stark, D.M., 80
Stein, C., 93
Steinberg, G.G., 158
Steiner, G.C., 123
Stern, P.J., 315
Stockelman, R.E., 136
Strafford, B., 193
Strecker, W.B., 8
Strom, B.L., 196
Stulberg, S.D., 149, 185
Summerville, D.A., 12
Suprenant, H.P., 148, 178
Suprenant, V.A., 148, 163, 178
Svalastoga, E., 117
Swann, M., 179
Swanson, S.A.V., 178
Swärd, L., 249
Symeonides, P.P., 107
Symmons, D.P.M., 229

T

Tait, G.R., 345
Takaoka, K., 189
Takatori, Y., 198
Talts, K.H., 83
Tanskanen, P., 268
Tartaglia, I., 352
Tarver, A.A., 356
Taylor, C.J., 156
Tefft, M., 292
Tegner, Y., 59
Tengborn, L., 169
Terho, P.H., 12
Terjesen, T., 39
Terrier, B., 46
Terry, G.C., 98
Tertti, M.O., 12
Thalgott, J.S., 356
Thomas, B.V., 199

Thomas, P., 292
Thomas, W.H., 79
Thompson, E., 287
Thorén, K., 369
Thornhill, T.S., 79, 137
Tiedeman, J., 368
Tillman, R.M., 145
Toby, E.B., 341
Tokuhashi, Y., 309
Tolo, V.T., 8
Tooms, R.E., 15
Toriyama, S., 309
Torres, M.M., 360
Traina, S., 151
Treves, S.T., 12
Tribukait, B., 298
Troup, J.D.G., 224
Truchon, R., 241
Trudell, D., 48
Tsao, A.K., 149
Tscherne, H., 355
Tsuji, H., 208
Tsukayama, D.T., 151
Tucci, J.J., 22
Tulipan, D.J., 325
Tullos, H.S., 80
Twyman, R.S., 108

U

Udén, A., 25
Ueda, T., 307
Urbaniak, J.R., 341
Urbanski, S.R., 199
Urmey, W.F., 83
Urvoy, P., 74

V

Vacanti, C.A., 190
Vacanti, J.P., 190
Vahvanen, V., 83
Vainionpää, S., 56
Valkenburg, H.A., 229
Vallee, B.L., 118
Vallier, G.T., 274
Vandenbroucke, J.P., 23, 229
Van Der Griend, R., 300
Vander Griend, R.A., 351
VanEnkevort, B.A., 38
Vangness, C.T., 48
Vangsness, C.T., Jr., 69
van Hemert, A.M., 229
Vanveicenaher, J., 74
Varecka, T.F., 373
Vargo, E., 218
Vaughan, C.L., 4
Vawter, G.F., 295
Venzon, D., 286
Vernon-Roberts, B., 222
Videman, T., 224

Vietti, T.J., 292
Vincent, K., 366
Viviano, D.M., 27
Vogl, T., 257
von Schulthess, G.K., 46
Vrbos, L., 253

W

Wada, R., 122
Waddell, J.P., 165
Wadenvik, H., 169
Walker, J.L., 32
Walker, P.S., 148
Walker, R.H., 134
Waller, B., 286
Wang, K.Y., 72
Ware, H.S., 142
Warren, R.F., 110
Wasilewski, S.A., 166
Watkinson, A.F., 105
Watt, J.M., 168
Weatherall, P.T., 10
Weaver-McClure, L., 286
Webb, P.G., 200
Wei, G., 122
Weightman, B., 178
Weiland, A.J., 329
Weiland, D.J., 252
Weinstein, J., 247

Weiss, H.C., 181
Weissman, B.N., 152
West, J.L., III, 251
Wetzel, R., 85
White, S.E., 131
Whiteside, L.A., 131
Whittle, T.B., 361
Wicklund, B., 151
Wiens, J.J., 213
Wiesel, S.W., 248
Wiklund, I., 185
Wiley, A.M., 72
Wilkinson, R.H., 295
Williams, J.L., 193
Wilsman, N.J., 38
Wilson, J., 262
Wingstrand, H., 212
Winkelmann, W., 289
Wirth, C.J., 73
Witt, J.D., 179
Wixson, R.L., 185
Wood, E.G., 351
Wood, M.J., 199
Woodward, C., 46
Woolson, S.T., 135, 168
Wright, T., 149
Wroblewski, B.M., 178
Wuh, H.C.K., 180
Wülker, N., 73
Wyman, E., 158
Wyss, U.P., 278

Y

Yamada, H., 208
Yamamuro, T., 122
Yamashita,K., 307
Yamaura, I., 234
Yang, K.H., 220
Yassouridis, A., 93
Yee, T., 367
Ylikoski, M., 268
Yonenobu, K., 307
Yoshii, I., 131
Young, D.C., 52, 61
Young, J.C., 106

Z

Zak, P.J., 5
Zelicof, S.B., 139
Zenz, P., 173
Zetterlund, B., 321
Zimmerman, R., 175
Zindrick, M., 253
Zingarelli, P., 371
Zlatkin, M.B., 47
Zollars, L., 10
Zuckerman, J.D., 77
Zuker, R.M., 34
Zwerling, C., 226